THE NURSING PROCESS
A scientific approach to nursing care

THE NURSING PROCESS

A scientific approach to nursing care

ANN MARRINER, R.N., Ph.D.

Associate Professor
University of Colorado School of Nursing
Denver, Colorado

SECOND EDITION

The C. V. Mosby Company

ST. LOUIS • TORONTO • LONDON   1979

To **JERRY**

SECOND EDITION

Copyright © 1979 by The C. V. Mosby Company

All rights reserved. No part of this book may be reproduced in any manner without written permission of the publisher.

Previous edition copyrighted 1975

Printed in the United States of America

The C. V. Mosby Company
11830 Westline Industrial Drive, St. Louis, Missouri 63141

Library of Congress Cataloging in Publication Data

Marriner, Ann, 1943-   comp.
   The nursing process.

   Bibliography: p.
   Includes index.
   1. Nursing—Addresses, essays, lectures.
I.   Title.
RT63.M37   1979   610.73   78-21093
ISBN 0-8016-3122-X

VT/M/M   9 8 7 6 5 4 3 2 1

PREFACE

In all nursing situations the proper utilization of the "nursing process" largely determines the degree of effectiveness and efficiency of nursing intervention. This book presents a compilation of various theoretical concepts concerning the four phases of the process: assessment, planning, implementation, and evaluation. Tools used in the implementation of each phase are discussed. Each chapter includes an annotated bibliography and selected readings to enrich and illustrate the chapter's content.

I wish to thank Carolyn Snidow-Smith for her assistance and my husband for editing and typing the manuscript.

Ann Marriner

CONTENTS

THE NURSING PROCESS
A scientific approach to nursing care

CHAPTER 1

THE NURSING PROCESS

Process is a method of doing something that generally involves a number of steps and is intended to bring about a particular result. The nursing process is the application of scientific problem solving to nursing care.[1] It is used to identify patient problems, to systematically plan and implement nursing care, and to evaluate the results of that care. The steps of the nursing process have been defined differently by various authors, probably because the phases of the process are often interrelated and sometimes overlapping. In the following chapters the steps of the nursing process are classified as (1) assessment, (2) planning, (3) implementation, and (4) evaluation.[2]

ASSESSMENT

Assessment is the first phase of the nursing process. Before the nurse can plan the patient's care, she must identify and define the patient's problems. Consequently, this phase includes collection of data about the health status of the patient and ends with the nursing diagnosis, a statement of the patient's problem.

Information is collected from a variety of sources to help the nurse understand the patient's situation. Observing and interviewing the patient and his family are two basic methods of gathering information. The nursing history provides a systematic format, usually in the form of a questionnaire or checklist that the nurse can follow to obtain relevant data about the patient through the interview method. Areas of assessment that should be included on the nursing history form include the patient's diagnosis and treatment, activities of daily living (cleanliness, defecation, eating, exercise, rest, relaxation, and sleep habits), physical condition, psychological status, and social-cultural-economic history—a factual recording of environmental, occupational, financial, educational, recreational, and spiritual habits. This written record of specific information about the patient provides facts on which to base an assessment of existing and potential patient problems. It also serves as a basis for planning and giving nursing care.

A survey of the patient's home and community is helpful in making an assessment but may be difficult to arrange. Secondary sources for the collection of information about the client include current and past medical and social records, developmental records, computer memories, nursing notes, the Kardex, nursing rounds, and change-of-shift reports. Because the nurse bases the planning of care on scientific principles and applies diverse theories while giving care, it may be useful to refer to books, journals, and experts for additional information.[3]

This assessment allows the nurse to make a diagnosis that is a statement of the patient's problems, including his strengths, limitations, and methods of adapting to that problem. It allows the nurse to develop a personalized plan for the care of the client.

PLANNING

The planning phase begins with the nursing diagnosis, which is made by collecting and evaluating data that have implications for nursing actions.[4] The nursing diagnosis is based on inferences, which are usually drawn from uncertain and incomplete data. In making inferences, the nurse considers a range of possibilities based on observation and, using the inductive method, predicts what will follow. Induction is the process of reasoning from the specific to the general or from a part to a whole. Sometimes inference, decision, and action are all completed within a few minutes. The level of inferences is dependent on the experiences, perceptivity, and theoretical knowledge of the nurse. Initial inferences, which are based on incomplete data about a patient, may be of low level. As the nurse continues to collect data and verify meaning with the patient, her inferences become more accurate.[5]

As soon as the patient's problems are identified, the nurse must establish priorities by determining which problems are most urgent. Immediate, intermediate, and long-term goals, or the ends to which one is striving, should be defined. Goals acceptable to the client and the nurse should be mutually defined. The client and his family should be active participants in the planning of patient care.

From the general goals the nurse may determine more specific objectives. Objectives should be stated in observable behavioral terms, such as "the patient will resume his normal bowel habits of one bowel movement every other day." The nursing actions directed toward the accomplishment of the objectives, which may be labeled nursing intervention, nursing treatments, or nursing therapy, should be listed explicitly on the nursing care plan; for example, "Give stewed prunes or prune juice for breakfast each day." "Sit on the toilet after breakfast at 9 A.M. each day." Instead of stating "force fluids," be more specific and state "force at least 2000 ml per day." Then list what types of fluids the patient likes at various times, such as fruit juice with breakfast, gelatin or ice cream for midmorning snack, hot tea midafternoon, and hot chocolate at bedtime. The nursing care plan should be so individualized that it cannot be used for any other patient. It should include the patient's problems, the goals and objectives, and the nursing intervention. Its development ends the planning phase.

IMPLEMENTATION

If planning is not put into action, it is useless. Thus once nursing intervention has been determined and the planning phase completed, implementation begins. The nurse continues to collect and assess data and plan and evaluate care while implementing the care plan.

Implementation is the actual giving of nursing care. A nursing care plan contributes to comprehensive nursing care because the plan takes into consideration the patient's physical, psychological, emotional, spiritual, social, cultural, economic, and rehabilitative needs. Care is personalized to be appropriate for a specific patient. Implementation of a care plan also contributes to continuity and coordination of care. Without planning and adequate communication about the plan, the patient could experience gaps and duplications in care. The plan guides the even flow of nursing care throughout the patient's stages of illness and coordinates the scheduling of diagnostic tests and various therapies from other health personnel into an adequate sequence of events for the patient. Health teaching, along with helping the client express his feelings and plan his own care, is an important nursing intervention. Completed nursing actions end the implementation phase.

EVALUATION

The final but continuous phase of the nursing process is evaluation or appraisal of the care given. Was the care given effective? If so, why? If not, why not? How could the care be improved? Evaluation of the patient's progress is based on a comparison of the outcome of care given with the outcome to be achieved by the nurse, health care team, patient, or family as stated in the objectives of the care plan. Evaluation of the patient's progress indicates which problems have been solved and which need to be reassessed and replanned.[6]

Evaluation of nursing care is a feedback mechanism for judging quality and is designed to improve nursing care by comparing actual care given with standards for that care. Phaneuf[7] has done extensive work with the nursing audit. She defines the nursing audit as the nurse's formal, systematic, written appraisal of the quality of nursing service as indicated in care records of discharged patients. The audit is a constructive review of practice and not of a practitioner. It should evaluate overall care and not just the care given by a particular nurse. It should not be punitive. The nursing audit indicates whether nursing care standards are being met and identifies areas in need of corrective action.

Although Phaneuf's audit is not designed for evaluation of patient care while the care is being given, other audits have been designed to be used at the bedside. They are usually checklists of nursing actions that are evaluated by a nurse from another ward in an effort to maintain objectivity. Sometimes the scores are posted to stimulate competition, increase motivation, and improve nursing care.

Although evaluation is considered to be the final phase of the nursing process, the process does not end there. Evaluation merely indicates which problems have been solved and which ones need to be reassessed, replanned, implemented, and reevaluated. The nursing process is a continuing cycle.

NOTES

1. Francis, G. M.: This thing called problem solving, J. Nurs. Educ. **6**:27-30, Nov. 19, 1967.
2. Beland, I. L.: Clinical nursing: pathophysiological and psychological approaches, ed. 2, New York, 1970, The Macmillan Publishing Co., Inc., pp. 14-18; Lewis, L.: This I believe . . . about the nursing process—key to care, Nurs. Outlook **16**(5):26-29, 1968. Two examples of different classifications of steps within the nursing process. Yura, H., and Walsh, M. B., editors: The nursing process, Washington, D.C., 1967, Catholic University of America Press. Identifies the same four phases as the author.
3. Prange, A. J., Jr., and Martin, H. W.: Aids to understanding patients, Am. J. Nurs. **62**(7):98-100, 1962.
4. Chambers, W.: Nursing diagnosis, Am. J. Nurs. **62**(11):102-104, 1962; Durand, M., and Prince, R.: Nursing diagnosis: process and decision, Nurs. Forum **5**(4):50-64, 1966; Komorita, N. I.: Nursing diagnosis, Am. J. Nurs. **63**(12):83-86, 1963.
5. Carrieri, V. K., and Sitzman, J.: Components of the nursing process, Nurs. Clin. North Am. **6**:115-124, March, 1971. Kelly, K.: Clinical inference in nursing, Nurs. Res. **15**:23-26, Winter, 1966.
6. Carlson, S.: A practical approach to the nursing process, Am. J. Nurs. **72**(9):1589-1591, 1972; Kneedler, J.: Nursing process is a continuing cycle, AORN J. **20**(8):245-248, 1974.
7. Phaneuf, M. C.: The nursing audit profile for excellence, New York, 1972, Appleton-Century-Crofts; Analysis of a nursing audit, Nurs. Outlook **16**(1):57-60, 1968; The nursing audit for evaluation of patient care, Nurs. Outlook **14**(6):51-54, 1966; A nursing audit method, Nurs. Outlook **12**(5):42-45, 1964; Quality of care: problems of measurement. I. How one public health nursing agency is using the nursing audit, Am. J. Public Health **59**(10):1827-1832, 1969.

Selected readings

The nursing process can be used by the nurse to help meet individual or group needs whether in hospital, school, industry, outpatient clinic, public health department, or neighborhood. The nursing process is basically the scientific method of problem solving applied to nursing. Gloria M. Francis succinctly describes five types of problem solving and explains how the scientific method is the most refined and efficient method for solving problems. She defines the six steps of the scientific method and relates them to the nursing process.

Authors have delineated the nursing process in as few as three or as many as six or more steps. Virginia Kohlman Carrieri and Judith Sitzman have identified the elements of the process as observation, inference, validation, assessment, action, and evaluation. Lorraine Hagar illustrates the nursing process with a case study.

Because the nursing process should involve an overriding concern for the patient, the "Patient's Bill of Rights" as prepared by the American Hospital Association is included in this selection of readings.

THIS THING CALLED PROBLEM SOLVING

Gloria M. Francis

Students of nursing have been known to question the amount of time given to the discussion of, and expectations in, so-called problem solving. They say that they have been solving problems all their lives. Why, they ask, do teachers make such an issue of problem solving?

No one will deny that among other considerations life is a process of satisfying needs. A need is a condition requiring supply or relief. As we move along the continuum from recognizing a need to relieving it, we encounter problems. Problems are unsettled questions. They may range from questions for simple inquiry to questions perplexingly vexatious. The procedure for overcoming difficulties of all kinds is called problem solving. Thus it is true that all of us have been solving problems all our lives. In fact, problem solving is also done by animals. The nature of the procedure varies with the difficulty of the problem, the intelligence of the solver, the extent of his experience and skill, and the method he uses. There are five methods or types of problem solving, and they can be ranked according to their efficacy in producing satisfactory effects.

UNLEARNED, INHERENT PROBLEM SOLVING

Unlearned, inherent problem solving is the lowest level and simplest kind of problem solving. Animals use it to a great extent. With this method one overcomes difficulties in blind, mechanical ways. The ways are determined largely by biological endowment. One reacts in fixed ways, without thought, whether or not the ways are appropriate for the occasion.

TRIAL AND ERROR PROBLEM SOLVING

Trial and error problem solving is the second most inefficient kind of problem solving. It is a pay-as-you-go method. While actually facing the difficulty, one tries different means of possible solution, with no forethought and by noting and eliminating means that failed. In this method, years may pass before a solution is reached. Having solved a problem in this manner does not guarantee the ability to repeat the attempt that finally worked because the problem solver was unaware of the relationship between the solution and the problem. It simply worked like magic.

INSIGHT PROBLEM SOLVING

Insight problem solving requires just enough intelligence to perceive the means of solution in relation to the goal either during or after the procedure. There is a belief that certain animals have this ability. Certainly human beings are able to see relationships. The solution is still arrived at through blind trial and error, but once the solution has been reached there is understanding as to why and how it worked. Unlike trial and error, it can be used again if an *identical* difficulty is encountered.

Reprinted from The Journal of Nursing Education 6:27-29, Nov., 1967. Used by permission of McGraw-Hill Book Company.

VICARIOUS PROBLEM SOLVING

Vicarious means "experienced or realized through imaginative participation." In vicarious problem solving, the problem solver extends his sensory range to predict consequences that may or may not occur. By description and prediction, one crosses his bridges before he comes to them. The possibility of error can be greatly reduced with this method. Animals, however, cannot engage in this procedure because they do not have language. Since one must be able to use concepts in order to conceptualize, or formulate ideas, a language is needed.

How does vicarious problem solving differ from the next and highest level of problem solving? It is based on assumptions rather than facts. It has its place when one must plan ahead, but it is only entirely successful if all the assumptions materialize.

SCIENTIFIC METHOD PROBLEM SOLVING

The most refined and efficient method of solving problems is by the scientific method. It has been said that perhaps man's greatest use of language is the way in which he applies it to his system of scientific problem solving. The method is distinctively characteristic of Western civilization, and its development and use account in large measure for Western technological advancement over the civilizations of the East. It has been defined variously as an orderly manner of thinking or of handling data, a systematic pursuit of knowledge, and discovering the logical whole from the component parts. The latter description is also the definition for induction or inductive reasoning, i.e., going from the parts to the whole. That is the direction in which scientific problem solving moves.

There are six steps in the formal scientific method of problem solving. They are (1) understanding the problem, which includes delimiting, defining, and describing it; (2) collecting data; (3) formulating an hypothesis; (4) evaluating the hypothesis; (5) testing the hypothesis; and (6) forming conclusions. A simplified and pragmatic version of the process has been adapted and adopted by medicine and nursing. The physician uses a modified, scientific method of problem solving when he engages in the process he calls *examination-diagnosis-treatment*. The nurse uses the method when she engages in the process she calls *facts-assumptions-action*. Nursing has not used the formal method as consciously as has the physician. The terms, therefore, are less universally accepted. For instance, some nurses refer to the first step as "observation," the middle step as "nursing diagnosis," and the last step as "nursing care," or intervention. In any case, the *first step* has to do with facts, data, reality, or the situation as it is. It is what there is, if you will. The *second step* is an analysis and interpretation of what the facts might mean, or what they might mean when put together into like categories, and giving meaning to, explaining, or translating the many facts or the several categories. It involves speculation or educated guessing. Having completed this step, one might detect recurring themes or patterns, some of which have very obvious implications for action. The *third step* has to do with what, if anything, one might do or try to do about the now more clearly understood facts. It is a plan of action based on one or more assumptions about the facts, and may include accessible opportunities, modifications of behavior, and choices and priorities of action.

Mentally healthy persons with reasonable intelligence tend to go about meeting difficulties in this manner, but it is a skill. It must be learned. One does not just do it naturally. Once well learned it can become second nature, but one still goes through the steps in conscious, orderly fashion. The concept is simply applied more rapidly, but it is always a

conscious operation. The individual who says he can do it unconsciously or without thinking is deluding himself or trying to delude his teacher. It is a consciously performed process.
One "knows" when he is measuring blood pressure. Similarly, one knows when he is using
the scientific method of problem solving.

A simple illustration of a modified, scientific method of problem solving as applied by a
nurse may be illustrated as follows, in the case of a former patient who continues to
complain of vague, generalized pain and asks for "shots" one year after his discharge from
the hospital.

There are, of course, many more facts and many more implications for action, but there
is no substitute for this relatively simple and orderly approach to solving nursing problems
and improving nursing care. This illustration has been kept simple (hopefully not decep-
tively simple) to encourage graduates and students who are often overwhelmed with more
sophisticated approaches calling for clinical inferences and nursing diagnosis based on very
elaborate systems of data collection. They have a very real place in nursing, but beginners
must begin at the beginning.

Facts	Assumptions	Action
Permanent colostomy for cancer 1 year ago. Medical exam 1 month ago—"no physical basis for pain, no metastasis."		
Calls PH nurse for "shot" every week.		Plan visits when he has not called for "shot."
70-year-old retired carpenter lives with wife; few visitors. Big, strong man physically able to be up and to do chores. Sleeps a lot, cries some; mood lowered.	Self-esteem decreased. Feels useless. Feelings of depression and despair.	Discuss feelings of depression with physician. New drugs may be indicated.
"Devout Baptist"—no church attendance for 5 years.	Some guilt over his standing with his church.	Call minister and share situation.
Frequently answers question "How are you?" with "I'll never work again."	Fears future.	Discover interests, provide opportunities for usefulness and satisfaction. What about small woodwork-ing—carving? Have wife designate chores and expect him to do them.
Grasps nurse's hand tightly when she arrives. Pulse rapid.	Afraid of dying. Anxious. He is saying, "Don't let me die or at least not alone."	Acknowledge recognition of fear of death with him. Share burden. Talk about it.

COMPONENTS OF THE NURSING PROCESS

Virginia Kohlman Carrieri and Judith Sitzman

Nursing care is a continuous process. It must have coordination of parts without interruption or cessation. It must be set in motion and progress toward the integration of the whole individual or his highest achievable level of wellness. To achieve these goals patient care must be deliberate, systematic, and individualized through the use of the nursing process.

Many theoretical frameworks could be used to examine process as a concept. Parker defines process as "that intellectual scheme whereby relationships are put together." According to Parker, this encompasses the procedures of analysis, synthesis, and reduction to practice. Analysis involves the accumulation of, the classification of, and the distinction between differences in data. Synthesis includes establishing relationships between data, deriving trends, performing deductive and inductive analysis, and creating operational devices. Reduction to practice involves operational devices used on particular occasions in specific settings and testing for the effectiveness and validity of the operational devices.[1]

These concepts and additional resources have been used by various workers to outline the unique elements of the nursing process.[3,4,5] These elements have often been identified as: observation, inference, validation, assessment, action, and evaluation.

This model of the nursing process was deliberately utilized by the present authors while caring for patients undergoing cardiac valve replacements. The process was initiated when data regarding a patient were obtained through interaction with the patient, from other health team members, or from patient records. Relationships with these patients usually began one week prior to surgery and were maintained until discharge.

OBSERVATION

The first step of the process, observation, is defined for this investigation as a deliberate search for relevant data about a patient with concurrent assignment of meaning to these data in light of the nurse's frame of reference.

It is realized that all observations are influenced by the nurse's previous experiences; however, what makes her observations scientific is the deliberateness and special care with which she makes reliable observations. The nurse is aware that observation is constantly subject to error and can be influenced by all past theoretical and experiential knowledge.

Kaplan contrasts scientific observation with casual everyday observations: "Observation is purposive behavior, directed toward ends that lie beyond the act of observation itself: the aim is to secure materials that will play a part in other phases of inquiry, like the formation and validation of hypotheses."[2]

Observation demanded the building of a trust relationship with the patient so that he felt free to verbalize all of his concerns. The relationship facilitated the collection of a wider range of observations about the physical and psychosocial status of the patient. Only through accumulation of significant information is the nurse able to progress beyond the first step of the process toward an accurate diagnosis and plan of care.

The authors utilized both a nursing history form and a nursing diagnosis as the format

Reprinted from Nursing Clinics of North America 6:115-124, March, 1971. Published by W. B. Saunders Company, Philadelphia.

for instituting the process, recording their findings, and retrieving information about the patient. All observations were categorized and coded using the following nursing history form unique to this report.

NURSING HISTORY FORM

Character of information:

1. Personal data, i.e., age, religion, marital status, etc.
2. Socio-economic and cultural influences
3. Concept or perception of self
4. Physiologic status
5. Adaptation to illness
   a. Current illness and life pattern of illness
   b. Hospital setting or health team
6. Understanding of treatments and procedures during hospitalization
7. Specific fears, i.e., fear of death, procedures, etc.

Source of information:

A. Observation or communication with the patient
B. Review of medical record
C. Communication with health team
D. Communication with significant others

Examples of selected observations and appropriate coding regarding one cardiac surgical patient are listed herewith:

Coding	*Observations*
(1B)	White male, 37, Protestant, divorced 3 years ago
(1B)	3 children with wife, many unskilled jobs
(4B)	Aortic stenosis, penicillin allergy, only sx "SOB"
(6A)	"All I know is they cut you open and sew you back together again."
(5aA)	"I came here for heart surgery, but they've had their fingers in everything I have"
(5bA)	"They're not going to throw something in my face and make me sign it"
(5aA)	"I've been having too much fun for the last 4 years to lie in bed for surgery"
(5A)	Moving constantly in bed
(1A)	Smoking frequently
(4A)	Skin color gray-white

These are examples of the significant information obtained during one interaction with a patient which had relevance for deliberate planning of nursing care, since they are clues about the patient as an individual. These are only a few of the many observations obtained during each interview with cardiac patients during the investigation of this interpersonal process.

INFERENCE

After coding all observations, the nurse initiated the second step in the process, that of inference. Inference is defined for purposes of this report as an interpretation of patient verbalization and behavior based on the nurse's prior theoretical knowledge of the type of problem with which the patient is confronted. The nurse infers, usually without sufficient data, that a certain type of problem exists for the patient. An awareness on the nurse's part that she is using the inference process with its reliance on intuition as well as theoretical knowledge, in making decisions about the nature of her patient's problems should be a caution to her that she may, in fact, be functioning without sufficient data, and thus lead her to seek additional information before acting on the problem as she first perceives it.

The following are exemplary observations and inferences taken from a lengthy list of patterns of observations received each day throughout one patient's hospitalization.

Observations	*Inferences*
Preop. Day #2	
"The only thing I hated was that tube down my nose—scared me to death"	Fear of suctioning
	Fear of nasogastric tube
Postop. Day #1	
"Froze all night, all I could think of was let me die warm"	Hypothermia mattress may be too high
	Fear of death
Rapid, shallow breathing. Rate 32/min. Flushed skin, restless	Atelectasis, consolidation, drug reaction
Postop. Day #4	
"I thought I was going to die or faint, all I could see was my open chest on that pissy floor"	Fear of death
"Now that I've gotten over the operation, I'll probably die of pneumonia"	Fear of pain
	Fear of body mutilation
"My heart went all to pieces, guess I'm coming all unglued"	
Postop. Day #7	
"Why don't they give me pain medication before the machine?"	Pain
"Now I know what pain is, it couldn't be worse"	
"All I can do is say, buddy, I'm here . . . sometimes I don't think they know it's you"	Hostility toward staff
	Impersonalization by staff
"I came here for heart surgery but they've had their fingers in everything I have"	Mistrust and resentment of staff
Postop. Day #8	
"My heart beats faster and makes more noise than it did before surgery"	
"I'm worse than before, weak as a cat, I'd rather give them their valve back and take mine; it was better"	Postoperative expectations of self not being met

VALIDATION

After the nurse formulated inferences as to the possibility of existing patient problems, she entered the third step of the nursing process, validation. Validation is defined as the corroboration of the patient's definition with that of the nurse's, and, when a discrepancy between the two occurs, attaining mutual agreement.

Agreement regarding definition of the problem can be achieved by various methods. If possible, verbal exploration of the situation with the patient should confirm the nurse's definition of the problem or necessitate its reformulation. The following exchange illustrates this method.

Patient discussing previous surgery: "The only thing I hated was that tube down my nose . . . scared me to death"

Based on the nurse's knowledge of the patient's previous appendectomy she inferred that he feared the nasogastric tube.

Nurse validating: "You're scared to death of which tube? The one put down your nose to make you cough or the tube which was inserted through your nose into your stomach for drainage?"
Patient response: "The one in my stomach that they put cold water down"

Thus, the patient confirmed the fact that in this case the nurse's definition and his own were the same. Further "hunches" explored by the authors were those based on their significance in terms of identification of patient problems.

If the problem cannot be confirmed verbally with the patient, the nurse has at her command alternate methods of identifying potential patient problems. Using all of her senses, available diagnostic tools, and/or actions on behalf of the patient, she indirectly validates her inferences.

For example, the authors observed that on the first postoperative day the patient had rapid, shallow respirations (32/min.), was restless, and had flushed skin. The following inferences were made: fever, atelectasis, consolidation, or possible drug reaction.

Nurse validating:
  1. Felt skin for temperature and took temperature
  2. Observed chest expansion, percussed chest, and used stethoscope to listen for quality and distribution of breath sounds
  3. Observed amount and character of sputum
  4. Examined chest films with M.D.
  5. Checked laboratory reports for lowered arterial Po_2

Through several sources the authors were able to confirm their inference that the patient had developed right lower lobe atelectasis.

ASSESSMENT

Validation of patient problems allows the nurse to direct her attention toward assessment, the fourth component of the nursing process. The authors used assessment and the concept of nursing diagnosis interchangeably. Both of these steps were defined as relating knowledge to patient problems and determining central problems, which led to the development of alternative mitigating actions.

Peplau has summarized some of the steps involved in the process of assessment. Thought processes might include: sorting and classifying, comparing, applying concepts and relationships, and summarizing or synthesizing data.[6] Review of the literature also indicates many suggestions for categories to be used in assessing data or making a nursing diagnosis.[3,7,8]

However, the authors chose to code daily patient observations using the categories described above in the nursing history form. Inferences were made from these observations and were subsequently recorded. Based on frequency and importance, only certain validated inferences were recognized as central problems, and functioned at the assessment of nursing diagnosis. Just as the physician's diagnosis may change, the nurse's diagnosis also may vary from day to day or minute to minute. As the nurse's understanding and knowledge of the patient increases and as the patient presents new problems, the diagnosis should be revised accordingly.

A deliberative approach to diagnosis leads the nurse to decisionmaking and priority-setting in the assessment of patient needs. The process enables formulation of nursing actions with a greater probability of success because more valid and comprehensive data are received.

The authors have included below one example of a preoperative nursing assessment or diagnosis. This assessment was formed by collecting many observations and inferences, similar to those shown above, during several interactions with the patient, family, or health team. Those validated inferences that demonstrated a pattern of frequency and importance were then established as the nursing diagnosis from which a plan of care was formulated.

ACTION

Nursing action, the next step in the process, is defined as the testing of alternatives and the carrying out of those considered the most suitable. The appropriate alternative actions chosen by the authors are listed below with the nursing diagnosis to illustrate these two steps in the process.

Nursing diagnosis
1. Decreased energy with dyspnea on exertion.
2. Possible reaction to antibiotics and other medications.
3. Apparent anxiety and need for tension release.
4. Need for knowledge of procedures as they relate to self.
5. Possible low self-esteem and low masculine self-image.
6. Possible denial of illness leading to self-destruction.
7. Fear of losing body intactness and death.
8. Unstable social environment.

Alternative nursing actions
1. Help patient to understand physical limitations prior to surgery in order to conserve energy; attempt to decrease environmental stressors.
2. Alert staff about possible drug reactions: observe for these reactions.
3. Assist patient to cope with illness by listening, focusing on what concerns him, and involving him in simple ward activities.
4. Investigate the patient's perception of the medical and nursing treatments in relation to himself; after investigation focus teaching on actual danger threats perceived by patient.
5a. Collect further data to validate low male identity.
5b. Allow patient to control his environment whenever possible.
5c. Involve patient in decision-making.
6a. Collect data to validate diagnosis of denial of illness and self-destructive behavior.
6b. Assist patient to develop a more realistic perception of postoperative self by focusing on realistic outcome of surgery.
6c. Help patient to gain understanding of rationale for M.D. order to stop smoking.
7a. Recognize nurse's behavior which may interfere with patient's ability to verbalize feelings about death.
7b. Listen for clues indicating patient's desire to express feelings about death.
8a. Collect more data to validate patient's life style and pattern of illness.
8b. Seek consultation from social workers and chaplain.

Nursing actions or interventions are in part dependent upon the nurse's theory of nursing. Such actions should encompass all activities from counseling and teaching to physical care and delegated medical therapy. Another important facet with which the nurse must concern herself is the priority of intervention. Although many factors beyond the scope of this report are significant, the patient's priority of needs primarily determines the type, level, and speed of intervention. Certainly, in particular patient situations, the nurse may need to act or intervene immediately after rapidly moving through the first steps of the process.

EVALUATION

The final step of these operational processes is that of evaluation. Evaluation is defined as a continuous process through which appraisal of the effectiveness of the previous steps in meeting the patient's needs is provided. Observation of patient behavior, communication with the patient, his family, and health team members, and diagnostic measurements were used to evaluate each step in the process and the total process. Because patient and nursing goals had been clearly defined, the authors were better able to determine the degree to which these goals had been achieved.

The following patient situations are presented to illustrate the process of evaluation. Previous steps in the process have been included in an attempt to describe more clearly the flow and developing nursing process for the reader.

Patient situation I

Postop. Day #2
   Observations:
      Flushed skin color, elevated temp., restless
      Rapid, shallow respirations, rate 32/min.
      Greater expansion of left chest than right
      Region of right lower lobe dull to percussion with diminished breath sounds
      Decreased sputum in last 24 hours
   Inferences:
      Possible atelectasis or drug reaction
   Validated Inference:
      Chest film and M.D. physical examination confirmed right lower lobe atelectasis
   Nursing Assessment/Diagnosis:
      Right Lower Lobe Atelectasis
   Nursing Actions:
      1. Frequent change in position
      2. Support incision during frequent deep breathing and coughing, clapping and vibrating, re-emphasize need for all procedures
      3. Contact physical therapist for chest therapy
      4. Administer IPPB with bronchodilator as ordered
      5. Observe for changes in expansion, rate, and breath sounds
      6. Observe laboratory reports of blood gases for possible changes in acidbase balance, hypoxia
      7. Force fluids
Postop. Day #5
   Nurse Evaluation:
      Chest film confirmed cessation of atelectatic process
      Blood gases within normal limits

Patient situation II

Postop. Days #8, 9
   Observations:
      "All I can do is say, buddy, I'm here . . . sometimes I don't think they know it's you."
      "They're not going to throw something in my face and make me sign it again."
      "That doctor is like a bull in a china shop."

Inference:
   Impersonalization of patient by staff
Validated Inference:
   Patient was asked his impressions of the health team, to which he replied, "They treat you like a guinea pig around here, sometimes I don't think they know it's you."
Nursing Assessment/Diagnosis:
   Impersonalization by staff
Nursing Actions:
   Discuss ways of personalizing care with nursing and medical staff.
   1. Patient decision-making whenever possible
   2. Possibility of one staff member caring for patient
   3. Explain rationale for procedures before acting
   4. Allow patient to express hostility
Postop. Day #13
   Nurse Evaluation:
      1. Patient's decreased frequency of negative comments about staff
      2. Also increased positive clues, such as:
         "Dr. B. didn't yank out those stitches so hard today."
         "Oh, I know that, Miss J. told me all about that pill this morning."

CONCLUSIONS

The authors formulated the following conclusions while putting this process into operation. The daily recording of all observations, inferences, diagnoses, actions, and evaluations in horizontal sequence within one notebook assisted the authors and the staff to see definite patterns of patient behavior and subsequent nursing actions for this group of patients. This method of recording and coding data also was practical, time-conserving, easy to use, and could actually be implemented in the patient setting.

It is apparent that this process requires the use of both theory and expert clinical practice in order that valid nursing actions can be derived and evaluated for effectiveness.

Continuity of care was necessarily increased as nurses gained an understanding of the process through discussions and care conferences. With increased knowledge of the process and recording designs they assisted the authors in establishing nursing histories, diagnoses, alternate actions, and evaluations. With such assistance a wider range of patient problems was identified and a unified plan of care achieved. Care plans were transferred with patients as they moved from preoperative to postoperative settings. These plans were easily communicated to other health team members and community agencies.

A trust relationship with the patient was the cornerstone of this process. The accumulation of data would have been impossible if the authors had not conveyed interest and concern, and used all their abilities to form relationships that became therapeutic catalysts.

One of the most important findings was that patients evaluated this process favorably. They expressed opinions that knowledge of procedures and potential danger threats, exposure to the intensive care unit preoperatively, and identification with one nurse throughout their hospitalization helped them to understand and anticipate events during hospitalization. Anxiety appeared to be reduced, and postoperative expectations seemed more realistic.

In conclusion, a more scientific approach to the nursing process has enabled the investigators to identify a wider range of patient problems, to apply theoretical knowledge toward the solution of identified patient needs, and to define a rationale for nursing action which has a higher probability of success. It is the authors' opinion that the use of this nursing process would help to increase understanding of individual patient problems and give insight into patterns of behavior to be used for future prediction.

REFERENCES

1. Parker, C. J., and Rubin, L. J.: Process as Content: Curriculum Design and the Application of Knowledge. Chicago, Rand McNally & Co., 1966.
2. Kaplan, Abraham: The Conduct of Inquiry: Methodology for Behavioral Science. San Francisco, Chandler Publishing Co., 1964, p. 127.
3. Lewis, L., Carozza, V., Carroll, M., Darragh, R., Patrick, M., and Schadt, E.: Defining Clinical Content Graduate Nursing Programs: Medical-Surgical Nursing. Colorado, Western Interstate Commission for Higher Education, 1967.
4. Wiedenbach, Ernestine: Clinical nursing—A Helping Art. New York, Springer Publishing Co., 1964.
5. Orlando, Ida Jean: The Dynamic Nurse-Patient Relationship. New York, G. P. Putnam's Sons, 1961.
6. Peplau, Hildegard E.: Process and Concept Learning. *In* Burd, Shirley, and Marshall, Margaret A., eds.: Some Clinical Approaches to Psychiatric Nursing. New York, The Macmillan Co., 1963, pp. 333-336.
7. McCain, R. Faye: Nursing by assessment—not intuition, Am. J. Nurs. **65**:82-84, April, 1965.
8. Little, Dolores E., and Carnevali, Doris L.: Nursing Care Planning. Philadelphia, J. B. Lippincott Co., 1969.

THE NURSING PROCESS:
A TOOL TO INDIVIDUALIZED CARE

Lorraine Hagar

In many ways, the nursing process is "common sense." It incorporates an approach that most of us use every day when we try to solve the problems we face. But each of us, from time to time, is guilty of sloppy thinking. We make assumptions about the problems we *think* a patient has; we think we know the solutions but never stop to evaluate their effectiveness; we fall into routine patterns of behavior—the old familiar "rut." Individualized nursing care, however, demands more than good intentions. It takes "common sense" to look at a patient's needs and problems in an organized and perceptive way and to use the time we have with a patient, no matter how limited, in the best way possible.

The use of the nursing process as a standard tool in all activities related to nursing has become a primary concern in our profession today. As a method that uses assessment, planning, implementation and evaluation as its formula, the nursing process is flexible and adaptable, applicable in any setting. It provides a deliberate, systematic and organized approach to nursing practice that accomplishes the main purposes of nursing—to promote wellness, to contribute to the quality of life and to maximize all resources.[1]

The nursing process requires the development of a therapeutic relationship between ourselves and our patients. We are past the day when nurses work with only one part of the patient—the part that is sick. Now, we are challenged to utilize all our knowledge to assess the patient's strengths as well as his weaknesses so that he can share in the assessment,

Reprinted with permission from The Canadian Nurse **73**(10):38-41, 1977.

planning and evaluation of his care. Familiarity with theories and disease entities is no longer enough. We need to know our patients as individuals. For example, to know that Mr. Smith in Room 401 has hypertension is to know only a small part of what is happening to Mr. Smith. If we plan our nursing care solely on that "classification", we will do a poor job of meeting Mr. Smith's needs. The nursing process provides a framework—a tool of the trade—that we can use to find out more about Mr. Smith's needs in a systematic rather than a haphazard way.

It is the relationship we develop with our patients—a relationship that allows him and his family to take part in the nursing process (that is, the assessment of unmet needs or problems, planning nursing activities to solve these problems, implementing the actions and then evaluating whether or not the actions did indeed meet these needs)—that constitutes the basis for our practice. As nurse educator and author Madeleine Leininger has said, "Nurses help people through a professional relationship that is learned. It is the use of the therapeutic relationship with patients that constitutes the heart of nursing practice and determines what is done to the patient and how it is done."[2]

In addition to information concerning the patient's personal history, capabilities and limitations, knowledge of current and traditional theories from various disciplines can help to provide a working basis for the nursing process. A basic knowledge of man/environment interactions in various cultural settings may be an asset in assisting the individual in the immediate situation. The nurse must make full use of her knowledge of physiology, pathology, psychology, hospital and community facilities, family interaction and support, as well as her own intuition. Use of her knowledge base and constant re-evaluation will help to develop the nursing process into a personalized device, tempered by personal experience as well as formal training. The nurse's efforts are aimed at helping the patient cope with his environment and society to their mutual benefit. It is often a tall order.

BRIAN—A CASE STUDY
Assessment

"The assessment phase begins with the nursing history and ends with a nursing diagnosis. The purpose of this phase is to identify and obtain data about the client that will enable the nurse and/or client and his family to designate problems relating to wellness or illness. If problems exist, then the first step toward a solution is to identify them."[3]

Brian, a four-year-old victim of child abuse and maternal deprivation, was admitted to hospital for treatment of a fractured femur sustained when he fell off his tricycle. Six months prior to the accident, he had been taken away from his parents and placed in a foster home. Little personal history was taken at the time of admission and his foster parents, living in another town, were rarely able to visit.

To the nursing staff, Brian appeared to be physically as well as mentally immature for his age. He did not speak intelligibly and his level of development was that of a one- or two-year old. Brian was originally diagnosed as an autistic child. Later it was recognized that maternal deprivation was the cause of his behavior.

Brian was immobilized in a hip spica cast and restrained on his stomach in his crib. He reacted to the pain in his leg, to immobilization and to the strange environment by crying, violently kicking his free leg and tearing the bed sheets and toys. When someone attempted to make contact with him, he would either withdraw or lash out. He mistrusted everyone who approached him.

In assessing Brian's needs, the threats to his wellness included not only his broken leg but all the ramifications that this injury caused in upsetting his physiological and psychological patterns of daily living. For example, he could not sit to eat and often vented his frustrations by throwing his food. Sometimes, he would refuse food altogether. If he was hungry enough, he would eat anything in sight. His dirty diaper proved to be no exception. Elimination was a problem—any gains made in toilet training had been lost. A case of diarrhea made matters worse. Brian's activity was largely curtailed by the cast and restraints. Rest was difficult because of his pain and agitation. These difficulties were compounded by an unfamiliar environment, and his great reluctance or inability to trust those trying to help him.

Generally, Brian dealt with his situation by aggression—by throwing or demolishing toys, food, bedding and attempting (sometimes successfully) to bite nurses. When very angry, Brian would destroy things with his teeth. When moderately upset, he would seem to find comfort in sucking on a diaper. It was interesting to note that in a calm state after Brian became used to me, he would examine and manipulate objects but made no attempt to put them in his mouth. He would sometimes even give the object back to me—a developmental task described by Erickson as "holding on" and "letting go."[4]

In this, he showed signs of having superseded Freud's oral gratification stage. He also demonstrated his ability to make choices, whether to let me have the object or not. Often, he changed his mind and decided to keep it himself.

But when Brian actually tried to put his fingers in my mouth, I decided that he trusted me more than I trusted him. I didn't dare let my hand go near those teeth of his.

In working with Brian, I felt that the establishment of a trusting relationship was the top priority. Without trust, all care was inflicted on Brian by force and he, in turn, used up all his energy in resisting it. Any effort to restrain him, even to hold his wrist to take his pulse, was violently resisted. The greater the force used to restrain him, the greater were his efforts to resist. For example, he proved this "heroically" when it took an orderly and two hefty nurses to hold Brian still for an X ray of his leg (already immobilized in the cast).

Planning and giving care

During the assessment, the unmet needs of the client have been identified. The purposes of the planning phase, the second step in the nursing process are:

1. to assign priority to the problems diagnosed
2. to differentiate among those problems that can be solved by the nurse, the health team and the client/family
3. to designate specific actions and their goals
4. to communicate the plan to others by writing it down in a nursing care plan.[5] The third step in the process is the implementation of the plan.

Brian's priorities differed radically from those of the health team in that he often did not want anyone to touch or come near him. When the goals of the patient and nurse are at odds, problems are compounded.

The abused child has an innate mistrust of those around him. In giving nursing care to Brian, I found that his mistrust of me could be overcome but that it reappeared with each contact. In establishing a trusting relationship with him, I had to follow a particular pattern of behavior each time. I did this by staying with him and letting him familiarize himself with me, by touching and speaking to him gently. I would let him handle the diaper I was going to put on him, put his fingers in the skin cream and touch anything used in his care. The music from a windup toy radio helped to soothe him and I would hold his hand on the knob to wind it up. Once a measure of trust had been developed, he would allow me to wash him and do cast care without too much fuss.

The importance of Brian's need to manipulate, explore and exert some control over his environment is emphasized by a review of the developmental tasks of the toddler stage. Although Brian was far behind developmentally, his capabilities seemed to vary with the degree of agitation he experienced. Using this rationale to plan activities and an environment conductive to successful achievement of these developmental tasks would, I hoped, prevent Brian from regressing to a great extent while hospitalized, and also provide him with sensory stimulation.

Brian became much more approachable and settled when freed from his restraints and placed on blankets on the floor. He soon learned to log roll over the cast and pull himself around to reach a desired toy. If the room was quiet, Brian could be encouraged to become interested in toys, instead of just throwing them around to release his frustration. It also became apparent that Brian could feed himself with a spoon and drink out of a cup. His ability to focus his attention and perform tasks varied with his level of anxiety.

Brian's cooperation could only be enlisted by a very slow, gentle approach, preferably by a familiar person. If he was given no opportunity to adjust to a new environment, procedure, or person, the result was a hysterical, kicking, screaming little monster, lashing out tooth and nail.

However, after he had tested out people and his environment, assuring himself that neither would harm him, his destructive tendencies disappeared (for a time) and he showed evidence of more advanced motor and social development such as feeding himself with a spoon, parallel play, interest in my book, pen, watch. This first step towards developing trust appeared to be the key to helping Brian achieve a sense of security and a balanced state from which he could progress.

Evaluation

"Evaluation is always in terms of how the client is expected to respond to the planned action . . . (It) is the natural intellectual activity completing the process phases because it indicates the degree to which the nursing diagnosis and nursing actions have been correct."[6]

My primary purpose during the short time I spent with Brian was to establish a therapeutic relationship which in itself would meet his basic need for someone to trust. Brian's mistrust of everyone appeared to stem from the damaging effect of his previous interactions with his parents as a victim of child abuse. In nursing Brian, I tried to concentrate on ways of caring for and assisting him rather than to accomplish or inflict set procedures such as taking vital signs, feeding, washing, giving skin care, and doing cast care. My aim was to involve him in his care, and find acceptable ways to acquaint him with the different procedures so that he would not find them so frightening.

Brian's problems appeared to be interrelated. In attempting to stabilize his food and fluid intake, by providing a quiet atmosphere and freeing him from his restraints, I hoped that his elimination would become more regular so that "bed pan training" might be initiated in the future. If the discomforts of indigestion, loss of bowel control and emotional turmoil were diminished, regular periods of rest and sleep could promote his recovery and perhaps improve his behavior.

Although Brian did not fit into any one developmental level, appreciation of the uniqueness of his personality and the effect of stress on the individual prevented me from vainly trying to categorize him. He presented the sad picture of what can happen when basic needs are not met early in life, and critical developmental tasks are not successfully accomplished. Brian had to repeatedly test out people and his environment, to gain confidence in his own ability to trust, or to decide not to trust.

In my attempts to focus Brian's attention, to promote familiarity, to provide a quiet atmosphere, and to reduce the barrage of incomprehensible stimuli, I was able to see Brian's progress, or rather his reattainment of a previous level of development. Unfortunately, in controlling his environment, I did not prepare or reconcile him with the changing circumstances he would face again the next day, when he would be open to the approaches of many different and unfamiliar people. He was considered a problem by most of the nursing staff on the floor and care was often given in the most expedient fashion, not necessarily tailored to Brian's unique needs. It would have been beneficial if the same nurse could have arranged to care for him on a regular basis.

Although I cared for Brian for only two days, this proved long enough to utilize and carry out the elements of the nursing process. At times, the process seemed to be reduced to a modified trial and error method, but its effectiveness was measured by the change observed in Brian's behavior. He began to respond to verbal commands and his destructive tendencies and wild behavior gave way to explorative interest in his environment.

I presented the approach I had used in caring for Brian to the staff nurses I came in contact with and also made explanatory nursing notes. The staff did substitute mats for his crib to eliminate the need for restraints and provide Brian with more sensory stimulation and freedom to explore his room.

In spite of this, however, my plan failed to maintain the element of continuity and pattern necessary to fulfill the purposes of care. It was reported that by the time of discharge, he had regressed further. The regular staff simply did not have the time to devote to Brian to make my plan a success.

Even so, this does not mean that the nursing process is bound to fail on a busy hospital floor. The key to the nursing process is continuity and consistency. Interaction that has proven to be effective needs to be continued and reevaluated by all nurses in contact with the patient. It takes a reorganization of thinking—to look at needs in an orderly, logical manner and to think things through. "What is this person's need? What actions can I take to help him meet these needs? Were my actions effective?"

STATEMENT ON A PATIENT'S BILL OF RIGHTS

The American Hospital Association presents a Patient's Bill of Rights with the expectation that observance of these rights will contribute to more effective patient care and greater satisfaction for the patient, his physician, and the hospital organization. Further, the Association presents these rights in the expectation that they will be supported by the hospital on behalf of its patients, as an integral part of the healing process. It is recognized that a personal relationship between the physician and the patient is essential for the provision of proper medical care. The traditional physician-patient relationship takes on a new dimension when care is rendered within an organizational structure. Legal precedent has established that the institution itself also has a responsibility to the patient. It is in recognition of these factors that these rights are affirmed.

1. The patient has the right to considerate and respectful care.
2. The patient has the right to obtain from his physician complete current information concerning his diagnosis, treatment, and prognosis in terms the patient can be reasonably expected to understand. When it is not medically advisable to give such information to the patient, the information should be made available to an appropriate person in his behalf. He has the right to know, by name, the physician responsible for coordinating his care.
3. The patient has the right to receive from his physician information necessary to give informed consent prior to the start of any procedure and/or treatment. Except in emergencies, such information for informed consent should include but not necessarily be limited to the specific procedure and/or treatment, the medically significant risks involved, and the probable duration of incapacitation. Where medically significant alternatives for care or treatment exist, or when the patient requests information concerning medical alternatives, the patient has the right to such information. The patient also has the right to know the name of the person responsible for the procedures and/or treatment.
4. The patient has the right to refuse treatment to the extent permitted by law and to be informed of the medical consequences of his action.
5. The patient has the right to every consideration of his privacy concerning his own medical care program. Case discussion, consultation, examination, and treatment are confidential and should be conducted discreetly. Those not directly involved in his care must have the permission of the patient to be present.
6. The patient has the right to expect that all communications and records pertaining to his care should be treated as confidential.
7. The patient has the right to expect that within its capacity a hospital must make reasonable response to the request of a patient for services. The hospital must provide evaluation, service, and/or referral as indicated by the urgency of the case. When medically permissible, a patient may be transferred to another facility only after he has received complete information and explanation concerning the needs for and alternatives to such a transfer. The institution to which the patient is to be transferred must first have accepted the patient for transfer.
8. The patient has the right to obtain information as to any relationship of his hospital to other health care and educational institutions insofar as his care is concerned. The patient has the right to obtain information as to the existence of any professional relationships among individuals, by name, who are treating him.
9. The patient has the right to be advised if the hospital proposes to engage in or perform human experimentation affecting his care or treatment. The patient has the right to refuse to participate in such research projects.
10. The patient has the right to expect reasonable continuity of care. He has the right to know in advance what appointment times and physicians are available and where.

The patient has the right to expect that the hospital will provide a mechanism whereby he is informed by his physician or a delegate of the physician of the patient's continuing health care requirements following discharge.

11. The patient has the right to examine and receive an explanation of his bill regardless of source of payment.
12. The patient has the right to know what hospital rules and regulations apply to his conduct as a patient.

No catalog of rights can guarantee for the patient the kind of treatment he has a right to expect. A hospital has many functions to perform, including the prevention and treatment of disease, the education of both health professionals and patients, and the conduct of clinical research. All these activities must be conducted with an overriding concern for the patient, and above all, the recognition of his dignity as a human being. Success in achieving this recognition assures success in the defense of the rights of the patient.

SUGGESTED READINGS for Chapter 1

BOOKS

Auld, M. E., and Birum, L. H., editors: The challenge of nursing, St. Louis, 1973, The C. V. Mosby Co. Unit III is a collection of articles related to nursing process.

Beland, I.: Clinical nursing: pathophysiological and psychological approaches, New York, 1970, The Macmillan Publishing Co., Inc. A medical-surgical textbook.

Readey, H., Teague, M., and Readey, W.: Introduction to nursing essentials: a handbook, St. Louis, 1977, The C. V. Mosby Co. The nursing process is discussed among other subjects.

Sundeen, S. J., Stuart, G. W., Rankin, E. D., and Cohen, S. P.: Nurse-client interaction: implementing the nursing process, St. Louis, 1976, The C. V. Mosby Co. The nursing process and nursing intervention are discussed.

Walter, J. B., Paradee, G. P., and Molbo, D. M.: Dynamics of problem-oriented approaches: patient care and documentation, Philadelphia, 1976, J. B. Lippincott Co. The nursing process, nursing diagnosis, and the problem-oriented system are discussed.

Yura, H., and Walsh, M. B., editors: The nursing process, Washington, D.C., 1967, The Catholic University of America Press. Discusses assessing patient needs, planning to meet those needs, implementing and evaluating plan of care.

Yura, H., and Walsh, M. B.: The nursing process: assessing, planning, implementing, evaluating, New York, 1973, Appleton-Century-Crofts. Discusses components of nursing process.

PERIODICALS
Nursing process

Altschul, A. T.: Use of the nursing process in psychiatric care, Nurs. Times 74(36):1412-1413, 1977. Describes the nursing process as a systematic way of planning individualized care.

Bloch, D.: Some crucial terms in nursing—what do they really mean? Nurs. Outlook 22(11):689-694, 1974, and in Nicholls, M. E., and Wessells, V. G., editors: Nursing standards and nursing process, Wakefield, Mass., Contemporary Publishing, Inc., 1977, pp. 3-11. Presents a five-step model of the nursing process.

Carlson, S.: A practical approach to the nursing process, Am. J. Nurs. 72(9):1589-1591, 1972. Compares medical and nursing processes.

Collins, R. D.: Problem solving: a tool for patients, too, Am. J. Nurs. 68(7):1483-1485, 1968. Discusses teaching patients how to do problem solving.

Dahlin, B.: Rehabilitation and the assessment of patient need, Nurs. Clin. North Am. 1:375-386, Sept., 1966. Relates nursing process to rehabilitation and stresses continuity of care.

Deininger, J. M.: The nursing process: implementation and evaluation, J. Pract. Nurs. 25(12):18, 32, 1975. Indicates that implementation is what the patient and his family see. Evaluation helps determine if the care plan was properly focused.

Deininger, J. M.: The nursing process: the history . . . the beginning, J. Pract. Nurs. 25(9):20-23, 1975. Presents the nursing history as the first component of the nursing process and as necessary for continuity and individualization of patient care.

Gahan, K. A.: Problem solving as a therapeutic process, J. Psychiatr. Nurs. 14(11):37-39, 43-44, 1976. Discusses the problem solving process and indicates it should be taught to people to help them assume control and responsibility for themselves.

Geach, B.: The problem-solving technique: as taught to psychiatric students, Perspect. Psychiatr. Care 12(1):9-12, 1974. Warns that automatism and omnipotence must be avoided if the helping relationship is to be preserved. The patient must be involved in solving his problems.

Geach, B.: The problem-solving technique: is it relevant to practice? Can. Nurse 70:21-22, Jan., 1974. Indicates that practicing nurses should inform educators if problem solving is not being used in nursing service.

Hargreaves, I.: The nursing process: the key to individuals care, Nurs. Times 71:89-91, Aug. 28, 1975. Presents a review of the literature about the nursing process and suggests that it can be used to assist the individual whether he is sick or well.

Jones, C.: The nursing process—individualized care, Nurs. Mirror 145(15):13-14, 1977. Describes the nursing process as a problem solving process.

Kelly, K.: Clinical inference in nursing, Nurs. Res. 15:23-26, Winter, 1966. Discusses observational, inferential, and decision-making roles of the nurse.

Kneedler, J.: Nursing process is continuing cycle, AORN J. **20**(8):245-248, 1974. Describes nursing process.

Knight, J. H.: Applying nursing process in the community, Nurs. Outlook **22**:708-711, Nov., 1974. Applies the nursing process to a remote community in Texas.

Lamy, M.: Is problem solving something that can be taught? Am. Lung. Assoc. Bull. **62**(10):8-9, 1976. A computerized model of the lung is used to teach problem solving to medical students at the University of Vermont College of Medicine.

Levenstein, A.: Problem solving technics for managing change, Hosp. Top. **52**(8):42-47, 1974. Discusses problem solving as it relates to supervision and management.

Lewis, L.: This I believe . . . about the nursing process—key to care, Nurs. Outlook **16**(5): 26-29, 1968. Discusses steps in nursing process and defines them as assessment, intervention, and evaluation.

McConnell, E. A.: What's the difference? Superv. Nurse **7**(11):20-22, 1976. Application of the nursing process is discussed.

Nolan, M. G.: Problem solving is research in action, AORN J. **20**(8):225-231, 1974. Outlines problem solving approach to nursing problems and maintains it is research in action.

Schaefer, J.: The interrelatedness of decision making and the nursing process, Am. J. Nurs. **74**(10):1852-1855, 1974. Argues that decision making is related to goals and nursing process is related to health results. The nurse should use both processes.

Silberstein, C. A.: Implementing and evaluating the nursing process in the occupational health unit, Occup. Health Nurs. **24**(11):14-19, 1976. Presents a conceptual model for an interdisciplinary approach, an industrial hazard reference file, and a sample nursing care plan for an industrial worker.

Wiedenbach, E.: The helping art of nursing, Am. J. Nurs. **63**(11):54-57, 1963. Describes nursing process through use of case study.

Wong, P., Doyle, M., and Straus, D.: Problem solving through "process management," J. Nurs. Admin. **5**(1):37-39, 1975. Lists ways to facilitate process management.

Patient's Bill of Rights

Annas, G. J.: The patient rights advocate: can nurses effectively fill the role? Superv. Nurse

5:21-25, July, 1974. Presents a proposed bill of rights and indicates that nurses should be patient advocates by promoting those rights.

Annas, G. J., and Healey, J.: The patient rights advocate, J. Nurs. Admin. **4**:25-31, May-June, 1974. Nature of rights are discussed and examples of how an advocate system can function are given.

Bandman, E., and Bandman, B.: There is nothing automatic about rights, Am. J. Nurs. **77**(5):867-872, 1977. Problems in implementing the patient's bill of rights are discussed.

Breitung, J.: The rights of patients, Nurs. Care **9**(9):30-32, 1976. Indicates that a right is enforceable in a court, and some states have set fines for violations of patient's rights. However, no document will ensure considerate care.

Carnegie, M. E.: The patient's bill of rights and the nurse, Nurs. Clin. North Am. **9**(3):557-562, 1974, and in Nicholls, M. C., and Wessells, V. G., editors: Nursing standards and nursing process, Wakefield, Mass., 1977, Contemporary Publishing, Inc., pp. 67-71. Lists patient rights in American Hospital Association and the NLN statements.

Glass, K.: Right to treatment: O'Connor v. Donaldson, Health and Social Work **2**(1):26-40, 1977. Supreme Court contended that confinement of a person who is not dangerous violates his right to liberty. Implications for the mental health system are explored.

Golodetz, A., Ruess, J., and Milhous, R. L.: The right to know: giving the patient his medical record, Arch. Phys. Med. Rehabil. **57**(2):78-81, 1976. Patients admitted to a 16-bed rehabilitation medicine service were allowed to read their charts and found them educational.

Kelly, L. Y.: The patient's right to know, Nurs. Outlook **24**(1):26-32, 1976. Presents the American Hospital Association's "A Patient's Bill of Rights." Discusses informed consent, sharing the record, and research implications.

Krant, Melvin J.: Rights of the cancer patient, Nurs. Digest **5**(2):32-33, 1977. Recommends that cancer patients be allowed to stay in control of their lives and to feel secure in rejecting what doctors and nurses want.

Nurses and informed consent: surgical permits, The Regan Report on Nursing Law **16**(8):1, 1975. When getting a surgical consent signed, the nurse should know "that the patient is: (1) Conscious and aware of what is being signed; (2) Informed regarding the nature and purpose as well as regarding the calculated risks of the proposed surgery; and (3) Ready and willing to execute the consent for surgery voluntarily and without duress." Presents a legal case.

The patient's right to know, The Regan Report on Nursing Law **16**(1):1, 1975. Indicates "the patient has a right to know (1) What's wrong with him; (2) What is being done about it; and (3) What the prospects are for physical recovery."

The pregnant patient's bill of rights, Keeping Abreast Journal **1**(3):253-255, 1976. The pregnant patient's bill of rights is presented.

Quinn, N., and Somers, A. R.: The patient's bill of rights: a significant aspect of the consumer revolution, Nurs. Outlook **22**(4):240-244, 1974. Discusses history and formalization of "The Patient's Bill of Rights."

CHAPTER 2

ASSESSMENT

To deal with a problem, one first must determine what the problem is. Therefore assessment is the first phase of the problem solving process. It begins with the collection of patient data that have implications for nursing actions and ends with the nursing diagnosis, a statement of the patient's problems.

Observing and interviewing the patient are basic methods of gathering information. The nursing history provides a systematic format from which to develop a written record about a client. It is usually in the form of a questionnaire or checklist. The nursing history provides the facts on which to assess existing and potential patient problems and serves as a basis for planning, implementing, and evaluating nursing care.

Taking a nursing history allows the nurse to establish a positive nurse-patient relationship, to observe the patient's behavior and condition, and to obtain information from the client. The use of a format helps ensure that necessary information will be obtained. Carefully worded questions may be read by the nurse who is not familiar with the interview technique; nurses who are more comfortable with it may paraphrase the questions. Interviewing with a purpose helps obtain satisfactory results.

Interviewing is a goal-directed method of communication. It should be as open-ended as possible, progressing from general to specific, and allowing the patient the opportunity for spontaneous expression. The client should be encouraged to express his feelings because during spontaneous discussions he is often likely to reveal useful information. The interviewer should focus on emotionally charged areas, since these are likely to be the areas where the patient is having difficulty adapting.

Interviewing is more than a question and answer session. It is an observational technique. The interviewer should listen most of the time. Verbal responses on the part of the interviewer tend to obstruct the client's responses. In making inferences it is necessary not merely to listen to the patient's words, but to watch for facial expressions and gestures and to listen to the way words are said.

Assessment through the use of the nursing history and secondary sources, such as medical records, nursing notes, nursing rounds, change-of-shift reports, and the Kardex, allows the nurse to make a nursing diagnosis that is a statement of the patient's problems. The nursing diagnosis is made by collecting and evaluating data that have implications for nursing actions.

OBSERVATION

An accurate description of what we observe is basic to care of the client. It requires use of all the senses. The nurse uses vision to perceive discoloration, swelling, color and amount of drainage, character of respirations, and nonverbal communications. Listening is another major means of observation. It is vitally important for the nurse to listen to what the patient says. Sounds such as choking, gasping, and sobbing may indicate patient distress. Hearing also aids in the evaluation of breath, heart, and bowel sounds. A sense of caring for and about the patient can be communicated by touching him; at the same time the nurse can determine if his skin is hot or cold, moist or dry. Through touch the size, shape, and texture of local swelling or an enlarged organ can be determined. The sense of smell can detect the fruity odor of diabetic acidosis, foul odor from drainage, or musty odor from beneath a cast—each of which might indicate an infection—or smoke from a patient's room.

Nurses must develop a proficiency for the observation of both overt and covert signs and symptoms of problems. Whereas the overt is obvious, the covert is more obscure and frequently is associated with psychosocial aspects. A symptom refers to any indicator of illness or change in the patient's condition that is perceived by the patient or observed by someone else. Symptoms are either objective or subjective. Objective symptoms (signs) are objective indications of disease that can be observed by others and measured by instruments that expand human capacities for observation. Subjective symptoms are apparent only to the patient. Inflammation and swelling are objective symptoms, or signs, since they may be observed by others. Subjective symptoms such as itching and pain are those felt by the patient.

Observation is essential for the planning of nursing care but is not adequate by itself. It is a continuous process accompanied by accurate inference and appropriate action. Although not solely responsible for observation, the nurse does have primary responsibility for it because of her knowledge, skills, and proximity to the patient.[1] Observation of the patient is most thorough if done systematically. A head-to-toe approach may be useful but tends to include only physical aspects. A more thorough approach is SELF-PACING, an acronym that represents a process developed for systematic assessment. SELF-PACING includes the following: S, socialization and special senses; E, elimination and exercise; L, liquids; F, foods; P, pain, personal hygiene, posture; A, aeration; C, circulation; I, integument; N, neuromuscular control and coordination; and G, general condition.[2] Ultimately each nurse may have to devise her own system.

Skill in observation is not readily acquired and requires regular, systematic practice. The novice needs to study what, when, and where to observe.

NURSING INTERVIEW

Interviewing is an observational technique. It is a method of learning about people through purposeful, goal-directed communication. The nursing interview was developed in an effort to give personalized care. Its purpose is to encourage the patient to express ideas, feelings, and facts that help identify his immediate and long-range needs. The nurse focuses on the patient and encourages him to identify his needs and goals. The nurse then gives the client an opportunity to explore his own solution for meeting his identified health needs. The information obtained is incorporated into the nursing care plan.[3]

The quality of the interview is influenced by the climate the nurse creates. Climate is the immediate conditions and circumstances that affect a person. The nurse should choose a time that will be most conducive to optimum communication—a time when there is minimal external stimuli. It is advisable for the nurse to allow sufficient time for the exploration of the patient's feelings, needs, goals, and solutions in meeting the identified health needs. If the interview is not adequately completed in the allotted time or if the interview is otherwise interrupted, the nurse should return to the client as soon as possible to continue the previous communication. The nurse should report progress made toward meeting interview goals to the nurse who replaces her and record pertinent observations on the patient's records as soon as possible.

Conditions such as heat, ventilation, humidity, odors, sounds, and furnishings should be taken into consideration when choosing a site for the interview. A private and confidential climate should be maintained. Physical privacy is desirable and can contribute to psychological privacy. The latter is the more important of the two and does not necessarily require physical privacy. The seats in a corridor, an isolated table in the cafeteria, or just pulling the curtains around the patient's bed may create physical privacy. The key to psychological privacy is attentiveness. The interviewer should express interest in the patient and his problems, conveying the impression that the patient is her only concern during the interview.

The nurse's attitudes can also affect the results of the interview. The attitude of warmth can be communicated through gentleness and thoughtfulness. It indicates a selflessness, a love of mankind, and implies a respect for oneself and others. The attitude of acceptance conveys to a person that his thoughts, feelings, and behaviors are important and worthy of attention. The client is treated as a person of worth and dignity. Compassion is a feeling of fellowship and an urge to help others. It is dependent on acceptance of one's own feelings, which implies a recognition of the feelings and an appreciation of their worth. Objectivity is the ability to evaluate a situation on the basis of what is actually happening without being influenced by one's biases and feelings. Knowledge of what is happening is determined by a person's perception of the situation. Perception is an individual experience affected by sensory receptors and one's history. The nurse needs to know herself before she can understand the patient.[4]

The level of competency in interviewing affects the results. The nurse should not concentrate on the interview guide so much that she is unable to listen to the answers. The questions should be prepared to flow easily and should not be so formalized that they indicate an impersonal manner. When asking questions, the interviewer should be careful to seek clarification of responses rather than to interpret the response in keeping with the nurse's expectations. The patient's description of his pain may not be the expected textbook picture of his diagnosis.

The nurse may use either a series of direct or open-ended questions. By allowing the patient to speak freely and by being a good listener, the nurse improves her relationship with the patient. The patient will more likely behave in his usual manner if he feels comfortable with the interviewer. He usually will offer all the information sought and more if given the opportunity to reveal his own story, in his own way, in an open manner. The facts may not be related in a precise, orderly fashion, but important information is less likely to be omitted than with a direct question technique.

The direct question technique elicits a reponse, but the patient is apt to reveal less about himself than he might by answering open-ended questions. A constant barrage of questions may satisfy the nursing history without allowing the patient to reveal what is of most concern to him. These questions tend to interrupt his chain of thought, diverting him into talking about topics he considers less important and possibly irrelevant. Although the direct question technique elicits answers, it is less effective for developing a positive nurse-patient relationship or for observation of the patient's behavior.

An interview should begin with a relatively broad question followed by progressively more detailed questions. Proceeding from general to specific helps reveal important and spontaneous patient attitudes. Sometimes, when the questions are of a personal nature, the patient resists the invasion of his privacy. If the nurse progresses from the less to more personal questions, the patient probably will be more relaxed and cooperative.

Closed questions elicit yes or no answers and should be avoided. Rather, questions should be worded in a manner that will elicit more than a one-word response. Even when asking specific questions, the nurse should try to keep the patient talking freely. "How are you feeling?" will elicit more information than "Do you have a stomachache?"

The interviewer should avoid biasing the patient's response. Asking a question in a manner that leads the patient to prefer one answer to another or using emotionally charged words are two methods of loading questions. "You have pain here too, don't you?" is a leading question that is more likely to receive a positive response than "Do you have pain here, too?" One is more likely to deny smoking if asked, "Are you inviting cancer by smoking?" than if asked, "Do you smoke?" Loaded questions tend to make the patient dependent on and subordinate to the nurse. The patient may become sensitive to the interviewer's language and give responses he thinks are expected. Loaded questions contribute to misunder-standing the patient's situation and to interfering with the nurse-patient relation-ship. They are, however, useful in a situation where the nurse thinks the patient is biased to the extent of avoiding a specific answer. "What are your favorite alco-holic refreshments?" or "How much can you hold?" implies the interviewer's acceptance of drinking. If the nurse had asked, "Do you drink and if so, how much?" the answer might vary according to the patient's perception of the nurse's approval of drinking.

The nurse should avoid double-barreled questions. When two separate ques-tions are asked in the same sentence, the answer is likely to be confusing. Did the patient's answer address the total question or was he answering only in part? If the patient answers yes to the question, "Are you having any problem with urination and defecation?" what does he really mean?—that he is having trouble with one, the other, or both? If the interviewer makes the question long and involved, the patient may answer only part of it and neglect the rest.

Obviously vocabulary not understood by the patient interferes with communi-cation. If the patient does not understand the direct question, he may answer yes or no simply to avoid appearing ignorant. Simplification is no panacea if it under-estimates the patient's capacity. Ultimately the interviewer must adjust his vo-cabulary to the patient's level of understanding.[5]

Listening

Good listening is a key to successful interviewing, to therapeutic communica-tion, and to being considered a stimulating conversationalist. Listening is a dif-ficult skill to learn. We think faster than we talk, so when we listen, we have time left over for thinking. The spare thinking time is frequently misused. The listener may think about an entirely different subject. He tends to be more interested in himself than in others, and his lack of interest in others leads to inattentiveness. His thoughts stray from the speaker to his own concerns; his prejudices block communication. When he hears a thought contrary to his own, he stops listening and starts formulating arguments to dispute that idea and support his own. He tends to use selective hearing, hearing only what he wants to hear.

Attentiveness is further reduced by hearing unfamiliar vocabulary or the fa-miliar, repetitive sounds or phrases found in pep talks and clichés. Hearing is also reduced by a congenital, infectious, or degenerative condition. Poor acoustics, noise, and poorly controlled room temperature and ventilation interfere with hearing. Irritating mannerisms of the speaker are also distracting. The good lis-tener concentrates a maximum amount of thought on what is being said, thus leaving less time for irrelevant thoughts. He can do this by thinking ahead of the speaker. Try to guess what points will be made next and what the conclusions will be. Evaluate the comments and supportive evidence. Periodically review and summarize the points made. Try to understand the speaker's frame of ref-erence. Listen between the lines. What thoughts are implied? What feelings are indirectly expressed? Does the nonverbal communication support the verbal communication?[6]

Nonverbal communication

Nonverbal language may be accidental or deliberate, and we do communicate our true feelings through nonverbal means. Body gestures, movements, posture, gait, facial expressions, and appearance offer clues. Body movements are culturally learned, mainly by an unconscious imitation of others. They usually accompany speech. Finger tapping, twisting and pulling hair, deep sighs, doodling, and foot swinging provide the nurse with additional information from means other than verbal communication.

Feelings are expressed in different ways by different people, and an expression does not always symbolize the same emotion in one person as it does in another. Expressions of pain vary according to the amount of pain, the patient's perception of his pain, and the patient's upbringing related to expression of discomfort. A person's posture is influenced by his body build, muscular development, occupation, health, attitude toward self, and consciousness of posture. One's selection of color, style, combinations, and cost of clothing are possible further indications of personality characteristics.

A nurse communicates with the patient by the manner in which she touches him while administering to his needs. The tone of the patient's voice may give an indication of his welfare. Other clues can be collected by classifying odors. Does the patient have nervous perspiration, concentrated urine, or is he expelling flatus?[7]

NURSING HISTORY

Taking a history by interviewing the client provides the nurse with an opportunity to establish a positive nurse-patient relationship, to extract information from the patient, and to observe the patient's condition and behavior. The nursing history is a written record of information about a patient. It provides data from which to assess existing and potential patient problems and is the basis for planning, implementing, and evaluating nursing care. The nurse should be able to collect the information quickly, avoiding duplicating information collected by other members of the health team. Some information can be recorded at the patient's bedside; other data can be added later. The best reports are concise and are organized into units of information that serve as foundations for realistic, individualized nursing care plans.

The nursing history form is usually developed by a committee within the institution. Members of the committee select the areas of inquiry such as physical, psychological, social, and cultural aspects. They also determine the categories of information within those areas that are needed to give individualized nursing care to the patient in a specific setting. What can be observed and what should be asked must be taken into consideration when planning the format. Each format can be expected to have advantages and disadvantages, should be evaluated as used, and revised periodically. Is the form used by the nursing staff? How long does it take to write the nursing history? Do the areas of inquiry thoroughly cover the information that is needed? Does the nurse obtain information through the use of the nursing history that would not be learned otherwise? Is the information used to develop individualized nursing care plans? How are priorities of nursing care affected? What is the patient's reaction to the nursing history?

Any format that contains or develops weaknesses needs to be revised from time to time. In addition, advances in technology, added knowledge, turnover in staff, and changes within individual nurses necessitate periodic review of the nursing history to maintain its usefulness.[8]

The nursing history needs to be adapted for the separate units within an institution. Information needed to individualize care for a patient in a maternity, pediatric, psychiatric, or intensive care unit will differ. In addition to the patient's name, age, medical diagnosis, and medical treatments, a basic nursing history might include the following:

Activities of daily living

Cleanliness
  Hair care
    Combing
    Shampoo
    Shaving
    Care of hair piece or wig
  Mouth care
    Usual brushing pattern (how often and
      when)
    Care of dentures
  Bathing
    Usual bathing pattern (type and time)
    Modifications
  Care of nails
Defecation habits
  Usual time
  Usual consistency
  Voiding habits
  Abnormalities
    Constipation
    Diarrhea
    Incontinence
    Urgency
  Dependent drainage
    Catheters
    Colostomy
    Ileostomy
    Draining wound
Eating habits
  Usual eating patterns
  Usual eating times
  Food preferences

  Food dislikes
  Allergies
Exercise
  Active or sedentary habits
  Usual sources of exercise
  Limits to exercise
    Diagnosis of current illness
    Paralysis
    Prosthesis
    Weakness
Rest, relaxation, and sleep habits
  Usual time for rising
  Usual time for retiring
  Naps or rest periods
  Favorite hobbies
  Modifications
Activities of daily living with which the patient
  requires assistance

Physical status

Level of consciousness
  Fully conscious
  Inattentive
  Drowsy
  Confused
  Stuporous
  Comatose
Senses
  Condition of eyes
  Vision
    Good
    Defective
    Blind

Contacts
Glasses
Prosthesis
Hearing
    Good
    Defective
    Hearing aid
Smell
Taste
Touch (numbness)
Teeth
    Quantity
    Quality
    Dentures
Skin
    Breaks or wounds
    Intact
    Bruised
    Rash
    Ulcers
    Sores
    Edematous
    Pale
    Flushed
    Jaundiced
    Dry
    Moist
    Tense
    Wrinkled
Body alignment

Psychological status

Agitated
Anxious
Apprehensive
Complies with suggestions
Demanding
Depressed
Discouraged

Eager to learn
Happy
Irritable
Restless
Shy
Withdrawn

Social-cultural-economic history

Present occupation:

    Hours per week _____

    Do you like your work? _____

Your work is

Regular	Crowded
Satisfying	Hot
Monotonous	Cold
Hazardous	Damp
Fatiguing	Seated
Indoors-outdoors	Standing
Odorous	Walking
Noisy	

Insurance
Educational level
Recreational habits
Language
    Spoken
    Understood
Religion
Position in family and community
Wishes for, and expectations of, contacts with
    family and friends during hospitalization or
    illness
Understanding of present health condition and
    events leading to it
Previous health care and reaction to it
Patient's and family's expectations of health
    care
Patient's resources or lack of resources[9]

Sources of information about the patient

The patient and his family. The patient and his family are key sources of information. By interviewing them, the nurse can learn about the patient's understanding of his illness, his thoughts and feelings about it, his normal daily activities, and his relationships with family and friends. The family may reveal what they know about the patient's condition, their feelings about it, and family resources.

Survey of patient's home and community. Much can be learned by making a home visit if this can be arranged. How do family members interact? What are the facilities and arrangements for sleeping, eating, toileting, bathing, dressing, and recreational activities? How are the lighting, ventilation, and heat controlled? How much space is there per person? Are there provisions for privacy?

The nurse can make many observations while driving to the patient's home. What is the residential area like—single family, duplex, multiple family, trailers, or vacant lots? What stores exist in the business area and how much do their prices vary? Are industries or empty buildings in the neighborhood? Are parks, playgrounds, or other recreational areas nearby? Is public transportation available? What cultural and educational institutions, such as schools, libraries, museums, and churches, are in the community? What are the population trends and living standards? What health organizations are available? How are their efforts coordinated?

Medical records. The medical records include the medical history, physician's examination report, medical diagnosis, prognosis, plan for medical management, physician's orders, and progress reports. The medical records also include reports of diagnostic studies, consultation, therapy, and surgical reports.

Social records. The social record usually includes such information as number of people in the family, occupations and incomes of family members, insurance information, and religious affiliation.

Developmental records. Developmental records may be available for some patients. They begin with a history of the individual's mother's pregnancy, labor, and delivery. When the infant first rolled over, sat unassisted, crept, crawled, pulled up on furniture, stood alone, walked alone, talked (one word, phrases, sentences), fed self, and achieved bowel control are standard items on a developmental history.[10]

Developmental records often do not go beyond early childhood, but the nurse should be aware of growth and development throughout the life cycle. School records may reveal a child's general health record, socialization, leadership abilities, progress in cognitive and physical skills. School records may also help evaluate the adolescent's developmental tasks. Is he achieving independence from parents, mature relationships with peers, preparation for college, work, and marriage?

The young adult usually establishes himself in an occupation, selects a mate, begins and manages a home, starts a family and rears children, and assumes some civic responsibilities. Middle-aged adults must adjust to teenage children, aging parents, and the physiological changes of middle age. A middle-aged couple may find more time to be together and to develop leisure-time activities. Elderly folks must adjust to retirement, reduced income, decreasing physical strength and health, and death of spouse and friends. The nurse will probably have to get much of the adult's developmental history through interviews with the patient and his family.[11]

Results of diagnostic tests. Diagnostic tests constitute much of the quantitative objective information about the patient. Each test has a normal range that establishes the area within which the patient is not considered to have a pathological condition. This range is necessary because tests are not accurate enough to have an absolute value and because of individual differences within the normal population. There are numerous laboratory tests available to assist in the assessment of the patient's condition. Specific tests may be used to confirm a diagnosis. Routine tests such as the complete blood count or urinalysis can reveal evidence of unsuspected disease. Results of diagnostic tests may redirect the diagnostic investigation as well as the nursing care. Coordination of laboratory work is a nursing responsibility. By efficient, effective scheduling the nurse can reduce the amount of time, discomfort, and cost to the patient.[12]

Computer systems. Computers have a massive storage capacity where, if the system is so programmed, information about a patient will be provided at any time on request. Computers can reduce the nurse's paperwork while providing all departments with a single source of information about a patient. Accessibility of information is increased. Quality of records is improved partially through a reduction of errors caused by transcription. Computers can facilitate quick development and updating of goals, treatments, and care plans in general. Standards of care can be incorporated into the care plans to control quality. Computers also can reduce clerical costs while improving operating and management tools.

The information being transmitted to the computer system should be as simple as possible. Input is the greatest source of error in the computer system. To reduce errors, input is verified by the person responsible for the information and is edited by the computer for such problems as incompatibilities, cumulative tolerance, and abnormal dosages. Information can be added to or deleted from the computer memory, and consequently the patient record input is expandable and can be combined with previous records. Programming should provide for patient emergencies, exceptions, and transactions on a priority basis. It is essential that the terminal device at the nursing station be operable by people with a minimum of training in computer usage.[13]

Nursing notes. Nursing notes should contain precise, objective comments about the patient's deviations from normal behavior. What are the signs and symptoms of the patient's condition, changes in his condition, reactions to tests and therapy, reasons for and results of pain medications, amounts and types of drainage, teaching accomplished, and reasons for omission of medications and treatments?[14]

Nurses have been criticized for repetitive, meaningless charting. Since most patient care is given by practical nurses and aids, some charting errors result from registered nurses trying to comment about patients with whom they have had little contact. Availability of the patient's chart as a source of information is also a problem, especially in teaching institutions where the charts are used by numerous people.[15]

Tape recording nurse's notes has improved their accuracy, precision, and pertinence at both hospitals and public health agenices.[16] New chart forms have improved nursing notes in other agencies. One agency found a checklist for routine care accompanying nursing notes to be satisfactory.[17] Others discovered that having all hospital personnel record notes about the patient's care and progress in chronological sequence on the same form improved interdisciplinary communications.[18]

Problem-oriented charting is becoming increasingly popular. It can be used to improve patient care through better charting, improved interdisciplinary communications, and as a teaching tool for the education of health personnel. The four basic parts of problem-oriented charting include (1) collection of a data base through assessment, (2) formulation of a problem list, (3) a plan for the management of each problem, and (4) plans for follow-up accompanied with progress notes.

The data base can be collected through the medical records and nursing history. The more complete the data base, the more comprehensive the identification of problems. For the problem list, it has been recommended that each problem be numbered, titled, and dealt with separately in the nursing notes.

SOAP is an acronym suggested to guide development plans for management of the problems: S for subjective data, a discussion of the patient's view of his situation; O for objective data, the nurse's observation; A for assessment or changes noticed; P for plan, the plan for intervention.[19]

University Hospital at the University of Washington developed a nurse's clinical record form with columns for time, identification of the problem, and progress notes. The nurse labels her progress notes "observation," "impression," "plan," "action," or "evaluation" as appropriate. Repetition of words and redundancy of thoughts are reduced because the nurse only comments on appropriate categories for the most pertinent problems at any one time. This facilitates reading about the progress of a problem and studying the relationship between problems.[20]

Problem-oriented charting has been adopted for community health nursing records too. Nurses at one agency divided their notes into four categories: observations, changes, actions, and future plans. Observations may be divided into subjective, what the patient reports, and objective, observations, tests, and measurements made by the nurse.

This new method saved nurses considerable charting time and allowed the charting to be done shortly after the visit was completed. It facilitated quick review before a follow-up visit. If the staff nurse was unable to visit the patient's family, another nurse could easily read what was to be done. Supervisors routinely reviewed staff records and quickly ascertained progress or lack of it with a specific family. Physicians found the nursing notes to be more comprehensive and useful to them.[21]

Not only do nursing notes help health personnel give and evaluate better health care, but they are important for the establishment of a reliable record of observation of the patient and therapy administered to patients in the event of litigation. The nurse is responsible for recording her observations and to use notes recorded by others.[22]

Nursing rounds. Nursing rounds are made by the staff nurse to assigned patients, and by the head nurse, the team leader, a combination of nursing leaders, or the whole nursing team. When rounds are conducted by the head nurse or team leader, they are usually intended to identify nursing care problems and to develop and revise nursing care plans. Rounds may also be used to develop leadership skills by having one nurse serve as a role model when a group of nursing leaders makes rounds together.

Careful planning is necessary if the whole nursing team makes rounds together. Will all patients be visited or only selected patients? When will rounds be conducted? How much time will be allowed? Will they be in addition to or a substitution for the team report or morning planning conference?

When rounds are the team report, the patient has an opportunity to help plan his care by expressing his preferences and recommendations for change. He has the opportunity to acquaint himself with the person responsible for his care during the next shift. Rounds allow the nurse to assess the patient's physical and emotional status, to learn the patient's desires for his care, to inform the patient of the physician's orders, to teach the patient about his condition and scheduled procedures and tests, and to plan his care with the patient.

It is not necessary to conduct rounds for every patient every day unless rounds replace the team report or morning planning conference. However, rounds should be conducted frequently enough that patients become comfortable participating in them. The patient and the whole nursing team should participate. It is helpful to make assignments before rounds so the staff member will take particular notice of her assigned patients, and the patient can be informed of who will be administering to his needs that day. When it is necessary to select patients for rounds, priority should be given to new patients, patients with complex nursing problems, the critically ill, and long-term patients.

Interruption of rounds should be avoided. It is preferable to schedule rounds when routine tasks are least likely to be disruptive and when arrangements can be made for emergency situations. If there are two or more teams on a unit, each can make rounds at a different time so they cover for each other. The head nurse may answer lights and give necessary medications while the team is making rounds.

Rounds are an opportunity for the patient and the staff to get involved in planning care for the patient. It is also a suitable time to discuss facts about the patient's care, such as use of special equipment, procedure for dressing change, or care of drainage tubes. Both the patients and staff may become disillusioned if the nursing care delivered is not consistent with plans made during nursing rounds.

Discussing the patient's diagnosis in his presence may be a problem. If the patient has been informed of his diagnosis, the medical terminology may be explained. The nursing history may inform the nurse of the patient's understanding of his condition. If the nurse does not think the patient knows his diagnosis or that he should be informed of it at this time, she may discuss the chief complaint instead of the diagnosis. Rather than saying the patient has muscular dystrophy, the nurse may explain that the patient has been having muscular weakness.[23]

Change-of-shift reports. Change-of-shift reports may be held in addition to or instead of nursing rounds. In some institutions the whole staff attends, where in others only the team leaders exchange reports. When the whole staff attends, everyone is able to be informed about all the patients. This is particularly useful when assisting another staff member or when answering call lights for patients assigned to others. Making assignments before report will encourage the staff to be attentive to their assigned patients and allow them to have their questions about their assigned patients answered. Tape-recorded reports have been useful in some situations and are especially helpful when the report needs to be given to numerous people throughout a shift because of staffing patterns. Another advantage is that the team leader can record the report during one of the more quiet times during the shift and just make necessary changes at the end of the shift. Pertinent information is less likely to be forgotten.

The change-of-shift report should discuss each patient and state the patient's name, room number, bed identification, age, diagnosis, physician, and patient care plan. Information such as vital signs, diagnostic tests, treatments, new tubes, dressings, quantity and quality of drainage, narcotics, special medications, intravenous infusions, and appetite is appropriate. Activities, emotional reactions, learning needs, teaching, and discharge planning should be included. Have there been changes in doctor's orders or the nursing care plan? What are the patient's symptoms? What are his major concerns? How is he responding to the nursing care? These and other questions can be answered at a change-of-shift report.

The nurse can start preparing her change-of-shift report when she receives the report by taking notes at that time. Some nurses use help sheets that list patients and have specific spaces for such information as vital signs, diet, and treatments. Jotting down reportable information during the shift is helpful. These techniques can help the nurse give an organized, succinct, yet complete report. The report should be given promptly as scheduled, since changes in the patient's condition will alter the nursing care required. The staff needs to be informed of the changes to ensure safe patient care. Delays in change-of-shift report can contribute to confusion and increase errors in nursing care. Pertinent information should be given quickly and efficiently to reduce reporting time and to allow the staff to get to the patient care. Gossiping should be avoided. It decreases the quality of the report and increases reporting time.[24]

Kardex. The Kardex contains pertinent information and a brief nursing care plan for each patient on the ward. It is revised continuously to serve as a quick, efficient means of obtaining information about patients.

Books and journals. Intelligent assessment of the patient is dependent on knowledge of the needs that are of particular importance in that patient's situation. What is the textbook discussion of that diagnosis and how do the patient's symptoms compare with it? The nurse refers to books, programmed instruction, and journals for initial information and to expand her knowledge of a particular topic.

Experts. At times the nurse may wish to consult with experts to plan specific aspects of the patient's care. What suggestions does the physical therapist have for performing a treatment with a patient having specific limitations? Can the nutritionist offer menu alternatives for a patient with a restricted diet?

Yourself. The nurse has a store of knowledge and is a major source of information. Much work is accomplished without the opportunity to look up facts. Basic nursing education provides the foundation for knowledge, and continuing education opportunities, such as workshops, seminars, institutes, speeches, study groups, and professional organizational activities, help keep the nurse abreast of the changes in nursing. The nurse should know how to use the library and should keep her personal library up to date. Of course, the nurse cannot learn and remember all she needs to know. The next best thing to knowing the information is knowing where to find it.[25]

IDENTIFICATION OF PATIENT PROBLEMS

Once the nurse has collected data about the patient's situation, present and potential nursing care problems must be considered. The present problems are those the patient has at the time of assessment. A potential problem is one for which a patient has a high risk such as the development of pneumonia after surgery or decubiti formations for a geriatric patient with a fractured hip. Usual problems are those normally expected for someone in the patient's situation and with which the patient copes satisfactorily. Unexpected and atypical problems are unique to the individual patient and not easily overcome. With these the patient has difficulty coping.

Deterrents to accurate identification of the patient's problems

Lack of skill in observation and faulty listening habits are major reasons for failing to understand a patient's problems. Erroneous interpretation confounds the problem. Value statements, clichés, and automatic responses indicate a lack of reflection on the meaning of what the patient has said. If the nurse does not understand what the patient has said and fails to interrupt him in order to question further, she hinders effective problem solving. Relying on patterned approaches, stereotypes, and preconceptions decreases her perceptiveness. Labeling is not effective. Facts do not exist in isolation and should be considered in relationship to other relevant data.

Paying attention to just a few characteristics yields only a partial understanding of the patient and, together with inadequate appreciation of social and cultural factors, decreases accurate assessment. Treating the patient as an object, a means for carrying out a work assignment, is not therapeutic. A lack of good intention on the nurse's part and use of the patient to meet the nurse's needs interfere with accurate identification of the patient's problems.[26]

NURSING DIAGNOSIS

After assessment, the nurse is able to make a diagnosis. The nurse must assess the patient's strengths and weaknesses as they relate to his overt and covert, present and potential problems. The nursing diagnosis is a statement of a conclusion based on scientific principles and indicating the patient's need for nursing care. It ends the assessment phase and begins the planning phase of the nursing process.

NOTES

1. Beland, I. L.: Clincal nursing: pathophysiological and psychosocial approaches, ed. 2, New York, 1970, The Macmillan Publishing Co., Inc., p. 15; Byers, V. B.: Nursing observation, Dubuque, Iowa, 1968, William C. Brown Co., Publishers, pp. 5-9; Johnson, M. J., Davis, M. L. C., and Bilitch, M. J.: Problem solving in nursing practice, Dubuque, Iowa, 1970, William C. Brown Co., Publishers, pp. 51-52; Seedor, M. M.: Aids to diagnosis: a programmed unit in fundamentals of nursing, New York, 1964, Teachers College Press, Columbia University, pp. 237, 240, 245, 254.
2. Geitgey, D. A.: Self-pacing—a guide to nursing care, Nurs. Outlook 71(8):48-49, 1969.
3. Bermosk, L. S., and Mordan, M. J.: Interviewing in nursing, New York, 1964, The Macmillan Publishing Co., Inc., pp. 1-11, 33; O'Brien, M. J.: Communications and relationships in nursing, St. Louis, 1974, The C. V. Mosby Co., pp. 94-96.
4. Bermosk and Mordan: Interviewing in nursing, pp. 46-61, 79-89; Bernstein, L., and Dana, R.: Interviewing and the health professions, New York, 1970, Appleton-Century-Crofts, pp. 30-32.
5. Bernstein and Dana: Interviewing and the health professions, pp. 85-98.
6. Kron, T.: Communicating in nursing, Philadelphia, 1972, W. B. Saunders Co., pp. 137-154. Devotes chapter to listening. Nichols, R. G., and Stevens, L. A.: Listening to people, Harvard Bus. Rev. 35:85-92, Sept.-Oct., 1957.
7. Lewis, G. L.: Nurse-patient communication, Dubuque, Iowa, 1969, William C. Brown Co., Publishers, pp. 21-48. Discusses nonverbal communication within framework of senses.
8. Little, D. E., and Carnevali, D. L.: Nursing care planning, Philadelphia, 1969, J. B. Lippincott Co., pp. 66-69.
9. Beland: Clinical nursing, pp. 18-22, offers an elaborate checklist; Byers: Nursing observation, is devoted to a discussion of observation of patients; Mayers, M. G.: A systematic approach to the nursing care plan, New York, 1972, Appleton-Century-Crofts. Contains examples of nursing history formats; Bower, F. L.: The process of planning nursing care, St. Louis, 1977, The C. V. Mosby Co., pp. 49-60. Discusses importance of content of nursing history.
10. Yura, H., and Walsh, M. B., editors: The nursing process, Washington, D.C., 1967, The Catholic University of America Press, p. 25.
11. Duvall, E. M.: Family development, Philadelphia, 1967, J. B. Lippincott Co. Discusses family developmental tasks; Havighurst, R. J.: Developmental tasks and education, New York, 1952, David McKay Co., Inc. Discusses developmental tasks of various stages of life cycle.
12. French, R. M.: The nurse's guide to diagnostic procedures, New York, 1971, McGraw-Hill Book Co., pp. 2, 7.
13. Flynn, E. D.: The computer: an aid to nursing communications, Nurs. Clin. North Am. 4:541-548, Sept., 1969; Price, E.: Data processing present and potential, Am. J. Nurs. 67(12):2558-2564, 1967; Weil, T. P., and Weil, J. W.: The use of computer systems in patient care, Nurs. Forum 4(2):207-217, 1967.
14. Healy, E. E., and McGurk, W.: Effectiveness and acceptance of nurses' notes, Nurs. Outlook 14(3):32-34, 1966.
15. Walker, V. H., McReynolds, D. A., and Patrick, E.: A care plan for ailing nurses' notes, Am. J. Nurs. 65(8):74-76, 1965.
16. Banks, A. W., McKee, M. E. A., and Moore, D. Y.: Tape recorded nurses' notes, Nurs. Outlook 14(10):42-44, 1966; Clark, J. H.: Instant recording, Nurs. Outlook 15(10):54-55, 1967.
17. Green, G., and Robins, L.: A rehabilitation nursing record, Am. J. Nurs. 61(3):82-85, 1961.
18. Morgan, E. M.: New chart forms solve old problems, Am. J. Nurs. 65(3):93-96, 1965.
19. Bonkowsky, M. L.: Adapting the POMR to community child health care, Nurs. Outlook 20(8):515-518, 1972; Schell, P. L., and Campbell, A. T.: POMR—not just another way to chart, Nurs. Outlook 20(8):510-514, 1972.
20. Bloom, J. T., et al.: Problem-oriented charting, Am. J. Nurs. 71(11): 2144-2148, 1971.

21. Field, F. W.: Communication between community nurse and physician, Nurs. Outlook **19**(11): 722-725, 1971; Lucido, P., et al.: Recording the home visit, Nurs. Outlook **15**(2):38-40, 1967.
22. Hershey, N.: Nurses notes—they can plan a critical role in court, Am. J. Nurs. **69**(11):2403-2405, 1969; Hershey, N.: Medical records and the nurse, Am. J. Nurs. **63**(3):96-97, 1963.
23. Sharp, B. H., and Cross, E.: Rounds and rounds, Nurs. Outlook **19**(6):419-420, 1971; Unangst, C.: The clinician's use of nursing rounds, Am. J. Nurs. **17**(8):1566-1567, 1971; Joy, P. M.: Maintaining continuity of care during shift change, J. Nurs. Adm. **5**(9):28-29, 1975.
24. Kron, T.: The management of patient care, Philadelphia, 1971, W. B. Saunders Co., pp. 131-134; Mezzanotte, E. J.: Getting it together for end of shift reports, Nursing '76 **6**(4):21-22, 1976; Wiley, L.: Whadda ya say at report? Nursing '75 **5**(10):73-78, 1975.
25. Johnson, Davis, and Bilitch, pp. 46-47.
26. Freeman, R. B.: Public health nursing practice, Philadelphia, 1957, W. B. Saunders Co., pp. 138-140; Travelbee, J.: Interpersonal aspects of nursing, Philadelphia, 1966, F. A. Davis Co., pp. 110-117; Yura and Walsh, editors, pp. 14-15.

Selected readings

In "Nursing by Assessment—Not Intuition," R. Faye McCain uses thirteen functional areas as a framework for a systematic collection of data about the patient. Her article offers one approach to assessment. Interviewing is a method of assessment used to identify patient problems. Jeanne B. Murray emphasizes the importance for the nurse to know and respect herself before she can understand others in her article, "Self-Knowledge and the Nursing Interview."

"The Problem-Oriented Record" by Rosemarian Berni illustrates the systematic method of organizing nurses' notes around the patient's problems. Pearl Lucido and co-workers offer another systematic method for recording nursing notes that has been used by health department personnel. Nursing notes are one source of information about the patient which the nurse uses to help formulate a nursing diagnosis. Examples of observation, inference, and diagnosis are presented by Mary Durand Thomas and Rosemary Prince Coombs in "Nursing Diagnosis: Process and Decision."

NURSING BY ASSESSMENT—NOT INTUITION
R. Faye McCain

Nursing, as it is taught and practiced today, is primarily intuitive. Unlike the professions of law, engineering, and medicine, nursing has not developed a precise method of determining when nursing intervention is needed. However, the need for a precise method has been recognized. Several years ago, Abdellah and associates described an approach to planning care, using as a guide "the twenty-one nursing problems".[1] More recently Bonney and Rothberg suggested a method of identifying the needs for nursing services of the chronically disabled person.[2] But, as yet, neither of these approaches have been widely accepted by nursing educators and practitioners.

Reprinted from American Journal of Nursing **65**(4):82-83, 1965. Copyright The American Journal of Nursing Company.

For the past three years graduate students in medical-surgical nursing at the University of Michigan have been evolving a method of systematically assessing functional abilities of patients. These assessments serve as the basis for making nursing diagnoses, for planning and evaluating the nursing therapy, and for writing the various nursing orders.

This method is far from precise and complete at this stage of its evolution. Some aspects of the method are developed to a higher degree than others; none have yet been developed in complete detail. We recognize that further experiential evidence is needed and that, ultimately, a controlled study should be done to validate the method. So far, we believe that it does have merit and does deserve further consideration by members of the nursing profession.

FUNCTIONAL ABILITIES APPROACH

The functional abilities of the patient were selected as the basis for assessment because such an approach agreed with our concept of nursing care. This concept incorporates the belief that the primary goal of nursing care is to assist a patient to attain and maintain a state of equilibrium as he reacts to internal and external stimuli. Equilibrium, as advanced by Johnson, represents a momentary balancing of opposing forces and does not imply a state of health or well-being.[3] To carry this concept further, the extent to which a patient does or does not achieve equilibrium is reflected in his physiological, psychological, and social behavior. Functional abilities, then, become another way of expressing behavior.

A patient, today, is expected to do for himself whatever he is capable of doing; in other words, he is expected to participate in his therapeutic regimen. But in order to help him be a participant, the nurse must know his functional abilities as well as his disabilities. When she plans nursing care and writes nursing orders, the nurse will capitalize on the patient's abilities but, at the same time, she will endeavor to assist him to live with his disabilities, whether they are temporary or permanent.

Before describing the proposed method of patient assessment, it is appropriate to consider some of the basic factors underlying the process. The systematic assessment of a patient's functional abilities is an orderly and precise method of collecting information about the physiological, psychological, and social behavior of a patient. The data collected from such an assessment provide a rationale for determining the patient's nursing needs and serve as a basis for planning and evaluating nursing therapy, writing nursing orders, and guiding and directing nursing activities. It is our working hypothesis that the nursing diagnosis, per se, is the identification of the patient's functional disabilities, or symptoms, as well as identification of his most important functional abilities. One can speculate, however, that with time, creativity, and sufficient precise data, symptoms that have a meaningful relationship in the nursing process can be grouped together, given a descriptive name, and be considered a nursing syndrome.

THE ASSESSMENT

Four resources are available for making an assessment: the patient, his family, health team members, and records. The primary resource, in most instances, is the patient; the other resources enlarge, clarify, and substantiate the information obtained from him. Interview and direct observation or inspection are the tools used by the nurse. Although these tools have long been recognized as essential to nursing care, in the patient assessment process they are used with direction and precision. Here again, one can speculate that with time, creativity, and sufficient precise data, specific nursing diagnostic tests could be evolved.

In assessing the patient's functional abilities, both objective and subjective data are collected and recorded. The time is long since past when the collection of only objective data should be advocated. Professional nurses can, do, and should make judgments. When professional nurses are more knowledgeable in the contributing sciences and become more competent in analytical thinking, some of these judgments probably will be independent judgments upon which nurses will make decisions without waiting for medical direction.

Patient assessment is the responsibility of the professional nurse. She initiates the assessment as soon as possible after the patient is admitted and continues to assess and evaluate, modifying the plan of care as the patient's behavior or functional abilities change.

In developing the method for systematic assessment of a patient's functional abilities, it was necessary to classify body functions. To date we have identified and used 13 functional areas: The patient's social, mental, emotional, body temperature, respiratory, circulatory, nutritional, elimination, and reproductive status; state of rest and comfort; state of skin and appendages; sensory perception; and motor ability. Although these functions are not mutually exclusive, for purposes of assessment we consider them separately. Social status may be questioned as a functional area, but after considerable thought and discussion, we decided it should be included. Our aim is to determine the patient's position in his family and community and discover, if possible, what social stimuli may be contributing to or detracting from his ability to function at an optimum level. In some instances, we decided to include a specific function under a category where the relationship cannot be validated by authorities, for example, placing the function of speech under sensory perception, and including intake and output in circulatory status.

ASSESSMENT FACTORS

Mental status

State of consciousness
  Alert and quick to respond to
  surroundings
  Drowsy and slow to respond
  Semiconscious and difficult to arouse
  Comatose and unable to arouse
  State of automatism
Orientation
  To time
  To place
  To person

Intellectual capacity
  Level of education
  Ability to recall events: recent; past
Attention span
Vocabulary level
  Use of simple, nontechnical words
  Use of complex, technical words
Ability to understand ideas
  Slow to learn meaning and make
  relationships
  Quick to gain meaning and make
  relationships
  Insight into health problems

MANY FACTORS, of which those listed above and on the following page are only a small sample, are taken into consideration when the graduate student first sees, talks with, and examines the patient.

ASSESSMENT FACTORS—cont'd

Emotional status

Emotional reactions
Mood
Presence or absence of anxiety
Defenses against anxiety; such as,
aggression; depression; fantasies;
identification; rationalization; regression;
repression; sublimation
Body image
Effect of illness on self-concept
Adaptation of self-concept to reality
demands
Ability to relate to others
To family
To other patients
To health team members

Sensory perception

Hearing
Sensitivity to sound
Voice tone that distinguishes sounds:
low; moderate; loud
Distance that sounds distinguished
Need to see speaker to distinguish
sounds
Presence of impairment
Partial or complete
Unilateral or bilateral
Ability to lip read
Use and effectiveness of supportive aid
Vision
Acuity
Presence of impairment
Partial or complete
Unilateral or bilateral
Type: hyperopia; myopia; astigmatism;
color-blindness; diplopia; photophobia;
nyctalopia; other
Use and effectiveness of supportive aid
Enucleation
Unilateral or bilateral
Use of prosthesis
Speech
Has auditory expression
Aphasia
Verbal defect
Syntactical defect
Nominal defect
Semantic defect
Anarthria
Mute
Laryngectomy
Use and effectiveness of esophageal
speech

Unusual speech patterns: such as, lisping;
repetitive; staccato; stammer; stutter
Touch
Hyperesthesia
Anesthesia
Paresthesia
Paralgesia
Smell
Anosmia
Hyperosmia
Kakosmia
Parosmia
Taste
Distinguishes: sweet; salt; sour; bitter
Aftertaste present

Motor ability

Mobility
Complete bed rest
Bed rest with bathroom privileges
Sit in chair
Ambulatory
Without assistance
With supportive aids: person; crutches;
walker
Use of wheel chair
Use of stretcher
Posture
In bed
Upright
Range of motion
Passive
Active
Gait
Equilibrium
Abnormal movement
Clonic
Tonic
Spastic
Flaccid
Tic
Ataxia
Muscle tone
Spasm
Contractures
Weakness
Paralysis
Hemiplegia
Paraplegia
Quadriplegia
Loss of extremity
Location
Extent
Use and effectiveness of prosthesis

SUGGESTIONS FOR USE OF GUIDE

Factors included in the guide we have developed are suggestive only. In a given patient, some factors will not be pertinent. The professional nurse in making the assessment, however, must consider all functional aspects and judge which ones do or do not apply.

We have included only those functional elements whose data can be collected by the professional nurse, using, primarily, the techniques of interview, direct observation, or inspection. It is well recognized, however, that more information will be needed before the nursing therapeutic regime for a specific patient can be planned and evaluated; for instance, findings from the medical history and physical examination, results of x-ray and laboratory tests, medical diagnosis, plan of medical management, medical prognosis, and data from hospitalizations will be needed. This information can be obtained from the patient's record or from his physician and should not be duplicated in the assessment done by the nurse.

The graduate student using the guide, approaches each patient much as a physician might in taking the patient's history and doing the physical examination—with a definite plan in mind of data to be collected. After the data are collected, she proceeds to analyze the data, make the nursing diagnosis, and decide upon a plan of care. This plan then is discussed with those who will be a part of the nursing team before it is implemented. Naturally, there will be instances when collecting data and carrying out care will be simultaneous, particularly when the patient is in acute need. At these times when symptoms are acute and may be changing rapidly, filling in the data collection forms comes after the emergency moment. However, nurses must, with the majority of patients, reach a point where their plans for care are not based on hunch alone.

Reactions to this method of patient assessment have been favorable, and there is general agreement on the wards that the nursing care plans based on the assessments take all of the nursing needs of the patients into consideration. Increased knowledge about patients and increased awareness of them have given graduate students greater satisfaction in carrying out their responsibilities. Further, we have noticed that whenever base line data are available, evaluation of the effectiveness of nursing therapy has improved.

In the beginning, we wondered how patients and physicians would react to this process. Our experiences so far indicate that patients are pleased that nurses take time to listen to their problems, demonstrate an interest in them, and obviously base nursing care on their expressed needs. Physicians' responses have been more general than those of patients, but they, too, have seen the value of the assessment process.

REFERENCES

1. Abdellah, Faye G., and others. Patient-Centered Approaches to Nursing. New York, Macmillan Co., 1960.
2. Bonney, Virginia, and Rothberg, June. Nursing Diagnosis and Therapy—An Instrument for Evaluation and Measurement. (League Exchange) New York, National League for Nursing, 1963.
3. Johnson, Dorothy E. The significance of nursing care. Amer. J. Nurs. **61**:63-66, Nov. 1961.

SELF-KNOWLEDGE AND THE NURSING INTERVIEW

Jeanne B. Murray

Every nurse knows the purposes of a bed bath, but how many of us would agree about the interview that occurs during the bathing process? To me, the main purpose of any nursing interview* is to provide the patient with an opportunity (which he may or may not use) to learn something about himself so that he may identify his health needs and decide if and how he wants to meet them. This opportunity is offered by the nurse through her responses to the patient. For the nurse to respond in this opportunity-providing way, it is essential that she listen and observe carefully. (Listening, of course, is one form of observation, and except in cases where the patient does not talk, occurs simultaneously with visual observation.) Accordingly, our beliefs about the main purpose of a nursing interview are intertwined with our beliefs about the purposes of our observations.

Sometimes we nurses seem to be observing only to get data for a record. However, I believe that most nurses would say that we must listen and observe carefully to learn more about the patient, and that such learning is important because the better we understand the patient the more success we shall have in getting him to follow our advice in matters of his health. We feel justified in this aim because we see ourselves as experts who have the ability to heal the patient (or to keep him well) by teaching him the facts of good health care.

Then we wonder why our advice so often goes unheeded. Could it be that our understanding of the patient does not necessarily help us to teach or to heal him? Lydia Hall, director of the Loeb Center for Nursing and Rehabilitation, has said that "the power to heal lies in the patient and not in the nurse unless she is healing herself." [1] If this is true, and I firmly believe that it is, then what the nurse learns about the patient is not nearly so important as what she can help him to learn about himself.

In my opinion then, the nurse observes carefully so that she can make those responses which will be most helpful to the patient. Such responses will provide the patient with an opportunity to become aware of what he is saying and doing. As the patient becomes aware of what he is saying and doing, he begins to know himself more fully.

To appreciate this type of learning experience we must first realize that much of what all of us say and do is said and done out of awareness. For example, a friend and I were once discussing a goal that I was trying to attain. She pointed out that while saying, "The pendulum swings from one extreme to the other," I had made a sweeping gesture with my hand. After I became aware of my words and gesture through my friend's reflection, I explored their significance for me and learned something about myself. The pendulum metaphor was an obvious reference to time, and I suddenly realized that I feared that time was growing so short that I might never be able to attain my goal. I had never before been aware of this fear, which was not based on the facts. I knew that I actually had about fifteen times as much time as was required. Once I became aware of my feeling, I was able to explore its meaning for me and to grow in self-awareness.

Reprinted from Nursing Forum 2(1):69-78, 1963.
*The term "nursing interview," as used here, denotes any interaction, either verbal or non-verbal, between a nurse and a patient which focuses on the health needs of the patient or his family. In this context, a bed bath would take place within the framework of an interview.

Obviously, then, listening and observing, in themselves, are not enough. Unless the nurse reflects her observations in her responses, she has not used them to help the patient to the greatest extent possible. For it is the nurse's response, guided by her observations, that invites her patient to learn about himself and to heal himself. The nurse must become such a good observer that she not only hears what the patient is saying but is aware of how he says it. In addition to the gist, or sense, of his statements, she must notice the particular words he chooses, his changing facial expressions, the gestures he makes with his hands, the tone of his voice, his posture and bodily movements. Moreover, she must be aware of any incongruities between his verbal and non-verbal communications—for example, smiling while saying, "I'm so unhappy."

Almost anyone can train himself to make these observations. The effective nurse learns how to make use of her observations in such a way as to help her patient learn from them, that is, through her responses to the patient's words and actions, she provides an opportunity for the patient to bring into awareness the feelings that motivated his words and actions. The nurse who simply listens and observes is like a sponge, absorbing what the patient pours out, but the nurse who responds without directing the course of the interview, who reflects the patient's words and actions, is like a sounding board which the patient can use to amplify his feelings and thus, to become aware of them.

It is true, of course, that the nurse who simply listens and allows her patient to talk things out may be helping him to some extent. "In general, catharsis through talking is more effective the more the disturbing emotion is related to a fairly recent experience, and it becomes of dubious value the more the feeling is due to repressed experiences."[2] All of us have gone through exasperating situations after which we have simply had to "sound off." Generally we do feel better after such catharsis, and as Annette Garrett points out, we find the most relief if we "blow off steam" immediately. This "sounding off" is not always possible, however, and even when it is, it probably won't help us to gain new insights, for catharsis results in plenty of expurgation but no inspiration. And it is the opportunity afforded for gaining new insights that constitutes the main value of the nursing interview.

It is always possible that the patient may not make use of the learning experience that the nursing interview provides. The nurse's role is simply to offer the opportunity—not to try to force it on the patient. The nurse needs to understand that before the patient can even decide (this is not usually a conscious process) whether or not he wants or is able to use the opportunity to learn something new about himself, he first has to find out who the nurse is. Until he feels safe with her, he may devote his efforts to testing her to see how well she will accept him and how far he can trust her. By the way the nurse responds to him the patient will know whether he is safe with her. If she is sincerely accepting of him and is able to use herself therapeutically, he will realize that she is someone who cares about him and wants to help.

For the nurse to be accepting of the patient, she must first accept herself. Such self-acceptance is built upon self-awareness. For example, when a patient says to his new nurse, "Are you sure you know how to dress my wound?" he is telling her that he doesn't yet feel safe with her. Whether he becomes more anxious or less anxious depends on the way in which she responds to this question, and the way in which she responds depends upon her image of self and her degree of self-awareness.

If the nurse feels unsure of herself, she will probably try to reassure the patient with words—actually, for the purpose of putting herself at ease. The patient will respond not to her words, but to her lack of confidence, and will become more anxious. On the other hand, if the nurse sees herself as somewhat of a superhuman Florence Nightingale, she will probably be indignant or angry. Her response will tell the patient that he has insulted her, and this information will increase his anxiety in her presence. If, however, the nurse is self-confident and is realistic in seeing herself as a human being who can make mistakes but who has mastered the arts and skills of nursing, she will feel neither threatened nor angry. She will be able to focus on the patient and his needs instead of unconsciously meeting her own needs for self-gratification.

The more the nurse grows in self-awareness, the better able she will be to help her patients. If the nurse is not aware of her own needs and they go unsatisfied, they will prevent her from helping the patient to meet *his* needs. If the nurse has feelings which she has never accepted or of which she is unaware, she will act out of her awareness on them and will be unable to help the patient focus on *his* feelings.

To return to our example, the patient has asked the nurse if she knows how to dress his wound. This happened to me on a first visit to a patient. I responded, "You want to know if I know how to dress your wound." The patient said, "Oh, I know they taught you how to do all that in nursing school." I replied, "You know they taught me, but you still feel unsure about having a new nurse do this for you." The patient admitted that this was true, and I commented that I could understand that he might feel this way—as indeed I could. As I changed the dressing, he gave me directions about the way the last nurse had done it. I didn't tell him (as I had done in the past) that every nurse has her own way of doing things. Instead, I accepted his information and used it. The next time I saw him, he seemed more at ease with me, and as I changed the dressing he offered no advice on how to do it. Instead, he talked about his hospitalization and what had happened to him. I took this behavior to mean that the patient's immediate need (to feel safe with the nurse) had been met, and that he now felt free to meet another need, namely, to talk about his experiences in the hospital. If we accept Ida Jean Orlando's definition of a need, it seems clear that my assumption was correct: ". . . need is situationally defined as a requirement of the patient which, if supplied, relieves or diminishes his immediate distress or improves his immediate sense of adequacy or well-being."[3]

If the nurse's purpose in interviewing is to provide the patient with an opportunity to learn more about himself so that he may correctly identify his health needs and decide how (or whether) he wants to meet them, it follows that she believes that the patient has the right and the ability to direct his own course. She realizes that she does not have the solutions to anyone's problems except her own and that actions that may appear good, right, or helpful to her may seem bad, wrong, or useless to another. She believes that all behavior has purpose and meaning and that only the patient can know what significance his behavior has for him.

The nurse's attitude is non-judgmental: she does not criticize her patient. She refrains from telling, urging, or advising. She gives praise with discretion, for she is aware that praise is often a means of reinforcing the behavior that *she* values; that is, she realizes that praise is often a subtle form of persuasion. She helps the patient to obtain any information for which *he* expresses a need. She plans referrals *with* him, if and when *he* feels a need for the assistance of another profession or of a nurse in another setting.

Martha Brown and Grace Fowler have pointed out, "The response of an individual in a specific situation is the best that he is capable of making at the given moment."[4] The nurse who understands this principle will find that she is able to accept her patient no matter what decisions he may make, including decisions to do nothing about situations she sees as health problems. The nurse who respects her patient's right to determine his own actions does not try to make decisions for him or to impose upon him her solutions to his problems.

In talking with nurses, however, I find that many of us are trying to make these decisions. It appears that nurses really don't believe that the patient has either the right or the ability to make the decisions about his actions in certain areas. We often find ourselves wondering how we can get a patient to do something that we think he ought to do. In these instances we are acting on our own feelings and satisfying our own needs.

To illustrate this observation with another example from my own experience: I used to visit a family in which the sixty-eight-year-old wife had suffered a stroke. She was bedridden and had an indwelling catheter. Her daughter irrigated the catheter daily until she fell and injured her shoulder and was temporarily unable to care for her mother. I tried to teach the patient's husband to irrigate the catheter, but he refused to do this although he assumed all the other tasks involved in the care of his wife. I began using interviewing techniques to find out why he was unwilling to do the irrigation. I didn't succeed in getting him to learn how to irrigate the catheter, nor did I discover why he refused. But, more important, I learned something about myself: I was trying to get this man to do what *I* thought he should do. If he would irrigate the catheter it would be less likely to plug up, and I wouldn't have to make a special trip to the home to reinsert it. Furthermore, I felt that it was his duty to accept responsibility for his wife's catheter. I was applying my values to him. When I realized these facts about myself and accepted them (and that was difficult!), I was able to accept this man's feelings also, even though I couldn't understand them and didn't know what was causing them.

This experience demonstrated to me that the nurse can learn to use the skills of listening, observing, and responding sincerely and disinterestedly to help the patient learn about himself, or she can memorize various techniques and devices to get the patient to open up and reveal information that she can use to attain her own goals. I believe that the nurse who sets goals for the patient and then practices interviewing skills designed to get him to attain these goals will not help her patient very much. If the nurse believes in her patient's worth as a human being, his powers of self-direction, and his right to make his own decisions, she can successfully use the skills she has learned. She will communicate her respect for him, and she will not feel the need or the desire for devices.

Carl Rogers asks several questions that we nurses would do well to ponder. I shall quote two of them: "Do we respect [the patient's] capacity and his right to self-direction, or do we basically believe that his life would be best guided by us? Are we willing for the individual to select and choose his own values, or are our actions guided by the conviction (usually unspoken) that he would be happiest if he permitted us to select for him his values and standards and goals?"[5]

The nurse probably cannot honestly answer these questions until she knows and accepts herself, for it is only as one grows in self-knowledge and self-acceptance that one becomes freer of the unmet needs and repressed emotions that make it so difficult for people to make decisons. Self-awareness and self-acceptance do not come all at once, nor do they come without effort. To obtain greater knowledge of ourselves we have to be constantly probing, and this probing can be painful. But as the nurse learns more about who she is and begins to have more respect for herself, she will be able to allow her patient to be himself and she will come to have greater respect for him as an individual. Interviewing will become easier for her and more successful for the patient.

The most important thing for the nurse to learn, then, is to know and accept herself, for, in the words of Erich Fromm: ". . . respect for one's own integrity, love for an understanding of one's own self, cannot be separated from respect and love and understanding for another individual."[6]

REFERENCES

1. Hall, Lydia E. "Nursing—What Is It", Virginia Nurse Quarterly, **27:**24, (1959).
2. Garrett, Annette. Interviewing: Its Principles and Methods, (New York: Family Service Association of America, 1942), p. 35.
3. Orlando, Ida Jean. The Dynamic Nurse-Patient Relationship, (New York: G. P. Putnam's Sons, 1961), p. 5.
4. Brown, Martha and Fowler, Grace. Psychodynamic Nursing, (Philadelphia: W. B. Saunders, 1954), p. 13.
5. Rogers, Carl R. Client-Centered Therapy, (Boston: Houghton Mifflin, 1951), p. 20.
6. Fromm, Erich. The Art of Loving, (New York: Harper and Brothers, 1956), p. 59.

THE PROBLEM-ORIENTED RECORD
Rosemarian Berni

Because nursing process involves patient problem identification and patient problem solving and because nursing practice includes accountability, there is a need to study the documentation of that problem solving process in many areas of nursing. Dr. Lawrence Weed has introduced a method of organizing the medical record or chart as an ongoing audit of the management of the patient's problems (Weed, 1970), and our book's purpose is to describe how to implement Weed's method.

NEED OF PERMANENT RECORDING OF NURSING PROCESS

Traditionally, written evidence of the many steps in the nursing process is described in pencil on the nursing care card file and erased as more current information is added. These steps may not appear on the chart or permanent medical record. Since the nurse is liable under the law to be called to give satisfactory reasons for nursing actions and since memory is not infallible, he is likely to need a permanent written record of the nursing process. The intent of the law is to protect the consumer, and the intent of nursing is the same since the nurse is striving to help the consumer to prevent or to solve his health care problems. The intent of the problem-oriented medical record is to monitor the health care team's progress with the consumer's problem solving process. The goal of the team is to help the consumer solve his problems (a problem is defined as any condition or situation in which the patient/client needs help). This problem solving system cannot be evaluated without a monitoring system.

Modified from Berni, R., and Readey, H.: Problem-oriented medical record implementation, St. Louis, 1978, The C. V. Mosby Co., pp. 1-15.

FRAMEWORK

The framework of the POMR will be described as the purpose, goals, and objectives of the people involved with it. The purpose is the result that health care personnel and the POMR should accomplish. The goals are broad behavioral outcomes necessary for the health care system to implement the POMR. The objectives are the intermediate steps in the realization of these goals of accountability and patient advocacy.

Purpose

The purpose of the POMR is to construct a detailed model of health care problem solving and recording that, once implemented, will be improved on and expanded by all health care personnel, a model that is a behavioral analysis system engineered to become a health care audit.

Goals

The goals that identify the four major behavioral outcomes necessary for POMR implementation are as follows:
1. Describe the need for the health care system to be accountable to the health care consumer.
2. Develop a written system of accountability to the health care consumer that also utilizes ongoing peer review by all disciplines.
3. Utilize a system of accountability to the health care consumer.
4. Reinforce health care personnel as they contribute to the accomplishment of goals one, two, and three.

Objectives

The behavioral steps toward meeting the aforementioned goals are as follows:
1. Read material and/or attend meetings covering the POMR and write a short summary of the need for and description of the POMR.*
2. Collect relevant and appropriate data base.
3. Identify patient's problems or potential problems (prevention). Number, label, and describe problems clearly.
4. Write initial plan for the solution or management of each problem identified in the progress notes, for example:
   a. Collection of more data for diagnosis or management.
   b. Treatments, programs, and/or drugs.
   c. Patient and/or family teaching about the illness, its management and prevention of complications and/or recurrences.
   d. Description of method of evaluating the plan, for example, flow sheet.
5. Write a numbered, labeled, dated, concise, and relevant progress note for each problem (as necessary) as a continuous evaluation.
   a. List subjective data under each problem when applicable.
   b. List objective data under each problem when applicable.
   c. Record assessment or interpretation of the data for each problem when applicable.

---

*Number 1 is usually applicable only once.

d. Write a plan for the solution or management of each problem. If goal is not implicit, state goal for which the plan is written. Include a plan for evaluation.
6. Apply the POMR technique to a temporary problem (omitting numbering) if problem seems minor but important enough to follow and evaluate. Include a listing or method by which to keep track of temporary problems.
7. Apply the POMR technique to problems identified by other team members.
8. Design or initiate flow sheets to record data graphically or more clearly.
9. Use flow sheets to record data graphically.
10. Write a numbered and labeled problem list at the beginning of the patient's progress notes or add numbered and labeled problems to an existing index when necessary.
11. Read other team members' information in the POMR.
12. Evaluate problems as necessary.
13. Modify plans as necessary.
14. Support health team's audit of patient care by initiating, attending, or supporting representation to meetings for the purpose of describing and implementing the POMR, appropriate standards of care, and audit tools.
15. Suggest that health team members computerize POMR data, analyze data collected by the audit, and correct deficiencies or support the team in these activities.
16. Teach team members POMR concepts and implementation.
17. Take part in facilitating publication of audit information and consequential health team behaviors on the patients' behalf (lay and professional publications).
18. Reinforce other health care team members' contributions and positive efforts toward an honest and complete POMR implementation and recognize accurate praise from others.

COMPONENTS

According to Hurst and Walker (1972), few professionals consider the POMR a punitive exercise. "The obstacles that occur are no different from those found when any new system or change is initiated." Therefore, in an attempt to eliminate some of these obstacles, let us explore the four components of the POMR—the four phases of clinical action involved in the inauguration of such a system. Each of the following elements will be discussed in detail.
A. Data base
B. Problem list
C. Initial plans or orders
   1. Diagnostic considerations or assessments
   2. Therapeutic plans
   3. Patient education
D. Progress notes
   1. Narrative
      a. Subjective statement by the patient and family or meaningful others
      b. Objective findings by health team
      c. Assessment(s)
      d. Plans
   2. Flow sheets
   3. Discharge summary

Data base

The data base simply refers to the sum total of information gathered in the admission workup. It may include a compilation of such pertinent data as the patient's chief complaint, the patient profile and related social data, present illness(es), the patient's past history and systems review, the physical examination, base-line laboratory data, special data collected by therapists, and the nursing history. Carefully prepared and refined questionnaires serve to gather this vital information.

It is essential that the data base be defined and that the patient's occupation and geographical location be considered. Hurst (1971) emphasized, however, that it is wise to inaugurate the system without trying to seek agreement from all the people possibly concerned, since this could act as a definite deterrent to getting the system in progress. Once in progress, feedback will be available to update the data base. The important issue is that the data base be so constructed that the guidelines built into the system demonstrate explicitly what is to be included and what is to be omitted. A very different problem list can evolve if each physician is permitted to create his own standards, particularly if, for example, one includes a proctoscopic examination as part of a routine physical examination and another does not. The relationship of the data base and problem list should be clearly evident. For example, from the systems review and the physical examination, an association between bleeding and anticoagulant therapy should be readily apparent.

If we are to take advantage of the patient education concept this system proposes, we must also consider the future implications of pathology—the future in light of genetic counseling of patients with sickle cell anemia or diabetes and the environmental factors that influence the patient with emphysema.

Proponents of the POMR have stressed the fact that the psychosocial data base, which is essential for comprehensive health care delivery, is one of the most neglected areas. Such factors as degree of indebtedness, degree of job security, educational achievement, previous psychological or psychiatric treatment, and use of tranquilizers, alcohol, etc. bear exploring since they may have serious implications in planning care for the patient. A patient who boasts of having at least six cocktails in any given day may experience a decided problem adjusting to a diabetic regime.

Paramedics have been used in the collection of the data base, but emphasis must be placed on the fact that they do not make decisions regarding patient care. Paramedics usually function in this capacity with specific, written behavioral steps (algorithms) as their guide.

The laboratory data base can be tailored to fit different patient populations. Because the incidence of diabetes is so high among Jewish people, it would seem practical to have a fasting blood sugar, 2-hour postprandial, or glucose tolerance test as part of the laboratory data base in a hospital in a basically Jewish community. Laboratory results may alter the problem list; therefore problems must be updated frequently. Since it is economically unsound to order a multiplicity of laboratory tests regardless of identified problems, it is important to follow data with action. It is a waste of time, then, to collect data unless action will be taken. Hurst and Walker (1972) place great emphasis on the need to update the POMR periodically after analyzing its contents for important omissions and redundant commissions.

"When the defined Data Base is not complete, then problem #1 becomes incomplete Data Base. In such a case an initial plan must be shown that will solve the problem" (Hurst and Walker, 1972). This approach is essential when a patient is admitted to the hospital in shock, for example, and priorities of care must be established. Stabilizing the patient's condition most assuredly takes precedence over collecting a complete defined data base.

Hurst and Walker (1972) feel that the readmission of any patient who has been evaluated previously with a POMR merely necessitates the writing of an interval note (a note that relates previous admission to current admission). An alternative is to update the information recorded on the previous POMR data base form. Unnecessary reexamination is usually looked on unfavorably by the patient.

A nursing history is collected by nursing service personnel at the time of admitting the patient to the hospital unit and is related to the personal habits and lifestyle of the patient.

A patient profile is compiled by nursing personnel from the information contained in the nursing history and is placed on the flip chart. It also becomes part of the nurse's admission note on the progress sheet. Such significant factors as the patient's ability to communicate and understand, the availability of his family, his way of life, his home situation, his personal habits that may be pertinent to treatment, and his behavior during the interview should be included.

An important concern regarding the collection of the information that becomes the data base is the need of health professionals to enhance their understanding of interviewing techniques while dialoguing with the patient. A good reference for interviewing is *Interacting with Patients* by Larson and Hays (1963).

The defined data base "assists the physician in identifying the problems that are already at a stage of high resolution and the problems that are at a stage of low resolution" (Hurst and Walker, 1972). A problem of high resolution would be entered as a diagnosis and a problem of low resolution may simply be identified as a physical finding. We would like to emphasize that the data base is the essence of the problem list. The problem list is the result of manipulation and interpretation of the raw biological information collected as the data base.

Problem list

"In assaying truth in the crucible of a problem or project we must be very careful about the ingredients which enter in, and the conclusions which are drawn forth" (Brubacker, 1962). The complete and well-defined data base, then, is essential to the identification of problems. The problem should be stated at a level of refinement in keeping with the recorder's understanding—a symptom, a finding, or a diagnosis. The need for truthful expression is inherent in this system of recording. "Truth is orderly and systematic, a web of closely intertwined relationships" (Dupuis, 1966). Truths, in this relation, are revealed only by disciplined study of the evidence collected in the data base. Thus the problem list is meaningful only if it emerges from an accurate and complete data base.

Because the problem list summarizes at a glance all the known problems of the patient and serves as an "index" for the patient's chart, it should always precede all other information in the patient's chart. Problems on this list should be dated and identified by Arabic numbers according to the order in which they emerge, with the chief complaint (what brought the patient to the hospital) always designated as problem No. 1 unless the problem numbers are maintained over multiple admissions into the health care system. The copy of a problem list found on p. 49 "is a 'table of contents' and an 'index' combined, and the care with which it is constructed determines the quality of the whole record" (Weed, 1971).

Problems are updated when evidence permits and an arrow is used to indicate that the problem is resolved. Examples follow:

6 P.M. 7/27/73 Dyspnea $\xrightarrow{7/28/73}$ Left-sided congestive heart failure

6 P.M. 7/27/73 Substernal chest pain $\xrightarrow{7/28/73}$ Myocardial infarction

The symptomatology initially entered may be the only way the problem can be truthfully stated without diagnostic laboratory results immediately at our disposal. A diagnosis is only used when there is supportive data. Hurst and Walker (1972) tell us it is better to state the problem as "hematocrit of 28" in lieu of "anemia" if a cause for the anemia is not established. Note that arrows are also dated to preserve the chronological order the system dictates. Needless to say, a highly resolved problem needs no arrow and the ultimate degree of resolution is a diagnosis.

Problems are classified by status: active and inactive or resolved problems. As active problems are resolved, a notation is made to this effect on the problem list. "Disorders such as diabetes and glaucoma should always be considered active problems regardless of how well-controlled they are at the present or how unrelated the current complaint of the patient may seem" (Weed, 1971). Inactive or resolved problems are included, since they may cause complications or exacerbations.

New problems as they develop are simply numbered, dated as to onset, and added to the original problem list. This problem list depicts all the patient's liabilities or weaknesses, so to speak. However, this data base should have room to define his assets or his strengths. The inclusion of social and demographic factors as well as psychiatric problems is strongly recommended. Referral to proper resource persons is imperative with problems that are not within the realm of the recorder to solve. Weed (1971) alerts us to the fact that "by many physicians, nonorganic problems encountered in the practice of medicine are regarded as alien, baffling, and perhaps not even interesting. Consequently, personality and adjustment problems are usually ignored in summaries of patient problems, even though they could have been described easily using clearly understood nontechnical formulations ('cries easily,' 'family difficulties')." For nursing, the pendulum has swung toward emphasizing the psychological as well as the physical problems of patients. Today we find that these problems are considered equally important by many nurses and therapists. Nursing personnel are asked, however, to identify psychological problems at a behavioral level such as "very quiet" or "withdrawn." Hay and Anderson's analysis of patient needs revealed that psychological problems took precedence over all other needs. Their study indicated that "the need most frequently mentioned by the patients was to be accepted with their illness and to belong to a group" (cited by Newman, 1966).

Noteworthy in this respect also are the observations of Skipper and associates who found "that the patients in their study hesitated to ask for information because they perceived the nurses as being too busy, because they feared negative reactions and subsequent rejection, and because of their prior experience with unsatisfactory answers" (cited by Newman, 1966). Cultural differences must also be given consideration because various people perceive health based on norms established in their own cultures. Many authorities in the health care field believe that it would seriously hinder a nurse's ability to administer to a patient if these cultural differences were disregarded.

Weed (1971) insists that "the problem list should not contain diagnostic guesses; it should simply state the problems at a level of refinement consistent with the physician's

St. V. 290 (3/72) (Old St. V. 1006)

ST. VINCENT'S HOSPITAL
Bridgeport, Connecticut

P R O B L E M   L I S T
(Attending and House Staff Physicians should
Formulate Single Problem List within 24 Hours)

Date Onset	ACTIVE PROBLEMS	Date Resolved	Inactive or Resolved Problems
	CHIEF COMPLAINT:		

STRUCTURED BY A:
1. Medical Problem:
   a. A "Diagnosis"
   b. Physiological Abnormality
   c. Symptom or Physical Finding

   d. Laboratory Abnormality
2. Psychiatric Problem
3. Socioeconomic Problem
4. Demographic Problem

understanding, running the gamut from the precise diagnosis to the isolated, unexplained finding." It is safer to underdefine than to overdefine a problem. With time, quantitative detail will help refine problems.

Weed (1971) strongly feels that "the word 'probable' should not be used in a problem list. Either the patient is suffering from a disease process or it should be stated clearly in terms of a symptom, or a sign, or an abnormal x-ray finding." The "rule outs" of the physician are of no importance here but become an integral part of the initial plan, which will be discussed later.

Whenever laboratory tests identify a problem, the results should be included with that problem, that is, "fatigue" identified at the nurse's intellectual level could be accompanied by a "hemoglobin value of 7 gm/100 ml." Nurses should be motivated to draw this type of association. The fact that this approach encourages nurses to reveal their innermost thoughts and to document their decisions is a plus factor for this system of records.

All allied members of the health team are encouraged to add to the problem list so long as it is expressed at their level of sophistication. "Dyspnea on exertion" at the nurse's level of understanding may be refined to "emphysema" by the physician. "The system is open-minded and allows for the simple and the complex, the ill-defined symptom and the well-established diagnosis" (Weed, 1971). Criticism regarding written expression should be of a constructive rather than of a critical nature lest the participants become prematurely discouraged with the system.

Minor episodes that are considered to be of a tentative or temporary nature are simply written as such in the progress notes and not given a problem number. If these tentative problems persist, they too should be added to the original problem list. This approach serves to eliminate cluttering of the problem list. The problem of diarrhea occasionally accompanying the dye given for a gallbladder series exemplifies a tentative problem. These problems may be listed on a separate worksheet so that they are not forgotten.

As the pathophysiology of a disease process progresses, problems should be anticipated. Preventive medicine is implicit in the patient education aspect of the POMR.

Weed (1971) emphasizes the fact that when "operative findings throw new light on the definition of problems, the problem list should be modified accordingly." For example:

2 P.M. 7/20/73 Problem No. 1: Anemia $\xrightarrow{7/24/73}$ Carcinoma of ascending colon

For the system to be truly effective, problems should be updated frequently in order to maintain an accurate account of the patient's progress. Weed suggests that complications following surgery be treated as new problems and that a note be included that reflects the specific problem that it relates to.

Proponents of the POMR tell us that "multiple problems may interact, and sophisticated understanding and management of any one of them requires at least an awareness of all of them" (Weed, 1971). This record-keeping approach should make clear the need for health care personnel to keep abreast of new knowledge and to review old knowledge continuously.

Significant, then, is the fact that proper problem identification depends on careful analysis of the data base and is considered the first step in the ultimate solution of problems. Only when we are made aware of all the patient's problems can we plan intelligent care that reflects consideration of all problems. It is not unusual to find that a medication that is specific for treating one problem is contraindicated for another problem.

Hurst and Walker (1972) found that "much of the remaining resistance to the POMR seems to stem from a desire to keep the patient's problems simple and therefore manageable by one man." They also reiterate the fact that it is not compulsory nor is it possible to solve all problems.

Fundamental to the POMR is the need to have all subsequent orders, plans, and progress notes related specifically to *each* problem and its accompanying number. *Each* is emphasized because it is imperative that the problems be considered individually. This brings us to the next phase of the system.

Initial plans

The goals for each patient should be stated explicitly in light of *diagnostic* considerations, *therapeutic* plans, and *patient education*. The familiar physician's "rule outs," or plan for the differential diagnosis, belong here. The manner in which these "rule outs" (R/O) will be treated should be precisely delineated, for example, "Hypertension, R/O pheochromocytoma." Physicians should be made cognizant of the economic factors regarding "ruling out" diagnoses. The following could exemplify the initial plans or doctor's orders for a patient admitted with substernal chest pain.

> *Diagnostic:* R/O Myocardial infarction (enzymes qd ×3)
> R/O Pericarditis (chest plate, EKG)
> *Therapeutic:* Coronary precautions, morphine sulfate gr ¼ q4h prn, O₂ via cannula, BP q½h ×6
> *Patient education:* Patient was told she may have had a "mild heart attack" and blood tests and EKG will be done to determine if this is so; was told not to get OOB until further notice and the importance of not straining with BM's. Patient has had EKG previously; accepted explanation given. Patient asked to repeat instructions given.

The initial plans are always formulated in accordance with the problem and number to which they relate. Each problem, then, has specific orders that relate to the three subsets of plan construction—the diagnostic, the therapeutic, and patient education. The educational tool provided by this system is truly priceless. The associations among drug therapy, nursing care measures, special therapies, and diagnostic tests are clearly evident. Weed (1969) substantiates this conclusion: "Too many serious omissions occur when sleeping pills, blood urea nitrogen orders, and siderails are all mixed up in a list of twenty items, which were spun off the top of the physician's head in a totally random fashion."

The last category, that of patient education, has not in the past been planned constructively so that all disciplines are aware of what the others have explored with the patient. Significant also is the response of the patient to the explanation. If the patient is not capable of participating in the management of his problems, other goals must be established to include family, neighbors, or appropriate health agencies. We all recognize that there is a place in education for repetition to cement concepts, but unnecessary duplication of efforts is costly to the patient, personnel, and institution.

The POMR makes us more aware of the patient's milieu and affords us the opportunity to share our observations in writing so all disciplines concerned with patient care will have access to this information. The POMR substitutes the opportunity for continuity of care for the old, basically verbal, and inconsistent means of helping a patient cope with his problems. We envision in the near future that all the post-hospital plans and expectations of the patient will be spelled out in written form so the patient can make reference to them as the need arises. So often patients fear seeking clarification of these orders or, because of the excitement of returning to their loved ones, forget about the orders. Weed (1971) states with compassion, "They should not expect the patient to grasp after one exposure, all the implications and details of the management of his disorders." Perhaps we have at our disposal another innovative way to utilize algorithms—protocols hitherto used for the short- or long-term management of certain chronic diseases.

Progress notes

Progress notes, numbered and titled so they coincide with the problem list, comprise the monitoring, plan modification, and follow-up phase of the problem-oriented process. The progress notes include narrative notes, flow sheets, and a discharge summary.

Narrative notes. The narrative aspect of the progress notes are written in SOAP fashion. Separate SOAP's are constructed for each problem. They should be dated and affixed with the author's credentials. The "S" stands for *subjective* and refers to the problem or symptomatology as the patient expresses it. Using quotations is helpful so that all other members of the health team may draw their own conclusions from what the patient stated. If the patient does not contribute to defining the problem, the "S" is simply followed by "none." Subjective data should describe symptomatology quantitatively and qualitatively.

"O" refers to *objective* or clinical findings, including astute observations related to the patient's problem. Relevant laboratory or other diagnostic findings should be included here. For example, a headache reported by the patient is a subjective finding, for he alone can relate this to you, but a rash clearly discernible on the patient's back may be unknown to him. Since you noticed the rash, you would chart this under "objective."

The "A" stands for *assessment,* which is expressed after you analyze the information and synthesize what the subjective and objective data together suggest to you. Has the status of the problem changed and by what criteria (Bonkowsky, 1972)? Assessment may also be thought of as a diagnosis, an impression, or a condition change for better or worse. Problems isolated in the history and physical data collection are used for the assessment. Donna Ganes, long an advocate of the POMR, states it rather clearly: "As with the other portions of SOAP, one need only to be honest. 'Assessment: don't know' is acceptable if it is true" (cited by Woody and Mallison, 1973).

The "P," or *plan,* relates to proposed solutions for the identified problems and, like initial plans, should be considered as a potential threefold program of action: diagnostic, therapeutic, and patient education. The diagnostic aspect is designed to obtain more information about the problem if necessary; the therapeutic aspect includes what has been suggested or proscribed to eliminate or control the problem; and the patient education plans reveal all the information the patient and his family has received or should receive in relation to his problem as well as the patient's role in managing his illness. The importance of sharing the patient's response to such guidance is a most essential aspect of the POMR.

All disciplines associated with patient care should contribute to the progress notes in a chronological sequence. "In this manner the medical and paramedical professions assume an integrated and easily audited role in solving the patient's problems, and each avoids establishing the kind of identity that permits or encourages the possibility of dealing with problems out of context" (Weed, 1971). Noteworthy is the fact that disciplines other than the medical profession contribute at their own level of understanding and should not attempt to state assessments that are not substantiated by evidence. In fact, the documentation of evidence that leads you to your decision clearly spells out for all concerned the reason why you said what you did. You may not always use the entire SOAP format. Weed suggests you use that which is pertinent. Most authorities agree that the progress notes are

ST. VINCENT'S HOSPITAL
BRIDGEPORT   CONNECTICUT

CLINICAL CARE FLOW SHEET   M-961

PROBLEM:

CRITICAL PARAMETERS (Including Clinical)																
DATE/TIME																

the most crucial aspect of the POMR. The progress notes provide the feedback about how realistic and successful the initial plans were.

Consultations should be requested in reference to a specific problem and its corresponding number. The consultation sheet should be structured so that the *conclusions, recommendations, discussion,* and *identification of new problems* are stated simply and directly so that it is not necessary to read the entire report to extract salient features.

A narrative note written in SOAP format is not deemed necessary regarding diagnostic tests or procedures performed on patients. A simple statement in the progress notes, including the patient's response, is ample. Assigning a time, date, problem number, and title to each notation made in the progress notes is essential if we expect the feedback from the auditing process to be accurate.

Flow sheets. Flow sheets, often referred to as shorthand for progress notes, are used to tabulate in graphic form parameters, or variables, unique to each patient. Duplication of effort can be avoided by requesting that the reader "see flow sheet" in respect to any problem that is being monitored, instead of repeating similar data in a SOAP format. The flow sheet serves as an excellent guide to ascertaining the source of a pathological process or to revealing relationships between many variables. When isolated parameters must be observed frequently, the flow sheet may be the only progress note necessary. The flow sheet often serves to eliminate a multitude of narrative notes and indicates the patient's progress at a glance. Weed (1971) suggests that parameters on flow sheets be filled in as the need arises, but in certain speciality areas where patients with specific problems are cared for, flow sheets with established parameters pertaining to those problems are used. For example, data regarding the diabetic patient's insulin coverage, urine tests, and blood sugar tests lends itself to flow sheet use rather than the narrative progress note. Specific flow sheets constructed to be used as a checklist often save considerable time in the event of a cardiac arrest. A chronological sequence is of essence in such critical situations. An analogy is readily evident between the format used for this flow sheet and the format used to graph any bits of information. (See flow sheet on p. 59.)

Discharge summary. The ultimate aspect of the progress notes is the discharge summary, which is usually written by the physician and other health care specialists and should always be problem oriented. Each problem should be summarized at a level of resolution assigned for it. Needless to say, the discharge summary is written so that it adheres to the principles inherent in the POMR—that of identifying each problem by its assigned number.

ADVANTAGES

In summary, both the consumer and the health team member benefit when POMR is implemented. It is possible for the consumer to have better and less expensive care, and the health team's documentation of their care process in the long run justifies their existence in the health care industry. The major impact is likely to be more progress in scientific health research because patient records become scientific documents instead of disorganized logs.

REFERENCES

Berni, R., and Readey, H.: Problem-oriented medical record implementation, St. Louis, 1978, The C. V. Mosby Co.

Bonkowsky, M. L.: Problem-oriented medical records, adapting the POMR to community child health care, Nurs. Outlook **20:**515-518, 1972.

Brubacker, J. S.: Modern philosophies of education, New York, 1962, McGraw-Hill Book Co.

Dupuis, A. M.: Philosophy of education in historical perspective, Chicago, 1966, Rand McNally & Co.

Hurst, J. W.: How to implement the Weed system, Arch. Intern. Med. **128:**456-462, Sept., 1971.

Hurst, J. W., and Walker, H. K.: The problem oriented system, New York, 1972, Medcom Books, Inc.

Larson, K., and Hays, J.: Interacting with patients, New York, 1963, Macmillan Publishing Co., Inc.

Newman, M. A.: Identifying and meeting patient needs in short-span nurse-patient relationships, Nurs. Forum **5**(1):76-86, 1966.

Weed, L. L.: Medical records, medical education, and patient care, Cleveland, 1971, The Press of Case Western Reserve University.

Woody, M., and Mallison, M.: The problem-oriented system for patient-centered care, Am. J. Nurs. **73**(7):1168-1175, 1973.

RECORDING THE HOME VISIT

Pearl Lucido, Nancy McDaniel, Leona Bryant, Frances McKenzie, Donna Chambers, Helen Lindberg, and Zelma Van Horne

If the gap between available nursing personnel and the public's demands for community nursing services is to be met, then new and creative approaches must be found to assess the effectiveness of nursing techniques and practices currently in use. One technique in need of such review is the method of recording home visits by public health nurses.

The traditional approach to establishing the family-nurse contact, which is the essence of public health nursing implementation, is through the home visit. There are other ways in which public health nurses engage in activities with or on behalf of a particular family or individual, but the home visit continues to be the chief method of nurse-patient contact. In addition, the number of home visits made is usually the barometer for measuring the nursing agency's service to the community. Recording these home visits on a patient or family case folder has become a major, time-consuming activity of every staff public health nurse.

In most agencies, the format and method of recording the home visit are much as they were decades ago. Recent improvements in office equipment (such as dictaphones and electric typewriters) have made little difference in recording techniques, and new machines are not the answer. Rather a new approach is needed to define the necessary content that should be included in the home visit record. The hours nurses spend handwriting, dictating, or typing long narrative records of home visits should be put to better use.

Practically all nurses decry the time and effort they must spend on writing up visits, but in general they have been too busy to experiment with new approaches or to review their present method of recording. Modifications of techniques handed down by planners far from the firing line have seldom been adopted by staff nurses on any wide scale.

Public health nurses have always believed the reasons for keeping family health records are that they provide the staff of a community nursing agency with a method for: (1) planning nursing care; (2) maintaining continuity of nursing care; (3) evaluating nursing services; and (4) collecting statistical data. Any modifications of these records should meet

Reprinted from Nursing Outlook **15**(2):38-40, 1967. Copyright The American Journal of Nursing Company.

these criteria. Freeman believes that if nursing records are to be effective tools they must have "accuracy and completeness," terms which have different meanings to different people and in different agencies.*

As the body of nursing knowledge grows, there will be changes in ideas as to what constitutes "accuracy and completeness." In practice, nurses' narrative recordings of home visits are highly individual in content and organization. Many contain masses of non-pertinent detail that is arbitrarily selective and subjective, and written in a style that might be described as "rambling rose" prose. Many of these details could be eliminated, thus saving both nursing and clerical time.

Beginning public health nurses usually write volumes, demonstrating completeness in accordance with their recent academic preparation. More experienced nurses tend to be brief, and vary in their skill in achieving succinctness and pertinence. Often their records are limited to the barest data about a patient or family, because they are able to augment whatever else needs to be known from the vast reservoirs of memory and knowledge they have acquired through years of experience.

RECORDS ARE TOOLS

Nursing records should be working tools, yet much of their present content has only transient interest. Few nurses would take issue in the typical jacket or family sheet, an agency record form which contains identifying data, medical reports and diagnosis, and records of inter- and intra-agency activity. What concerns nursing is the narrative recording of home visits.

Each nurse has her own style and point of view, and when she is assigned to a family previously visited by another nurse, she must reassess the situation through a review of the total family record. If the last nurse's recordings are objective or at least exhibit "disciplined subjectivity," this will facilitate the assessment program. As nursing grows in its professional knowledges and skills, it seems doubtful that the narrative recording is suitable to describe and maintain present nursing practice. We must ask ourselves: For whom are we composing these records? Can we not find some more organized approach to recording the home visit?

PROBLEM-SOLVING

The Oakley public health nurses raised these questions and, with the consent of their nursing administrator, embarked on a search for a better way to record home visits in family records.

Many staff discussions took place and a number of ways to record home visits were tried. After six weeks of experimentation with trial methods, the nurses met as a workshop group. From this group action a method evolved that was based on a problem-solving approach and it appeared to have possibilities.

The home visit was defined by the nurses as "a data gathering, interactional process from which could come the implementation of action toward improving health of an individual or family in relation to the community." The nurses then defined the data that should be included in a record and how this material should be classified.

Areas discussed—The group agreed that an essential part of the data was a record of

---

*Freeman, Ruth B. Public Health Nursing Practice, 3rd ed. Philadelphia, Pa., W. B. Saunders Co., 1963.

the person with whom the nurse visited, and the areas they discussed. It was considered unnecessary to record details of the suggestions made by the nurse, when the agency had available clearly defined, up-to-date manuals on nursing practices. Recording, therefore, could be made through the use of key words—almost telegraphic in nature.

Observations—After reviewing many traditionally recorded home visits, the nurses realized that much of what the nurse actually observed was not clear and that often her observations were entangled in reams of hearsay and generalizations. The staff believed observations, as part of the recording, should include only that which is actually seen, heard, or perceived *during the time* of the visit. If a patient or a condition under discussion is *not* seen, then this should be noted.

Changes—The members of the unit agreed that changes recorded should include only those that have occurred since the last home visit, and are perceived by the nurse as pertinent to the patient's or family's health and are a result of action by the family or the nurse. If there have been no changes, this too should be noted.

Action—The next step after classifying the data is synthesizing the material, developing a nursing care plan, and then putting it into operation. This part of the recording includes actions taken by the family or the public health nurse or both during the time of the home visit. Typical examples are: "bath demonstration"; "referral to mental health clinic"; "mother practiced injection technique"; "patient phoned for mental health appointment."

Future plans—This is a list of items that describe measures to be taken by family members, the nurse, or both in order to achieve mutually agreed upon health goals.

EXAMPLES OF RECORDINGS

The following are examples of recording techniques that demonstrate the problem-solving approach.

The first is a record of a home visit to an 18-month-old child suffering from mental retardation due to cerebral trauma, a condition severe enough to have required surgery several weeks earlier. The mother of the child is separated from the child's father and works in a nearby town. The grandparents care for the child.

Arthur 11/16/65 H.V. with child and grandparents.

   Discussed—"Severe" reaction to smallpox vac. (rash); private medical care; progress with ambulation; fluctuations of mood; demanding; difficulties in "keeping up with child's care."

   Observed—Fretful child with small amount of rash on legs; living space crowded with a number of boxes and multiple toys; attempts to walk, but crawling is chief form of locomotion; is demanding, with swift changes of mood. Grandparents continually involved in child's activities; seem incapable of setting limits.

   Changes—Says a few words distinctly, mimics sounds and tones of grandfather; will obey some simple commands.

   Action—Examined rash; reassured grandparents; suggested ways to set limits; gave them child training pamphlet, marking areas to be read.

   Plans—Continue attempts to guide grandparents in child's care. Observation of recovery from surgery and growth patterns. Mother now pregnant, plans to work four months longer. AP supervision when she returns.

This second example is a recording of a home visit to a young primipara who was referred to the agency by the private physician during her last trimester of pregnancy.

Carrie 10/27/65 H.V. with patient.

    Discussed—EDC 11/22/65; "rooming in" policy at hospital; danger signs to be reported to M.D.; processes of labor and delivery; nutrition; breast feeding; layette and supplies; false and true labor—differences between; help at home after delivery; hospital admittance, articles needed; plans for well baby care.

    Observed—Happy, slender girl, anxious for baby to arrive—appears nervous (severely bitten fingernails, constantly twisting ball of tissue).

    Action—Reviewed birth atlas; left literature on breast feeding; demonstrated arrangement of nursery needs for efficiency; reassured.

    Changes—Pregnancy appears at term. PMD (private medical doctor) has stated that "baby has dropped down as far as it can." Occasional Braxton Hicks' contractions last month or so.

    Plan—Return once more before delivery to reinforce teaching and allow patient to discuss any questions she may have in regard to impending delivery. Assist mother in infant care and arrange well-baby care if desired. Introduce subject of family planning six weeks postpartum if mother interested.

From review of the third family record, we saw that the public health nurse prior to the home visit had a conference with the psychiatrist about the negative interaction of the young mother and her 18-month-old son. The mother had demonstrated aversion to all male physical contact and had a poor concept of herself as a person. The child exhibited disturbed behavior and his activities in the home had been limited and controlled by barriers created by the mother. The psychiatrist recommended that the nurse: (1) give special recognition to the mother's need for ego support; (2) communicate to her that she has a crucial influence in the child's emotional behavior; (3) gently integrate beginning positive interactional behavior; (4) assist the mother in verbalizing her perceived problems; (5) reinforce any valid contribution mother may make; and (6) demonstrate loving attitude toward child.

Davy 11/4/65 H.V. with mother and son.

    Discussed—Continued "insomnia" with severe crying spells; parents professed inability to cope with his actions; mother's disagreement with physician's suggestions to let child play and eat as he wishes ("can't stand messes") bowel changes ("runny-loose"); refuses all solid food ("holds in mouth and spits out behind furniture"); need for love and security by increased positive attention; consistent discipline with limit setting; continuance of medical attention.

    Observed—Ate eagerly. Fed without difficulty (not allow to feed self); mother never holds him; when ignored or thwarted, lies on floor in fetal position sucking thumb; mother yells and screams in attempt to regulate his behavior.

    Action—PHN initiated physical contact with baby (held on lap) to demonstrate love and affection; directed attention to his positive response and attempts to communicate; mother spontaneously followed this with small pat on head.

    Changes—Mother allows more freedom than on earlier visits; some gate barriers removed, others left open; mother's beginning perception of child's problem leads to increased anxiety; not as pre-occupied with own feedings as usual; out of night clothes for first time.

    Plan—Continue integrating and supporting beginnings of positive behavior toward child. Continue physical contact and attention to baby to demonstrate that positive interaction is mutually satisfying. Allow opportunities for continued verbalization of problems mother identifies. Anticipatory guidance as mother's receptiveness permits.

EVALUATING THE METHOD

After several months of using this method of recording, the nurses pooled their impressions, evaluated the method, and identified its advantages. An unexpected but professionally satisfying outcome was an upgrading of the quality of each nurse's service to a family. The new recording format was regarded from the beginning as a guideline or framework for recording data, but soon the nurses realized they were using the method "in reverse"—more action seemed to be observed in a home visit; more changes were defined; more nursing and family action was taken; and better plans were made.

All staff members agreed that the greatest saving was time—50 percent less time was needed to record home visits through the new technique. The time saved permitted the nurses to record the home visit soon after it had taken place, thus insuring greater accuracy in the recording. Current recordkeeping became an actuality, and large backlogs of unwritten records disappeared. Unbelievable! The staff nurses were able now to devote time to reviewing patient problems, developing new ways to potentiate families toward solutions, and augmenting their skills and knowledge through reading professional literature.

The staff nurses were not alone in benefiting from the new recording system; the clerical staff did too. Typing time for transcribing the nurses' notes to the records was reduced to half.

To test the exact differences in typing time, the nurses at the beginning of the experiment recorded visits in the traditional narrative style and then reconstructed the data into the new outline. Both types of records were typed, and the differences in the time were noted.

The clerical personnel find the organized information easier to transcribe, whether it is taken from written notes or dictated tapes. Records return from the clerical service promptly and this in turn has made it unnecessary for the nurses to type their own records when the swamped clerical staff could not keep up with them.

Another feature of the method is the speed with which the record can be reviewed by the professional staff and physician. Prior to a repeat home visit the public health nurse can quickly review the problems, actions, and future plans. If a staff nurse is ill or unable to visit her family, another nurse can see at a glance what needs to be done.

The supervisor finds her time shortened in routine review of staff records and can more accurately assess movement or nonmovement in a particular family. Physicians who sometimes have occasion to review family records, as in the well baby conference, report the new nursing notes are more comprehensive and useful to them.

The consensus of the nurses in our agency is that the problem-solving approach to recording home visits has many advantages. It is one way to lessen the time spent "nursing the desk," and it provides guides for a means of better planning for patient care.

NURSING DIAGNOSIS: PROCESS AND DECISION

Mary Durand Thomas and Rosemary Prince Coombs

The diagnostic process is not unique to any one occupation or profession. The medical history, the physical examination, and the laboratory tests which lead to the physician's diagnosis have been compared to the work of the police detective, who asks questions, examines clues and submits material to a crime lab for the data he needs to identify a criminal accurately.[1] When a student is not achieving at the expected level, educators seek out the strengths and weaknesses of his performance so as to make an educational diagnosis.[2] A social worker gathers facts from the client and the client's family "to make as exact a definition as possible of the situation and personality of a human being in some social need."[3] In recent nursing literature, the term "nursing diagnosis" has occurred with increasing frequency.[4]

If everyone is diagnosing, how is nursing diagnosis similar to and different from the diagnoses made by other professions and occupations? There are similarities. Every diagnosis begins with the gathering of facts. The facts may be a hematocrit of 30 percent, the location of a stray bullet, the inability to add a column of figures, or the report that the father of a large family has lost his job. At some time during or at the completion of the fact-gathering, the practitioner in a given field recognizes a pattern. He then states his conclusion.

Differences in diagnoses arise from each practitioner's view of his role behaviors and responsibilities and from the knowledge necessary for the practice of each profession. The nurse's definition of nursing determines both her view of nursing responsibilities and the knowledge those responsibilities require. Our definition of nursing is consistent with Hall's conception of nursing as a professional process involving three over-lapping aspects: (1) *the nurturing aspect—a close interpersonal relationship concerned with the intimate bodily care of patients;* (2) *the medical aspect shared with the medical profession and concerned with assisting the patient through his medical, surgical, and rehabilitative care;* and (3) *the helping aspect, shared with all professional persons and involving therapeutic interpersonal skills to assist the patient in self-actualization.*[5]

With a working definition of nursing in mind, a nurse can make a nursing diagnosis which specifies an aspect of the patient's condition that requires nursing care. How does a nurse make a nursing diagnosis? What is a nursing diagnosis?

We define a nursing diagnosis as *a statement of a conclusion resulting from a recognition of a pattern derived from a nursing investigation of the patient.* We visualize this definition as implying the two aspects of diagnosis—(1) *the process of diagnosing* and (2) *the decision, or actual diagnosis.* (Fig. 1). We will explain this definition as we have used it to make nursing diagnoses. In practice, the process of diagnosing, including the nursing investigation and the thought process leading to the recognition of a pattern precedes the actual diagnosis.

NURSING INVESTIGATION

The nursing investigation begins with a collection of facts. Some of these facts are gained from members of the health team through written and spoken communication. The

---

Reprinted from Nursing Forum 5(4):50-64, 1966.

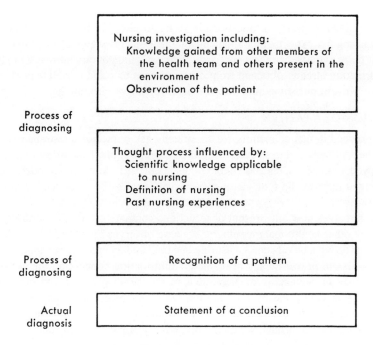

Fig. 1. The steps to nursing diagnosis.

patient's chart is the major means of written communication. The admission, or face, sheet gives us facts regarding the patient's age, sex, marital status, occupation, religion, and place of residence. The medical history and physical examination provide us with the patient's past and present experiences of illness. In the physician's progress notes we find an overview of changes in the patient's condition since hospitalization. The physician's orders outline the plan for diagnostic studies and therapy. Reports of diagnostic studies add to our information about the patient's present illness. The nurses' notes are reviewed for nursing observations of the patient.

Spoken communication with nurses who have cared or are caring for the patient complement the information gained from the chart. These nurses may be asked such questions as: "Tell me about Mr. G. What is he like as a person?" and "What signs and symptoms did you observe?" Other health team members, such as the medical social worker, the physical therapist, the occupational therapist, and the inhalation therapist, may be asked questions relevant to their information about the patient.

Communication with the patient's family and friends may yield information regarding the patient's prehospitalization habits. A question such as "What was he like before he became ill?" may elicit facts not obtained from the health team members.

A major source of fact collection is our own observation of the patient. Observation, as we use it, implies the use of four of the five senses. We visually observe the patient to detect overt physical and psychological signs of illness. We talk to the patient and listen to his responses, and we may listen to sounds from the heart or chest or abdomen. We may touch the patient at the site of a subjective complaint, such as pain. We may smell discharges from body orifices or from a wound.

We make statements or ask questions in order to elicit further information from the patient regarding his expectations about hospitalization, his views of his illness, and his prehospital daily activities concerning food, exercise, elimination and rest and sleep. We utilize information already obtained from other sources to guide our statements or questions and to prevent our subjecting the patient to repetitive questioning.

RECOGNITION OF A PATTERN

As we proceed in fact collection, we continually ask ourselves questions to determine the relatedness of facts and to structure our data collection. Mr. T mentions that his barium enema showed a "mass" in his abdomen. On his history it is noted that he had a cancerous lesion removed from his lip four years previously. Could he be concerned about a recurrence of cancer?

We ask ourselves how our present observations compare or contrast with those made previously by other health team members. A nurse observes that Mrs. E's newly applied cast is saturated with a blood stain measuring one inch in diameter. Fifteen minutes later we find the blood stain is two inches in diameter. Information concerning the possibility of hemorrhage may be sought by measurement of the blood pressure and heart beat, by inspection of skin color, and by consultation with the physician about his expectations regarding bleeding. Thus, one fact helps us to structure further observations.

The thought process through which the relatedness of facts is seen is influenced by our background of scientific knowledge, by past nursing experiences, and by our definition of nursing.

Scientific knowledge applicable to nursing may be drawn from such sciences as psychology, sociology, anthropology, anatomy, physiology, pathology, and bacteriology. Our education in these sciences forms our background working knowledge. Referral to new scientific findings keeps us informed about changing trends. Scientific knowledge is reinforced and expanded by our past nursing experiences with patients exhibiting similar signs and symptoms. Together, scientific knowledge and past experiences provide a mental card file of facts and principles to which we refer as we seek the significance of our observations.

Thus, as we seek the relationship of facts, we are influenced by these considerations: a certain scientific mechanism may be present; an observation from past experiences is similar to that seen in this patient; a nurse has a responsibility in this area. Gradually or suddenly our thought process draws the facts into a pattern. The end result of this process we have named the recognition of a pattern.

STATEMENT OF A CONCLUSION

The actual nursing diagnosis is the statement of a conclusion. The diagnosis may be descriptive as "Communicates exclusively through gestures" or "Limited response to auditory and tactile stimuli." The diagnosis may be etiological as "Lessened intestinal peristalsis" or "Inadequate understanding of hospital environment because he does not speak English." As more facts are obtained through nursing investigation, a descriptive diagnosis may become an etiological diagnosis. Knowledge of the etiology may suggest more pertinent nursing care.

We have made diagnoses which are primarily physiological ("Lessened intestinal peristalsis") and others which are primarily psychological ("Feelings of powerlessness").

Some nursing diagnoses—for example, "Nausea"—imply both physiological and psychological aspects. "Nausea" is also an example of the use of a major medical symptom as suitable terminology for a nursing diagnosis.

A nursing diagnosis might be anticipated in a certain medical diagnosis; for example, "Pain" may be the nursing diagnosis in a patient with a myocardial infarction. Or, a nursing diagnosis may be distinct from the medical diagnosis; it may describe a condition due to hospitalization ("Lonesomeness") or to a complication of the primary illness ("Urinary retention" in a patient with benign prostatic hypertrophy).

We have made the same nursing diagnoses in patients with different medical diagnoses, since the same physiological or psychological processes may be present even when the total patterns as viewed by the physician are different. "Inadequate oxygenation" may be a nursing diagnosis in patients whose medical diagnosis is "asthma," "postoperative pneumonectomy," or "congestive heart failure."

The nursing diagnosis may be the same as the medical diagnosis. This occurrence is most likely in emergency situations when the nurse's therapeutic actions are the same as the physician's. An initial diagnosis of "Cardiac arrest" may be both a medical and a nursing diagnosis calling for immediate respiratory and cardiac resuscitation. Following emergency treatment the medical diagnosis may become "Ventricular fibrillation" or "Myocardial infarction" and the nursing diagnosis may become "Ineffective cardiac output" or "Fear of pain."

With the exception of such an emergency, a nursing diagnosis is not a medical diagnosis. A nursing diagnosis tends to be more individualized. Where a medical diagnosis serves to summarize a group of signs and symptoms, a nursing diagnosis may consist of one sign or symptom that focuses on the patient's particular response to his illness. A nursing diagnosis tends to reflect the progress of the patient. Whereas a medical diagnosis may remain the same until the patient has recovered or died, a nursing diagnosis indicates the significant responses the patient makes at the stages of his illness and therefore may change with daily changes in the patient. This individualization and reflection of patient progress make a nursing diagnosis useful in the round-the-clock performance of hospital nursing as well as in community nursing. Both are situations in which medical diagnosis is made, but in which there are many hours of nursing responsibilities in the absence of the medical practitioner.

The process of diagnosing begins as soon as the patient comes under nursing care, and it continues until he no longer needs nursing care. As the nurse learns more about the patient, she may revise the nursing diagnosis. The diagnosis may become more specific; "Fear and anxiety concerning the surgical procedure" may become "Fear and anxiety concerning the possibility of cancer." Or the diagnosis may become more generalized; "Cyanosis" may become "Inadequate oxygenation."

In some instances, because of interruptions or masking of physiological or psychological cues, the nurse does not have sufficient facts to recognize a clear-cut pattern. The facts merely suggest a pattern. The decision, or diagnosis, then becomes what we call a rule-out, or tentative nursing diagnosis. This diagnosis is, in fact, a hypothesis which structures and stimulates the nurse's search for more information. We seek this information, usually by returning to the patient, to determine the accuracy or inaccuracy of the tentative nursing diagnosis.

At this point we do not believe that all nursing diagnoses can or should be of a given degree of specificity or generalization. It may be possible to organize nursing diagnoses into a classification system comparable to the classifications used by medicine. Such a system will not be possible until nurses are skilled in diagnosing and agree about the meaning and implication of the nursing diagnosis.

What is the value of a nursing diagnosis? Nursing is seeking a scientific basis for practice. The process of diagnosing necessitates the use of scientific knowledge and requires the relation and application of this knowledge to nursing. The actual diagnosis establishes a point of departure, a basis for nursing care. George B. Shaw has been credited with saying "Diagnosis should mean the finding out of all there is wrong with a particular patient."[6] We believe a nursing diagnosis could mean the finding out of all that is necessary to know to begin a plan of nursing care.

Examples of nursing diagnosis

Mr. A was a 55-year-old man hospitalized for a pneumonectomy complicated by a cerebral embolus, which in turn necessitated a tracheotomy and a gastrostomy.

Facts obtained during nursing investigation	*Major points in the thought process leading to recognition of a pattern*	*Nursing diagnosis*
Vocal cords bypassed by tracheotomy		
Had difficulty covering the opening of the tracheotomy tube with his finger	Physical discomfort and physical disability when attempting spoken or written communication	
Said "It hurts there (pointing to gastrostomy) when I talk."		
Had difficulty holding tablet while writing because of paresis of left arm		Limited ability to communicate 1) by vocal sounds 2) by writing
Nodded or shook head		
Exaggerated changes in facial expression	He is trying to express himself in the way in which he experiences the least frustration— usually through gestures or changes of facial expression	
Rubbed his stomach		
Pointed to his hip		
Shook his finger		
Held out his hand to shake hands		
Waved		
When he does speak, he says only one or two words		

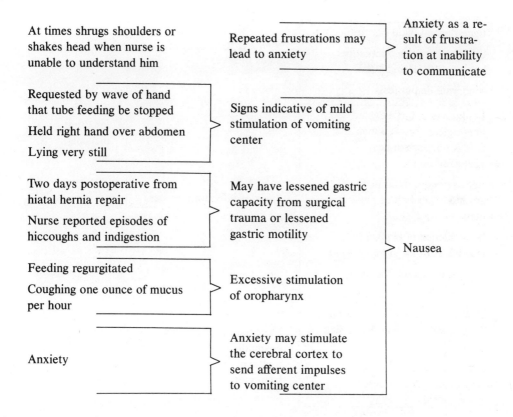

At times shrugs shoulders or shakes head when nurse is unable to understand him	Repeated frustrations may lead to anxiety	Anxiety as a result of frustration at inability to communicate
Requested by wave of hand that tube feeding be stopped Held right hand over abdomen Lying very still	Signs indicative of mild stimulation of vomiting center	
Two days postoperative from hiatal hernia repair Nurse reported episodes of hiccoughs and indigestion	May have lessened gastric capacity from surgical trauma or lessened gastric motility	Nausea
Feeding regurgitated Coughing one ounce of mucus per hour	Excessive stimulation of oropharynx	
Anxiety	Anxiety may stimulate the cerebral cortex to send afferent impulses to vomiting center	

Mrs. B. was a 65-year-old woman hospitalized for polypectomy of the descending colon.

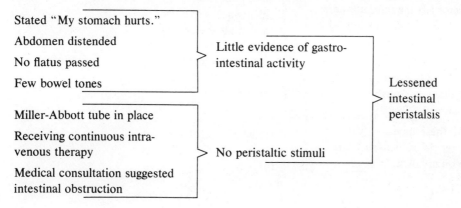

Stated "My stomach hurts." Abdomen distended No flatus passed Few bowel tones	Little evidence of gastro-intestinal activity	Lessened intestinal peristalsis
Miller-Abbott tube in place Receiving continuous intra-venous therapy Medical consultation suggested intestinal obstruction	No peristaltic stimuli	

Continued.

Face flushed, skin hot to touch

Oral temperature fluctuating between 100°F and 102°F

Moderate diaphoresis

> Signs of fever

Leukocyte count elevated
Presurgical: 7000/cu.mm.
One week postsurgical:
12,000/cu.mm.

Red, swollen, indurated area around lower half of midline incision site

No evidence of healing in lower half of incisional wound

Serosanguineous discharge from wound

> Signs of infectious process

> Pathogenic bacteria infecting incision site

Talked of coming into hospital feeling well and now being sick

Said she had expected that the polyps could be removed by way of the proctoscope and "now all this"

> Expectations regarding hospitalization and treatment have not been met

"I'm told it will take time to get well. But I don't know what they mean by time— a day, a week, a month."

"I don't understand why the doctor left the inhalator here. He knows. I don't know why he left it, but he knows."

> Does not feel she can plan what is to come and what she can do

"I don't know why I have to have the intravenous tubes. The doctor probably knows best."

> Does not understand or feel in control of her environment

"All these tubes—I just want to get rid of them so I can be on my own."

> Feelings of powerlessness

One week later:

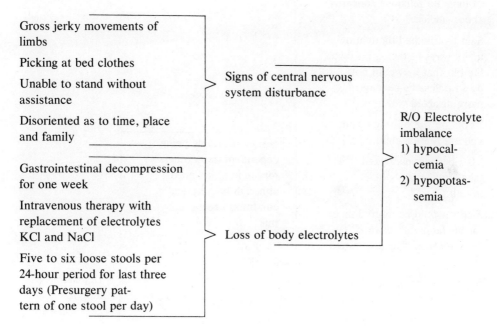

Gross jerky movements of limbs

Picking at bed clothes

Unable to stand without assistance

Disoriented as to time, place and family

> Signs of central nervous system disturbance

Gastrointestinal decompression for one week

Intravenous therapy with replacement of electrolytes KCl and NaCl

Five to six loose stools per 24-hour period for last three days (Presurgery pattern of one stool per day)

> Loss of body electrolytes

> R/O Electrolyte imbalance
> 1) hypocalcemia
> 2) hypopotassemia

Mr. C. was a 44-year-old man hospitalized for thrombophlebitis of the right leg and headaches in the left frontal region.

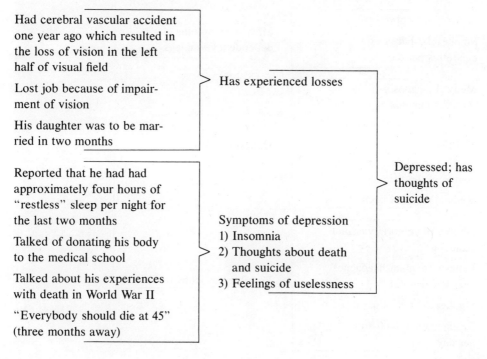

Had cerebral vascular accident one year ago which resulted in the loss of vision in the left half of visual field

Lost job because of impairment of vision

His daughter was to be married in two months

> Has experienced losses

Reported that he had had approximately four hours of "restless" sleep per night for the last two months

Talked of donating his body to the medical school

Talked about his experiences with death in World War II

"Everybody should die at 45" (three months away)

> Symptoms of depression
> 1) Insomnia
> 2) Thoughts about death and suicide
> 3) Feelings of uselessness

> Depressed; has thoughts of suicide

Continued.

"I have no religious concerns about suicide."

Said that he had thought of many ways of taking his own life but that he would not do so unless he became more disabled

"You are useful only when you are rearing children."

"If I become paralyzed, I'll take a gun and shoot myself."

Said it would be more difficult for his family if he were disabled than if he committed suicide

Repeatedly emphasized that he did not want to be a burden

Up to the bathroom against the doctor's orders

Unwraps leg against the doctor's orders

> Not comfortable being dependent upon others for some of his needs, although his physical condition necessitates this

History of alcoholism

Smokes 2-3 packs of cigarettes per day

> May be symptoms of dependency longings

> Dependency longings

Medical diagnosis of thrombophlebitis

Veins in left thigh slightly engorged

Skin inflamed over the course of the vein

Medical order of bedrest

> Danger of emboli

History of cerebral vascular accident

Reports frequent headaches over left temple

Smokes 2-3 packs per day

Drinks coffee, 8-10 cups per day

> Possible vasoconstriction

> R/O Vascular insufficiency
> 1) cerebral
> 2) lower limbs

REFERENCES

1. John A. Prior and Jack S. Silberstein, *Physical Diagnosis: The History and Examination of the Patient.* St. Louis: The C. V. Mosby Company. 1959. pp. 17-18.
2. Leo J. Brueckner, "Introduction" Educational Diagnosis. *Thirty-fourth Yearbook of the National Society for the Study of Education.* Guy Montrose Whipple (ed.). Bloomington, Ill. Public School Publishing Company. 1935. p. 2.
3. Mary E. Richmond, *Social Diagnosis.* New York: Russell Sage Foundation. 1917. p. 357.
4. Virginia Bonney and June Rothberg, *Nursing Diagnosis and Therapy.* New York: National League for Nursing. 1963.
5. Lydia E. Hall, "Nursing—What Is It?" Revised, Mimeographed. Loeb Center, New York, April 26, 1963, p. 1-5.
6. F. G. Crookshank, "The Importance of a Theory of Signs and a Critique of Language in the Study of Medicine" Supplement to C. K. Ogden and I. A. Richards, *The Meaning of Meaning.* 10th edition, London: Routledge and Kegan Paul, Inc. 1949. p. 343.

SUGGESTED READINGS for Chapter 2

BOOKS

Auld, M. E., and Birum, L. H., editors: The challenge of nursing, St. Louis, 1973, The C. V. Mosby Co. Unit III is collection of articles related to the nursing process.

Beland, I.: Clinical nursing: pathophysiological and psychological approaches, ed. 2, New York, 1970, Macmillan Publishing Co., Inc. A medical-surgical textbook.

Benjamin, A.: The helping interview, Boston, 1969, Houghton Mifflin Co. Discusses conditions, stages, and philosophies of interviewing, recording, types of questions and communication, responses and leads.

Bermosk, L. S., and Mordan, M. J.: Interviewing in nursing, New York, 1964, Macmillan Publishing Co., Inc. Discusses interviewing, the climate for interviewing, and the role of the nurse.

Berni, R., and Readey, H.: Problem-oriented medical record implementation: allied health peer review, St. Louis, 1978, The C. V. Mosby Co. Describes the POMR system and discusses system implementation, evaluation, modification, and computerization. Presents a system implementation model.

Bernstein, L., and Dana, R. H.: Interviewing and the health professions, New York, 1970, Appleton-Century-Crofts. Discusses interviewing techniques, evaluative, hostile, reassuring, probing, and understanding responses, emotional reactions to illness, death, and dying.

Bird, B.: Talking with patients, Philadelphia, 1955, J. B. Lippincott Co. Discusses communication with adults and children.

Bower, F. L.: The process of planning nursing care, St. Louis, 1977, The C. V. Mosby Co. Discusses planning individualized nursing care, identifying nursing problems, selecting nursing actions, formulating evaluative criteria, and implementing the nursing care plan.

Byers, V. B.: Nursing observation, Dubuque, Iowa, 1968, William C. Brown Co., Publishers. Discusses the role of observation in nursing practice; observation of patients in their environment—voice, eyes, gait, appetite, elimination, sleep; observation of signs and symptoms—pain, hemorrhage, edema, dizziness; observations related to nursing activities—admitting and bathing the patient; and applications of observation to patient situations.

Byrne, M. L., and Thompson, L. F.: Key concepts for the study and practice of nursing, St. Louis, 1978, The C. V. Mosby Co. Discusses the following concepts: organismic behavior, basic human needs, level of wellness, adaptation, behavioral patterning, steady state, stress, behavioral stability continuum, structural variable, and consequences of an act. Presents a working model for assessing patient's needs and predicting the effects of nursing care.

Easton, R.: Problem-oriented medical record concepts, New York, 1974, Appleton-Century-Crofts. Discusses the difference between the source-oriented and problem-oriented patient care record, problem list and data base concepts, components of the patient care note, problem types, flow sheets, problem-oriented patient care instruction, nonproblem data, and audit concepts.

Fowkes, W. C., and Hunn, V. K.: Clinical assessment for the nurse practitioner, St. Louis, 1973, The C. V. Mosby Co. Taking a medical history, examining the patient, and use of laboratory studies are explained.

French, R. M.: The nurse's guide to diagnostic procedures, New York, 1971, McGraw-Hill Book Co. Discusses numerous diagnostic tests.

Froelich, R. E., and Bishop, F. M.: Clinical interviewing skills, St. Louis, 1977, The C. V. Mosby Co. Conducting the interview, interview techniques, and influences upon the interview are discussed. Practice interviews and simulations are presented.

Gebbie, K. M., and Lavin, M. A.: Classification of nursing diagnosis, St. Louis, 1975, The C. V. Mosby Co. Classification is discussed and diagnoses are identified.

Hays, J. S., and Larson, K. H.: Interacting with patients, New York, 1963, Macmillan Publishing Co., Inc. Identifies, illustrates, and discusses 25 therapeutic techniques and 19 nontherapeutic techniques. Most of book consists of process recordings of case studies that illustrate therapeutic and nontherapeutic communication.

Hein, E. C.: Communication in nursing practice, Boston, 1973, Little, Brown & Co. Discusses therapeutic communication, channels of communication, and feedback.

Johnson, M. M., Davis, M. L. C., and Bilitch, M. J.: Problem solving in nursing practice, Dubuque, Iowa, 1970, William C. Brown Co., Publishers. Discusses an overview of problem solving, patient problems vs. nursing problems, problem assessment, problem statement, and solving the problem.

Kahn, R. L., and Cannell, C. F.: The dynamics of interviewing: theory, technique, and cases, New York, 1957, John Wiley & Sons, Inc. Various types of interviewing are discussed.

Kron, T.: Communication in nursing, Philadelphia, 1972, W. B. Saunders Co. Discusses elements of communication, thinking, perceiving, doing, listening, speaking, reading, writing, and keys to effective communication.

Larkin, P. D., and Backer, B. A.: Problem-oriented nursing assessment, New York, 1977, McGraw-Hill Book Co. Basic interviewing, taking histories, beginning physical examinations, and mental health assessments are discussed.

Lewis, G.: Nurse-patient communication, Dubuque, Iowa, 1969, William C. Brown Co., Publishers. An introduction to study of communication. Emphasizes nonverbal communication within the framework of senses.

Little, D. E., and Carnevali, D.: Nursing care planning, Philadelphia, 1969, J. B. Lippincott Co. Discusses current concepts and rationale for planning patient care, the relationship of philosophy of patient care to nursing care plans, processes used in care planning, nursing history, nursing care plans, revisions of nursing care plans, nursing care plan forms, activating a nursing care plan system, and teaching planning of nursing care.

Lockerby, F.: Communication for nurses, St. Louis, 1968, The C. V. Mosby Co. Discusses communication, observation, listening, speaking, and writing.

Malasanos, L., Barkauskas, V., Moss, M., and Allen, K. S.: Health assessment, St. Louis, 1977, The C. V. Mosby Co. Describes how to obtain a health history and how to do a physical examination using the organ-system format.

Maloney, E., editor: Interpersonal relations, Dubuque, Iowa, 1966, William C. Brown Co., Publishers. A collection of articles on interpersonal relations.

Mayers, M. G.: A systematic approach to the nursing care plan, New York, 1972, Appleton-Century-Crofts. Discusses systematic problem solving, the problem as basis for care planning, the expected outcome as standard for evaluation, nursing action as strategy for solving problems, patient's response as test of good planning, nursing history, communicating patient care information, implementing nursing care planning and current trends for improved patient care. Care planning in hospitals, in-

stitutions, community agencies, and nursing education are considered.

O'Brien, M.: Communications and relationships in nursing, St. Louis, 1978, The C. V. Mosby Co. Discusses verbal and nonverbal communication, effective communication, perception, writing, and communication as it relates to patient care and administration.

Orlando, I. J.: The dynamic nurse-patient relationship, New York, 1961, G. P. Putnam's Sons. Discusses function, process, and principles of the nurse-patient relationship. It is rich with illustrations.

Peplau, H. E.: Interpersonal relations in nursing, New York, 1952, G. P. Putnam's Sons. Studies nursing as interpersonal process. Discusses the phases of nurse-patient relationship and roles in nursing. Discusses influences of human needs, interferences to achievement of goals, opposing goals, and unexplained discomfort in nursing situations. Identifies psychological tasks of the sick role.

Peplau, H. E.: Basic principles of patient counseling, Philadelphia, 1964, Smith, Kline & French Laboratories. Extracts from two clinical nursing workshops in psychiatric hospitals. Discusses the form of counseling interviews and the principles for nurse-counselor. Principles discussed in detail include setting an example for the patient, maintaining a professional attitude, respecting the patient, assessing the patient's intellectual competence, guiding the patient to reinterpret his experiences rationally, asking sensible questions to aid description, studying and applying theory in counseling.

Readey, H., Teague, M., and Readey, W.: Introduction to nursing essentials: a handbook, St. Louis, 1977, The C. V. Mosby Co. Charting and the problem-oriented record system are discussed.

Seedor, M. M.: Aids to diagnosis: a programmed unit in fundamentals of nursing, New York, 1964, Teachers College Press, Columbia University. A programmed unit in fundamentals of nursing. Discusses vital signs, observation, physical examination, and laboratory tests.

Skipper, J. K., Jr., and Leonard, R. C., editors: Social interaction and patient care, Philadelphia, 1965, J. B. Lippincott Co. A collection of articles about social and psychological aspects of a nurse's role, importance of communication, patient's view of his situation, structural and cultural content of patient care, and role and status relationships between doctor, nurse, and patient.

Skydell, B., and Crowder, A. S.: Diagnostic procedures: a reference for health practitioners and a guide for patient counseling, Boston, 1975, Little, Brown & Co. A general description of the purposes and means of conducting nearly seventy clinical tests and suggestions on what to tell the patient to expect are presented.

Sullivan, H. S.: The psychiatric interview, New York, 1954, W. W. Norton & Co., Inc. Discusses basic concepts, technical considerations, structuring, early stages, detailed inquiry, and termination of interview process.

Travelbee, J.: Interpersonal aspects of nursing, Philadelphia, 1971, F. A. Davis Co. Discusses the nature of nursing, nurse-patient relationships, and nursing intervention. The concepts human being, patient, nurse, illness, suffering, and communication are explored.

Vitale, B. A., Latterner, N. S., and Nugent, P. M.: A problem solving approach to nursing care plans: a program, St. Louis, 1978, The C. V. Mosby Co. Stresses data collection and classification, making deductions, nursing diagnosis and hypothesis, and hypothesis implementation and evaluation in a programmed text form. Presents numerous case studies.

Walter, J. B., Paradee, G. P., and Molbo, D. M.: Dynamics of problem-oriented approaches: patient care and documentation, Philadelphia, 1976, J. B. Lippincott Co. Includes a discussion of nursing diagnosis.

Weed, L. L.: Medical records, medical education, and patient care, Chicago, 1971, Year Book Medical Publishers, Inc. Discusses data base, problem list, initial plan, progress notes, flow sheets, and discharge summary. Presents implications of problem-oriented record and computerization of medical record. Appendices include questionnaire for obtaining patient's medical history by computer.

Woolley, F. R., et al.: Problem-oriented nursing, New York, 1974, Springer Publishing Co., Inc. Identifies the POR system and explains how data base, problem list, progress notes, and flow sheets are used. Stresses POR as it relates to education, implementation, and application in various settings. Presents three case studies for review exercises.

Yura, H., and Walsh, M. B., editors: The nursing process, Washington, D.C., 1967, The Catholic University of America Press. Discusses assessing patient needs, planning to meet those needs, implementing, and evaluating the plan of care.

Yura, H., and Walsh, M. B.: The nursing process: assessing, planning, implementing, evaluating, New York, 1973, Appleton-Century-Crofts. Discusses components of the nursing process.

PERIODICALS
Assessment

Abbey, J. C.: Nursing observations of fluid imbalance, Nurs. Clin. North Am.**3:**77-86, March, 1968. Discusses criteria for determining fluid balance, types of fluid and electrolyte imbalance, and acid-base phenomena.

American Journal of Nursing: Patient assessment: taking a patient's history, Am. J. Nurs. **74**(2):293-324, 1974. A programmed instruction about taking patient's history as part of patient assessment.

Aspinall, M. J.: Development of a patient-completed admission questionnaire and its comparison with the nursing interview, Nurs. Res. **24**(5):377-381, 1975. Research report indicates that nurses made significantly more errors of omission in an unstructured interview than patients made in completing a questionnaire. It took less time to explain the reason for the questionnaire and get the patient's consent than to do an interview. A nursing history questionnaire is presented.

Barger, R. C., and Barger, J.: Pharmacist, nurse cooperate in taking drug histories, Hospitals **50**(17):93-94, 1977. Task Force on the Pharmacists' Clinical Role has stated that the pharmacist's involvement in drug and allergy history taking is a desirable goal. They also recommend that the pharmacist teach nurses to take drug histories and receive a copy of all drug histories in the pharmacy.

Bermosk, L. S.: Interviewing in nursing: a key to effective supervisor-staff relationships. Superv. Nurse **4**(3):46-56, 1973. Indicates that better communication could reduce errors in patient care, decrease staff conflict, dissipate rumors, and elevate staff morale. Discusses principles of interviewing and actions of the interviewer.

Burgess, A. W., and Laszlo, A. T.: Courtroom use of hospital records in sexual assault cases, Am. J. Nurs. **77**(1):64-68, 1977. Discusses assessment of sexual assault victims and stresses importance of the record in the legal process.

Burtt, E. A.: Employee assessment of the young and the older worker, Nurs. Clin. North Am. **7:**109-119, March, 1972. Discusses the importance of assessing developmental and situational factors and attitudes.

Cahill, A. S.: Principles and practice: dual-purpose tool for assessing maternal needs and nursing care, JOGN Nurs. **4**(1):28-32, 1975.

Presents a six-part assessment form including maternal history, maternal characteristics and behaviors, infant characteristics and behaviors, parental-infant interaction, maternal physical condition, and knowledge and education needs. Discusses the function of the form.

Calnan, M. F., and Hanron, J. B.: Nursing assessment—dialogue with meaning, Superv. Nurse 2(7):18-21, 1971. Discusses development, implementation, and evaluation of nursing assessment.

Coates, L.: Nursing by assessment, AORN J. 19(5):1091-1104, 1974. Stresses the importance of preoperative assessment.

Deininger, J. M.: The nursing process: how to assess your patients' needs, J. Pract. Nurs. 25(10):32-34, 1975. Suggests Henderson's fourteen principles and Maslow's hierarchy of needs as frameworks for assessment.

Ford, L.: Head to toe, Can. Nurse 72(9):26-27, 1976. Outlines what to observe and chart about the head, neck and chest, abdomen, extremities, skin, and equipment.

Fuller, D., and Rosenaur, J. A.: A patient assessment guide, Nurs. Outlook 22(7):460-462, 1974. Presents a nursing assessment tool that addresses general information, basic needs for adults and children, and observations made during history taking.

Garant, C.: A basis for care, Am. J. Nurs. 72(4):699-701, 1972. Suggests how to systematically observe and document patient's behavior as a basis for a care plan.

Geitgey, D. A.: SELF-PACING—a guide to nursing care, Nurs. Outlook 17(8):48-49, 1969. Discusses "SELF-PACING" as an acronym for systematic assessment.

Giblin, E. C.: Symposium on assessment as part of the nursing process, Nurs. Clin. North Am. 6:113-114, March, 1971. Discusses purposes of the nursing process and systematic assessment.

Gilbo, D.: Nursing assessment of circulatory function, Nurs. Clin. North Am. 3:53-63, March, 1968. Discusses normal circulatory function, cardiovascular changes, and nursing observations of abnormal cardiovascular performance.

Haferkorn, V.: Assessing individual learning needs as a basis for patient teaching, Nurs. Clin. North Am. 6:199-209, March, 1971. Presents plan for assessment and discusses teaching the myocardial infarction patient about his disease and its therapy.

Hamdi, M. E., and Hutelmyer, C. M.: A study of the effectiveness of an assessment tool in the identification of nursing care problems, Nurs. Res. 19:354-359, July-August, 1970. The authors modified Faye McCain's Guide to the systematic assessment of the functional abilities of a patient for use in assessing the needs of patients with diabetes mellitus and studied the reliability of the instrument.

Hamilton, C., Pratt, M. K., and Groen, M.: The nurse's active role in assessment, Nurs. Clin. North Am. 4:249-262, June, 1969. Discusses principles of nursing assessment, an assessment tool, a nursing care plan, and a nurse's role in the rehabilitation evaluation unit.

Hefferin, E. A., and Hunter, R. E.: Nursing assessment and care plan statements, Nurs. Res. 24(5):360-366, 1975. Research report of scope, specificity, and interrelationship of patient problems and nursing intervention statements on ninety nursing care plans in relation to the use of an observation checklist or a nursing history form. Reports that care plans reflect less than half of the patient problems identified on nursing histories.

Hegarty, J.: Passing on assessment skills to charge nurses, Nurs. Mirror 141(23):62-63, 1975. Stresses the importance of preparing nurses to assess mentally handicapped adults.

Heinemann, E., and Estes, N.: Assessing alcoholic patients, Am. J. Nurs. 76(5):785-789, 1976. Presents and discusses a nursing history form to be used with alcoholic patients.

Hobart, C. L.: The interview as a management skill, Superv. Nurse 2(10):56-59, 1971. Stresses the importance of listening to gain an understanding of what is being said as a basis for nursing actions.

Jones, M.: Principles and practice: antepartum assessment in high-risk pregnancy, JOGN Nurs. 4(6):23-27, 1975. Discusses amniocentesis, ultrasonography, and the oxytocin challenge test and the importance of being responsive to the socioeconomic and cultural needs of clients.

Karch, A. M.: This assessment habit saves lives, RN 39(3):42, 44, 1976. Describes a cardiovascular-pulmonary assessment.

Kimball, C. P.: Interviewing, diagnosis, and therapy. Postgrad. Med. 47:88-93, May, 1970. Discusses components of an interview and identifies psychotherapeutic maneuvers.

Kurihara, M.: Assessment and maintenance of adequate respiration, Nurs. Clin. North Am. 3:65-76, March, 1968. Discusses pulmonary physiology and pathology, nursing and laboratory assessment of respiration, and respiratory problems and their treatment.

Langelaan, D. G.: Neurological assessment,

Nurs. Times **70**:70-72, Jan. 17, 1974. Discusses the assessment of the consciousness level, mental state, speech, pupils, temperature, pulse, respirations, and blood pressure on the neurological patient.

Langner, S. R.: The nursing process and the interview, Occup. Health Nurs. **21**(12):19-23, 1973. Presents principles of interviewing, and a nursing history form.

Linkert, M.: Nurses can improve data collection, Dimens. Health Serv. **52**(9):32-34, 1975. Itemizes ways to collect data.

Lynaugh, J. E., and Bates, B.: Physical diagnosis: a skill for all nurses? Am. J. Nurs. **74**(1):58-59, 1974. Who should know physical assessment skills? Who is qualified to teach them? How can they be maintained before program development?

Manthey, M. E.: A guide for interviewing, Am. J. Nurs. **67**(10):2088-2090, 1967. Presents admission interview guide of twelve questions.

Mayers, M. G.: A search for assessment criteria, Nurs. Outlook **20**(5):323-326, 1972. A study to identify tangible and significant indicators of achievement in community health nursing.

McFarland, G. K., and Apostoles, F. E.: The nursing history in a psychiatric setting: adaptations to a variety of nursing care patterns and patient populations, J. Psychiatr. Nurs. **13**(4): 12-17, 1975. Presents a psychiatric history form and indicates the need for an objective attitude by staff and validation of observations.

The nurse's role in health assessment and promotion, Can. Nurse **73**(3):40-41, 1977. Board of Directors of the Registered Nurses' Association of British Columbia position paper about health assessment and promotion.

Patient assessment: taking a patient's history, Am. J. Nurs. **74**(2):293-324, 1974. Programmed instruction for taking a history.

Serafini, P.: Nursing assessment in industry, Am. J. Public Health **66**(8):755-760, 1976. Identifies six areas from which information should be obtained to assess an industry. Presents an annotated assessment guide.

Snyder, M., and Baum, R.: Assessing station and gait, Am. J. Nurs. **74**(7):1256-1257, 1974. Presents a checklist to evaluate neurological patient's station and gait.

Steckel, S. B.: Utilization of reinforcement contracts to increase written evidence of the nursing assessment, Nurs. Res. **25**(1):58-61, 1976. Research report reveals an increase in charting with systematic reinforcement.

Talabere, L., and Graves, P.: A tool for assessing families of burned children, Am. J. Nurs. **76**(2): 225-227, 1976. Presents and discusses a tool for assessing families of burned children.

Tapia, J. A.: The nursing process in family health, Nurs. Outlook **20**(4):267-270, 1972. Presents a system for assessing family's level of functioning to determine appropriate nursing activities.

Thomas, B. J.: Clues to patients' behavior, Am. J. Nurs. **63**(7):100-102, 1963. Discusses application of psychiatric nursing principles to medical-surgical nursing.

Ungvarski, P. J.: Nursing assessment in hypertension, Occup. Health Nurs. **23**:9-15, Nov., 1975. Discusses the results of a survey of public awareness of high blood pressure, definition and measurement of hypertension, pharmacological and dietary management in hypertension, and the nursing assessment and intervention.

Valencius, J. C.: Guidelines for neuro assessment, AORN J. **20**(3):442-450, 1974. Discusses assessment of auditory-visual responses, tactile-painful stimuli, motor activity, pupil responses, and vital signs.

Vincent, P. A., Broad, J. E., and Dilworth, L.: Developing a mental health assessment form, J. Nurs. Adm. **6**(4):25-28, 1976. Presents a mental health assessment form, including physical, psychological, social, medical, and household member's behaviors with suggestions for development of the tool.

Computer systems

Adams, R. P.: Selecting a data abstracting service, Med. Record News **48**(1):38-40, 1977. Gives directions for selecting a data abstracting service.

Ashcroft, J.: Computers in intensive care units, Nurs. Mirror **138**(14):50-52, 1974. Discusses reasons for having a computerized system, the system, intercom terminals, required staff, how the system was introduced, and the initial reaction.

Austin, C. J.: Planning and selecting an information system, Hospitals **51**(20):95-100, 202, 1977. Details how to plan and select an information system.

Birckhead, L. M.: Automation of the health care system: implications for nursing; part I: dangers to nursing practice in the automation of the health care system, Int. Nurs. Rev. **22**(1): 28-31, 1975. Warns about the dehumanizing effects of automation. Stresses the importance of professional nurses defining their relationships with machines.

Brown, R. L.: Computerized nursing, Nurs. Mirror **142**(6):56, 1976. Reports that patient records were accurate and more complete, medication errors decreased, direct patient care and job satisfaction increased with the use of a computer system. Confidence in the system and enthusiasm affect use of the system more than age.

Burfeind, R.: Schoitz Memorial inaugurates on-line computer system to cope with rapid increase in outpatient service needs, Hosp. Top. **55**(3):20-23, 1977. Describes an on-line system.

Cook, M., and McDowell, W.: Changing to an automated information system, Am. J. Nurs. **75**(1):46-51, 1975. Discusses changing from a manual to a computerized system for handling paper work.

Cornell, S. A., and Carrick, A. G.: Computerized schedules and care plans, Nurs. Outlook **21**(12):781-784, 1973. Describes and evaluates an automated system. Presents a care plan system functional flow chart and a bedside printout.

Crook, W. J., and Syrett, D.: Computerized admissions mean automatic efficiency, Dimens. Health Serv. **52**(9):26-30, 1975. Describes a system that can produce the daily admission list, transfer list, discharge list, and daily census.

Flynn, E. D.: The computer: an aid to nursing communications, Nurs. Clin. North Am. **4:**541-547, Sept., 1969. Discusses the computer as an asset to patient care.

Goodwin, J. O., and Edwards, B. S.: Developing a computer program to assist the nursing process: phase I—from systems analysis to an expandable program, Nurs. Res. **24**(4):299-305, 1975. Defines nursing. Constructs a systems model of the nursing process. A computer program is written and processed to formulate a nursing diagnosis based on collected patient data.

Hannah, K. J.: The computer and nursing practice, Nurs. Outlook **24**(9):555-558, 1976. Encourages nurses to get involved with computer technology to improve nursing practice.

Hill, P. A.: Medical information and patient care, Nurs. Mirror **139**(12):52-53, 1974. Discusses information media and loss, purposes of storing information, the historical background of medical information, and the unit system.

Holbrook, F. K.: Computerization aids utilization review, Hospitals **49**(17):53-55, 1975. Computer is used to develop a profile for length of stay by diagnosis and to help physicians evaluate their performance.

Holland, B., Holland, P. M., and Hsieh, R. K. C.: Automated multiphasic health testing, Public Health Rep. **90**(2):133-139, 1975. Research report about the diagnostic and testing results of a multiphasic screening program.

Hosking, D. J.: The computer assisted school health program (CASH): a field unit's viewpoint, Can. J. Public Health **64:**521-537, Nov.-Dec., 1973. Describes a computer system and discusses advantages and problems.

Jelinek, R. C., Zinn, T. K., and Brya, J. R.: Tell the computer how sick the patients are and it will tell how many nurses they need, Mod. Hosp. **121**(6):81-85, 1973. Describes an automated system that does workload monitoring, personnel scheduling, and management reporting.

Johansen, S., and Orthoefer, J. E.: Development of a school health information system, Am. J. Public Health **65**(11):1203-1207, 1975. Describes a computer system for school nursing records.

Meldman, M. J., and Mcleod, D.: A goal list and a treatment methods index in an automated record system, Hosp. Community Psychiatry **26**(6):365-370, 1975. Five hundred goal statements, 1500 treatment method statements, and all drugs and activity therapies used in the hospital were indexed and stored in a computer. Comprehensive treatment plan can be developed by entering the numbers of the appropriate goals and treatments.

Miller, S. I.: A multidimensional problem-oriented review and evaluation system for psychiatric patient care, Med. Record News **48**(1):9-12, 1977. Describes a multifunctional system that helps review standards in addition to costs.

Moll, D. B., Lande, M. A., and Buckley, J. J.: O.R. information system implemented, Hospitals **49**(1):55-60, 1975. Explains how a computer-based information system was used to improve operating room utilization.

Monte Carlo theory and probability applications in medicine, Respir. Care **22**(2):200-202, 1977. Recommends use of computer for applications of probability theory.

Norwood, D. D., Hawkins, R. E., and Gall, J. E.: Information system benefits hospital, improves patient care, Hospitals **50**(18):79-83, 1976. Reports that an automated communications system affected the quality of patient care by improving the use of hospital resources.

O'Desky, R. I., and Ball, M. J.: Ten rules to bridge the communication gap between the health-care professional and his computer systems department, Hosp. Top. **54**(5):53-54, 1976. Lists and discusses ten rules for integrating computer systems into health care systems.

Oldfield, N.: The LP/VN and the computer, Nurs. Care **10**(4):18-19, 31, 1977. Describes an automated multiphasic health testing system.

Price, E.: Data processing: present and potential, Am. J. Nurs. **67**(12):2558-2564, 1967. Defines differences between manual, semiautomated, and fully automated computer systems and discusses the nurse's role in developing these systems.

Proctor, T. D., and Cutts, N. J.: A novel method of collecting information, Occup. Health **28**(6): 302-307, 1976. Describes an automated system used in occupational health.

Schmitz, H. H.: The anatomy of a successful system implementation, Hospitals **51**(20):105-106, 110-115, 1977. Alerts the reader to potential problems with information systems.

Schmitz, H. H., Ellerbrake, R. P., and Williams, T. M.: Study evaluates effects of new communications system, Hospitals **50**(21):129-134, 1976. Research report reveals a significant increase in the amount of time personnel conversed in the form of instruction. Time spent telephoning, requisitioning items and services, and transporting patients and equipment decreased significantly after the introduction of a computer system.

Siegel, J. H., et al.: Computer-based consultation in "care" of the critically ill patient, Surgery **80**(3):350-364, 1976. Discusses Clinical Assessment, Research, and Education System (CARE), a national time-shared computer system designed to provide management and education aid for the treatment of critically ill surgical patients.

Smith, E. J.: The computer and nursing practice, Superv. Nurse **5**(9):55-62, 1974. Discusses planning for and implementing a computer system. Lists goals of the system and nursing care benefits.

Straitiff, P. A.: Antibiotic surveillance, Med. Record News **48**(3):58-62, 1977. A computer abstracting service aids study of infection control.

Tate, S. P.: Automation of the health care system: implications for nursing, part 2—change strategies for nurses, Int. Nurs. Rev. **22**(2):39-42, 1975. Discusses strategies for effecting change.

Taylor, J. D.: Control system ensures documentation of care, Med. Record News **48**(2):25-30, 1977. This computerized control system improved the manageability of medical record documentation.

Tobin, G.: The computer—an aid to intensive therapy nursing, Nurs. Mirror **140**(5):72-73, 1975. Describes how a computer is used in intensive care.

Van Cura, L. J., et al.: Venereal disease: interviewing and teaching by computer, Am. J. Public Health **65**(11):1159-1164, 1975. Discusses the use of a computer for obtaining medical histories and teaching about venereal disease.

Wasserman, A. I.: Minicomputers may maximize data processing, Hospitals **51**(20):119-128, 1977. Discusses how a decentralized information network may be economical for some hospitals.

Weil, T. P., and Weil, J. W.: The use of computer systems in patient care, Nurs. Forum **6**(2):206-217, 1967. Covers the history of computers in hospitals, medical information system, terminal devices, and physiological monitoring.

Wilson, N. C., and Mumpower, J. L.: Automated evaluation of goal-attainment ratings, Hosp. Community Psychiatry **26**(3):163-164, 1975. Describes an automated system for evaluating treatment effectiveness. Patients, relatives, and staff specify treatment goals from 703 standardized statements. They rate the importance of the goal and the degree of its attainment.

Zielstorff, R. D.: The planning and evaluation of automated systems: a nurse's point of view, J. Nurs. Adm. **5**(6):22-25, 1975. Elements of automated information systems are discussed.

Zielstorff, R. D.: Orienting personnel to automated systems, J. Nurs. Adm. **6**(3):14-16, 1976. Discusses orienting all personnel to an automated system and orienting new personnel to an established system.

Listening

Brunner, N. A.: Communications in nursing service administration, J. Nurs. Adm. **7**(8):29-32, 1977. Emphasizes the importance of feedback to evaluate accurate transfer, correct interpretation, and desired behavioral change related to the communication process.

Burkhardt, M.: Response to anxiety, Am. J. Nurs. **69**(10):2153-2154, 1969. Stresses listening and tolerance of silence as interventions for anxiety.

Edwards, P. J.: Listening comprehension test for nurses, Int. Nurs. Rev. **23**(3):88-91, 1976. Describes a listening comprehension test.

Haggerty, V.: Listening: an experiment in nursing, Nurs. Forum **10**(4):383-391, 1971. Study supports hypothesis that patients will talk about what concerns them, regardless of nurse's stated purpose of visit.

Hein, E. C.: Listening, Nursing '75 **5**(3):93-102, 1975. Stresses the importance of listening for themes to assess patient's needs.

Johnston, R.: Listen nurse, Am. J. Nurs. **71**(2): 303, 1971. A poem about listening.

Martin, I. C. A.: A strident silence, Nurs. Times **73**(20):754-755, 1977. Encourages the judicious use of silence.

Meir, E.: Nursing is . . . listening. II. Nurs. Mirror and Midwives Journal **135**:24, July, 1972. Mentions listening as it relates to paranoid behavior.

Nichols, R. G., and Stevens, L. A.: Listening to people, Harvard Bus. Rev. **35**:85-92, Sept.-Oct., 1957. Discusses gap in listening training, rules for reception, listening for ideas, emotional filters, and benefits in business.

Rubin, D.: "Listen to me!" Helping children develop listening skills, Children Today **3**(5):7-9, 1974. Describes activities for auditory discrimination, concentration exercises, and interpretive, creative, and critical listening.

Schweitzer, B.: Miss Pinet knew? Nursing '75 **5**(4):18, 1975. Case study of a woman whose communication indicated she knew she was going to die and the nurse's response.

Suhrie, E. B.: The importance of listening, Nurs. Outlook **8**(12):686-687, 1960. Discusses intelligent listening.

Van Dersal, W. R.: How to be a good communicator—and a better nurse, Nursing '74 **4**(12):57-64, 1974. Lists rules about talking and listening, discusses the reading-writing process, and gives the "Fog Index" to determine the reading level necessary for written material.

Walke, M. A. K.: When a patient needs to unburden his feelings, Am. J. Nurs. **77**(7):1164-1166, 1977. Suggests how the nurse can create an atmosphere in which a patient can feel free to express his feelings.

Wallston, K. A., and Wallston, B. S.: A role-playing approach toward studying nurses' decisions to listen to patients, Nurs. Res. **24**(1): 16-22, 1975. Uses role playing to simulate patient disclosures and finds that nurses are able to give considerable information and interpretive data.

Westhoff, M. E.: Listening to relieve the fear of death, Superv. Nurse **3**(3):80-83, 85, 87, 1972. Stresses importance of listening to patient to help relieve his anxiety about death.

Nursing diagnosis

Aspinall, M. J.: Nursing diagnosis—the weak link, Nurs. Outlook **24**(7):433-437, 1976. Main- tains that the effectiveness of nursing intervention depends on an accurate nursing diagnosis.

Bircher, A. U.: On the development and classification of diagnosis, Nurs. Forum **14**(1): 11-29, 1975. Stresses the need for a taxonomy. Discusses categorization and identifies steps in the diagnostic process.

Brown, M. M.: The epidemiologic approach to the study of clinical nursing diagnoses, Nurs. Forum **13**(4):346-359, 1974. Uses epidemiology as the framework for determining the nursing diagnosis.

Chambers, W.: Nursing diagnosis, Am. J. Nurs. **62**(11):102-104, 1962. Discusses process of making nursing diagnosis.

Gebbie, K., and Lavin, M. A.: Classifying nursing diagnosis, Am. J. Nurs. **74**(2):250-253, 1974; and in Nicholls, M. E., and Wessells, V. G., editors: Nursing standards and nursing process, Wakefield, Mass., 1977, Contemporary Publishing Co., pp. 13-18. Classification process is discussed, and nursing diagnoses are listed.

Gordon, M.: Nursing diagnoses and the diagnostic process, Am. J. Nurs. **76**(8):1298-1300, 1976. Components of diagnoses, nomenclature of diagnostic categories, and the diagnostic process are discussed.

Komorita, N.: Nursing diagnosis, Am. J. Nurs. **63**(12):83-86, 1963. Discusses objections to and advantages of nursing diagnosis.

Mahomet, A. D.: Nursing diagnosis for the OR nurse, AORN J. **22**(5):709-711, 1975. Discusses the operating room nurse's responsibility with nursing diagnosis.

Mundinger, M. O., and Jauron, G. D.: Developing a nursing diagnosis, Nurs. Outlook **23**(2): 94-98, 1975. Indicates that a nursing diagnosis is a statement of a patient's actual or potential unhealthful response which should identify contributing factors and objectives for the patient and the nurse.

Myers, N.: Nursing diagnosis, Nurs. Times **69** (38):1229-1230, 1973. Suggests drawing conclusions from observations to determine the nursing diagnosis.

Prange, A. J., Jr., and Martin, H. W.: Aids to understanding patients, Am. J. Nurs. **62**(7): 98-100, 1962. Stresses that the nurse selects what is important about available information and gives it meaning.

Reflections on nursing diagnosis, Mo. Nurse **42**:10-11, June, 1973. Presents working definition of nursing diagnosis and clinical situations in which nursing diagnoses were utilized; analyzes current status of nursing diagnosis in order to make recommendations for future.

Rothberg, J. S.: Why nursing diagnosis? Am. J. Nurs. 67(5):1040-1042, 1967. Discusses elements of nursing diagnosis.

Roy, C.: A diagnostic classification system for nursing, Nurs. Outlook 23(2):90-94, 1975. Recommends a standardized typology of nursing diagnoses and discusses categorization.

Roy, C.: The impact of nursing diagnosis, AORN J. 21(6):1023-1030, 1975. Discusses the nursing diagnosis as it relates to practice and education.

Nurses' notes

Ademowore, A. S., and Myers, E.: Use of the problem-oriented medical record by nurses caring for high-risk antepartum patients, JOGN Nurs. 6(1):17-22, 1977. Discusses how the problem-oriented medical record is used for antepartal care for high-risk gravidas. Presents a case history.

Ansley, B.: Patient-oriented recording: a better system for ambulatory settings, Nursing '75 5(8):52-53, 1975. Presents a family history, problem list, progress notes, and a POR checklist.

Atwood, J., Mitchell, P. H., and Yarnall, S. R.: The POR: a system for communication, Nurs. Clin. North Am. 9(2):229-234, 1974. Lists questions about POR, identifies areas of communication difficulties and considerations for implementations, and lists advantages of the POR system.

Badgley, R. F., et al.: How good are the records your agency keeps? Nurs. Outlook 10(2):118-119, 1962. Study of an agency's records revealed incompleteness in recording, inconsistencies in use of the family folder, and ambiguity in definition of terms.

Banks, A. W., McKee, M. E. A., and Moore, D. Y.: Tape recorded nurses' notes, Nurs. Outlook 14(10):42-44, 1966. Using tape recording system on a nursing unit gave nurses more time for direct patient care and improved the quality of nurses' notes.

Bashook, P. G., Sandlow, L. J., and Hammett, W. H.: Education plan key to POMR success, Hospitals 49(8):54-58, 1975. Stresses the importance of orienting staff to the problem-oriented record system. Presents a flow chart for introducing the record system.

Baumann, B. A.: The integrated progress record, Superv. Nurse 8:29-35, Aug., 1977. Discusses the implementation of an integrated progress record and presents the forms.

Berni, R., and Hicholson, C.: The POR as a tool in rehabilitation and patient teaching, Nurs. Clin. North Am. 9(2):265-270, 1974. Describes how POR was used by a rehabilitation team as a tool for patient teaching.

Best, R., et al.: POMR for operating and recovery room, Superv. Nurse 7(8):18-22, 1976. Presents record forms and examples of OR-SOAP notes.

Biron, R., and Goodman, P.: The problem-oriented medical record as a training tool for staff, Hosp. Community Psychiatry 28(12):909-910, 1977. Describes use of orientation to problem-oriented medical records to improve record keeping, clinical thinking, and logical treatment planning.

Bloom, J. T., et al.: Problem-oriented charting, Am. J. Nurs. 71 (11):2144-2148, 1971. Discusses systematic method of organizing nurses' notes around patients' problems by commenting on objective and subjective observations, nurses' impressions, goals, action taken, and evaluations.

Bloom, J., Molbo, D., and Pardee, G.: Implementing the problem oriented process in nursing, Superv. Nurse 5:24-38, Aug., 1974. Discusses implementation of a problem-oriented record system pilot project.

Bonkowsky, M. L.: Adapting the POMR to community child health care, Nurs. Outlook 20(8):515-518, 1972. Describes use of problem-oriented medical records in community health setting.

Burgess, A. W., and Laszlo, A. T.: Courtroom use of hospital records in sexual assault cases, Am. J. Nurs. 77(1):64-68, 1977. Assessment of sexual assault cases is discussed, stressing the importance of the record in the legal process.

Charting: meaningful and accurate nurses' notes, The Regan Report on Nursing Law 15(10):2, 1975. Presents a legal case about the postoperative development of decubitus ulcers. Stresses the importance of notations.

Charting: nurses' notes as evidence, The Regan Report on Nursing Law 16(8):2, 1976. Presents a case that demonstrates the importance of accurate, inclusive information related to physician's orders and medications.

Christie, R. W.: Periodic comprehensive health assessment and a problem-oriented medical record for public school students, J. Sch. Health 46(5):256-262, 1976. Describes a comprehensive health assessment pilot study and presents the history questionnaire and problem-oriented school health record.

Clark, J. H.: Instant recording, Nurs. Outlook

15(12):54-55, 1967. Public health nurse uses portable tape recorder for dictating nurse's notes.

Cohn, S., Fulcher, A., and Gustafson, N.: Reliability study of a nursing flow sheet, J. Nurs. Adm. 5(9):30-33, 1975. Research report reveals a high inter-rater reliability for dyspnea, chest pain, fatigue, and leg or ankle edema, but depression needs more sensitive indicators.

Corbett, P. D.: Simplified records for a unit-dose system, Hospitals 49(10):93-94, 1975. Presents and discusses a chart-sized pressure-sensitive medication administration record.

Countersignatures on charts: legal aspects, The Regan Report on Nursing Law 17(7):2, 1976. Presents a legal case and stresses the importance of each agency developing a consistent policy about countersignatures.

Creighton, H.: Medical records: patient access, Superv. Nurse 7(9):64-65, 1976. Advises nurses to record firsthand factual information. Charts should not be given to patients without appropriate medical supervision. Presents a legal case.

Davis, B. C., et al.: Implementation of problem oriented charting in a large, regional community hospital, J. Nurs. Adm. 4:33-41, Nov.-Dec., 1974. Discusses implementation of problem-oriented charting at the Western Pennsylvania Hospital. Several chart forms are presented.

Do your records really fit your needs? Patient Care 10(12):100-119, 1976. Records a round table discussion about the functions of records, hints for organizing records, who should have access to office records, pros and cons of dictation, and suggestions about recording telephone calls.

Fahrner, B. G., et al.: Record-keeping in a state hospital: a modification of the Weed system, Hosp. Community Psychiatry 28(12):907-908, 1977. Describes the adaptation of the Weed problem-oriented medical record system to an interdisciplinary team approach to long-term psychiatric care.

Fay, H., and Norman, A.: Modifying the problem-oriented record for an inpatient program for children, Hosp. Community Psychiatry 25(1):28-30, 1974. Each section of a problem-oriented record and benefits of its use are discussed. Outline of the data base is presented.

Field, F. W.: Communication between community nurse and physician, Nurs. Outlook 19(11):722-725, 1971. Marginal headings on new progress notes form include subjective, objective, impression, discussion, treatment, and plan.

Foss, B., and Magill, K.: A pilot study of problem-oriented nurses notes, Superv. Nurse 5:47-53, Aug., 1974. Phases of the pilot project are described.

Frost, M.: Ward reports—sense or nonsense? Nurs. Mirror 140(18):67-68, 1975. Stresses the importance of clarity in nursing notes.

Gansheroff, N., Boszormenyi-Nagy, I., and Matrullo, J.: Clinical and legal issues in the family therapy record, Hosp. Community Psychiatry 28(12):911-913, 1977. Offers guidelines for writing family therapy records. Advises omitting potentially damaging or embarrassing material.

Gerken, B., Molitor, A. M., and Reardon, J. D.: Problem-oriented records in psychiatry, Nurs. Clin. North Am. 9(2):289-300, 1974. Implementation of POR in a state mental hospital and components of the system are discussed.

Gilandas, A. J.: Implications of the problem-oriented record for utilization review and continuing education, Hosp. Community Psychiatry 25(1):22-24, 1974. Describes a chart-review checklist and discusses its use.

Goodman, R. D., et al.: A uniform medical record system for ambulatory services, Med. Record News 48(9):6-16, 1977. Describes the parts of a record for ambulatory services.

Greene, G., and Robins, L.: A rehabilitation nursing record, Am. J. Nurs. 61(3):82-85, 1961. New form combines a checklist and nursing notes on the same page.

Healy, E. E., and McGurk, W.: Effectiveness and acceptance of nurses' notes, Nurs. Outlook 14(3):32-34, 1966. Study to determine who reads nurses' notes, how helpful they are, on which patients they should be kept, how detailed they should be, and what behavioral indexes should be included.

Hershey, N.: Medical records and the nurse, Am. J. Nurs. 63(3):96-97, 1963. The nurse is liable for making entries on nursing notes and for making use of entries made by others.

Hershey, N.: Nurses notes—they can play a critical role in court, Am. J. Nurs. 69(11):2403-2405, 1969. Nursing notes can be used as evidence to find nurses negligent and hospitals liable. Major questions in a complex court case include "Was the physician's order proper? Did the nurses carry it out properly? Did the nurses keep proper records?"

Hershey, N.: The influence of charting upon liability determinations, J. Nurs. Adm. 6(3):35-37, 1976. Cites several case reports to emphasize the importance of accurate charting for evidence in malpractice and negligence cases.

Hospital records, Nurs. Mirror 141(20):67-71, 1975. Presents an array of standard record forms available from the Department of Health and Social Security.

Howard, F., and Jessop, P. I.: Problem-oriented charting—a nursing viewpoint, Can. Nurse **69**(8):34-37, 1973. Maintains charting is more meaningful when related to patient's problems.

Hull, E. H.: Nursing records of patients' operations, Am. J. Nurs. **71**(6):1156-1157, 1971. New operating room record and recovery room record are illustrated and discussed.

Jessee, W. F., et al.: PSRO: an educational force for improving quality of care, N. Engl. J. Med. **292**(13):668-671, 1975. Recommends PSRO to improve medical care and encourages peer review.

Johansen, S., and Orthoefer, J. E.: Development of a school health information system, Am. J. Public Health **65**(11):1203-1207, 1975. Describes computerized school nursing records.

Johnstone, E. E., Allen, R. H., and Webb, L. J.: Problem-oriented charting: innovations at a psychiatric institute, Med. Record News **48**(5): 22-35, 1977. Describes the use of problem-oriented charting in a psychiatric setting.

Keliher, P.: The standardized form, Superv. Nurse **6**:40-41, Nov., 1975. A seven-part computer form saves considerable repetitive writing.

Kelly, M. E., and McNutt, H.: Implementation of problem-oriented charting in a public health agency, Nurs. Clin. North Am. **9**(2):281-287, 1974. Implementation of the POR system at Tacoma-Pierce County Health Department at Tacoma, Washington, is discussed.

Kelly, M. E., and Roessler, L. M.: Development of interdisciplinary problem-oriented recording in a public health nursing agency, J. Nurs. Adm. **6**:24-31, Dec., 1976. Several chart forms are presented.

Kerr, A.: Nurse's notes: making them more meaningful, Nursing '72 **2**(9):7-11, 1972. Discusses what information should be included in nurses' notes.

Kerr, A. H.: Nurses' notes: "that's where the goodies are!" Nursing '75 **5**(2):34-41, 1975. Discusses what should be recorded in the nursing notes and how it should be recorded.

Kinney, L., Smith, C., and Barnes, R. H.: The problem-oriented record: a community hospital approach, Nurs. Clin. North Am. **9**(2):247-254, 1974. Evaluates the implementation of the problem-oriented record system at the Doctors Hospital in Seattle, Washington. Presents the initial data base and progress notes, nursing care plan, problem list, and activities of daily living flow sheet.

Kuhn, I. M.: Looking at outpatient medical record systems, Hospitals **51**(20):145-152, 1977. Re-

search report about the use of an automated medical record system in an outpatient setting.

Lee, L. S.: R_x for record problems, Med. Record News **47**(2):70-76, 1977. Describes a record conversion process.

Leonard, P., Cowan, D. B., and Mattingly, P. H.: The POR as a means of collaboration between the pediatric nurse practitioner and other health team members, Nurs. Clin. North Am. **9**(2): 271-279, 1974. Discusses how POR can promote collaboration among health team members in ambulatory pediatric settings.

Luttman, P. A.: OR/RR nursing record improves care, AORN J. **22**(6):909-912, 1975. Presents an OR/RR record and discusses communication theory.

Miller, M. B., and Elliott, D. F.: Errors and omissions in diagnostic records on admission of patients to a nursing home, J. Am. Geriatr. Soc. **24**(3):108-116, 1976. Research report indicates that 64% of primary admitting diagnoses were inaccurate and 84% of secondary diagnoses were either lacking or inaccurate in patients admitted to a nursing home.

Morgan, E. M.: New chart forms solve old problems, Am. J. Nurs. **65**(3):93-96, 1965. Interdisciplinary communications improved when doctors, nurses, and other hospital personnel started recording notes about patient care and progress in chronological sequence on the same chart form.

Niland, M. B., and Bentz, P. M.: A problem-oriented approach to planning nursing care, Nurs. Clin. North Am. **9**(2):235-245, 1974. Discusses how POR system can be used to implement the nursing process.

Opp, M.: The confidentiality dilemma, Nurs. Digest **4**(4):17-19, 1976. Confidentiality problem with computerized records is discussed.

Park, W.: Patient transfer form, Am. J. Nurs. **67**(8):1665-1668, 1967. Illustrates and discusses a form designed to include patient information required under Medicare and to aid continuity of care.

Payne, S., McBarron, R. A., and O'Connor, E. J.: Implementation of a problem-oriented system in CCU, Nurs. Clin. North Am. **9**(2):255-263, 1974. Implementation of the problem-oriented record system at Evergreen General Hospital in Kirkland, Washington, is discussed. Coronary Care Unit forms are presented.

Phillips, D. F.: Some POMR criticism clearly misdirected, Hospitals **49**(8):58-61, 1975. Criticisms of the POMR system are discussed.

Robinson, A. M.: Problem oriented record: uniting the team for total care, RN **38**(6):23-28, 1975.

Describes how the POR system is implemented at the Medical Center Hospital of Vermont and gives guidelines for establishing the system on a traditional unit.

Ross, D.: A medical record system, Occup. Health Nurs. 27(12):516-523, 1975. Chart forms are presented.

Sandlow, L. J., Bashook, P. G., and Hammett, W. H.: Is the problem-oriented medical record really being used? Hospitals 51(21):137-140, 1977. Indicates that use of POMR will increase as students are taught the process.

Scales, E. J., and Johnson, M. S.: A psychiatric POMR for use by a multidisciplinary team, Hosp. Community Psychiatry 26(6):371-373, 1975. Describes the forms that compose the POMR.

Schell, P. L., and Campbell, A. T.: POMR—not just another way to chart, Nurs. Outlook 20(8):510-514, 1972. Describes problem-oriented medical records in general and their use in a hospital setting.

Sehdev, H. S.: Adapting the Weed system to child psychiatric records, Hosp. Community Psychiatry 25(1):31-32, 1974. Reports that problem-oriented records promote a holistic approach to patient care, provide clear treatment guidelines, and facilitate a team approach. Disadvantages are also discussed.

Smith, L. C., Hawley, C. J., and Grant, R. L.: Questions frequently asked about the problem-oriented record in psychiatry, Hosp. Community Psychiatry 25(1):17-22, 1974. Lists questions and answers about the data base, problem list, plans, and progress notes. Presents sample progress notes.

Walker, V. H., McReynolds, D. A., and Patrick, E.: A care plan for ailing nurses' notes, Am. J. Nurs. 65(8):74-76, 1965. A study revealed very little time spent during day writing nursing notes.

Williams, D. H., et al.: Introducing the problem-oriented record on a psychiatric inpatient unit, Hosp. Community Psychiatry 25(1):25-28, 1974. Introduction and use of problem-oriented record for a psychiatric unit are discussed. Staff skills and treatment planning improved.

Woody, M., and Mallison, M.: The problem-oriented system for patient-centered care, Am. J. Nurs. 73(7):1168-1175, 1973. Describes a system of problem-oriented records and their use for auditing.

Woolley, F. R., and Kane, R. L.: Telling it like it is through problem orientation, Nurs. Care 9(6):25-27, 1976. The problem-oriented system is discussed as a means of improving recording.

Yarnall, S. R., and Atwood, J.: Problem-oriented practice for nurses and physicians, Nurs. Clin. North Am. 9(2):215-228, 1974. Components of the problem-oriented record are identified and discussed.

Nursing reports

Copp, L. A.: Improvement of care through evaluation: change of shift report, Bedside Nurse 5(2):19-23, 1972. A study of change-of-shift reports shows 53.5% of the comments indicate nursing needs perceived and 46.5% indicate no nursing needs perceived.

Georgopoulos, B. S., and Sana, J. M.: Clinical nursing specialization and intershift report behavior, Am. J. Nurs. 71(3):538-545, 1971. Study indicated hospital units led by clinical nurse specialists outperformed those led by traditional head nurses in respect to evaluative nurse reporting.

Mezzanotte, E. J.: Getting it together for end-of-shift reports, Nursing '76 6(4):21-22, 1976. Lists information that should be included in reports.

Mitchell, M.: Inter-shift reports—to tape or not to tape, Superv. Nurse 7(10):38-39, 1976. Supports the oral report over the taped report in specialized areas.

Rait, A.: A Kardex system, Nurs. Times 71(42) NATN supplement, iii, 1975. Presents a Kardex for the operating room.

Roberts, G.: Patient reporting, Nurs. Mirror 140(4):68-69, 1975. Presents a unit statement chart and explains the coding system. Can be used for unit reports and for determining nurse-patient ratio.

Wiley, L.: Whadda ya say at report? Nursing '75 5(10):73-78, 1975. Discusses different structures for report and lists guidelines.

Nursing rounds

Copp, L. A.: Improving nursing care through evaluation. II. As you make nursing rounds, Bedside Nurse 5(6):25-28, 1972. Discusses nursing rounds as a means of planning, supervising, assessing, problem-solving, teaching, and evaluating patient care.

Eitel, D. J.: Head-nurse grand rounds provide many benefits, RN 37(3):33, 1974. Grand rounds are used to teach head nurses to function more effectively with physicians.

Janz, N., et al.: How shared nursing rounds pay off, RN 40(3):45-48, 1977. Discusses advantages of nursing rounds and gives a format for the presentations.

Joy, P. M.: Maintaining continuity of care during shift change, J. Nurs. Adm. **5**(9):28-29, 1975. Discusses the use of nursing rounds for assessment and evaluation of nursing care at the change of shift.

Sharp, B. H., and Cross, E.: Rounds and rounds, Nurs. Outlook **19**(6):419-420, 1971. Discusses plans for techniques, benefits, and potential pitfalls of nursing rounds.

Unangst, C.: The clinician's use of nursing rounds, Am. J. Nurs. **71**(8):1566-1567, 1967. Describes rounds and lists their benefits.

CHAPTER 3

PLANNING

The planning phase of the nursing process begins with the nursing diagnosis, which is made by collecting and evaluating data that have implications for nursing actions. After the patient's needs have been identified, they should be ranked in order of priority to establish a preferential order for the delivery of nursing care.

If the patient is in a life-threatening situation, a quick assessment limited to breathing and circulation and necessary emergency measures is implemented. Further assessment is delayed until physiological stability is achieved. If the patient is in acute physical or psychological distress, the nature of the distress should be determined, and the situation controlled before further assessment is attempted. However, most patients with whom the nurse works are not in acute states. Many patients are capable of identifying their own needs, setting their goals, and collaborating in setting priorities.

Maslow's theory of the hierarchy of needs may guide the setting of priorities. He identified five basic human needs as physiological, safety, love, esteem, and self-actualization and maintains that they are arranged in a hierarchy beginning with physiological needs and progressing upward to self-actualization. According to Maslow's theory, the higher-level needs arise after satisfaction of more fundamental ones. Consequently, the nurse may anticipate that as the lower-level needs are met, the patient's priority will shift upward.

A nursing care plan based on assessment and nursing diagnosis should be developed. It would ordinarily include the patient's problems, nursing care goals and objectives, and nursing intervention. Nursing care conferences and multidisciplinary team conferences may be used to develop and revise nursing care plans. The sharing of information increases precision in the identification of problems. The development of the nursing care plan ends the planning phase.

SETTING PRIORITIES

After the patient's needs have been identified, the nurse should rank them in order of priority. Priority setting is the process of establishing a preferential order in the delivery of nursing care. To set priorities a nurse must decide which problems—both present and potential—are usual and which are unusual. By dealing only with the problems with which the patient is having difficulty, the nurse is able to reduce the number of problems with which she must work. With an awareness of potential problems, the nurse can take preventive actions. Having carefully considered actual and potential, usual and unusual problems, she sets priorities for attention. She can decide which problems the patient can handle by himself, with which he will need assistance and what assistance, and the relative urgency of the patient's needs.[1] Identification of patient needs, establishment of goals, and selection of appropriate nursing action is the planning phase of the nursing process.

Hierarchy of needs

Maslow's theory of the hierarchy of needs may guide the nurse in setting priorities. Maslow maintains that physiological needs, safety, love, esteem, and self-actualization are the five goals of basic human needs. These goals are related and arranged in a hierarchy, beginning with physiological needs and progressing upward to self-actualization. The most basic need will monopolize consciousness while the less urgent ones are minimized, forgotten, or denied. As one need becomes satisfied, there is a gradual emergence of the next on the hierarchy that in turn dominates the conscious life and serves as the center of organization for behavior. The gratified needs are not active motivators and are likely to become unconscious. Human beings may be only partially satisfied because occurrences of nonsatisfaction increase with progress up the hierarchy. The higher the need, (1) the less necessary it is for survival, (2) the longer gratification can be delayed, and (3) the easier it is for the need to disappear.

Satisfaction of physical needs is the primary motivation for the extremely deprived. Physical needs include the need for oxygen, food, water, and sex. A person lacking food, safety, love, esteem, and self-actualization will probably want food and water more than anything else. All human capacities are used to satisfy hunger. When hunger is satisfied, a new need emerges, and hunger becomes unimportant in the current dynamics of the individual. It is believed that those individuals in whom a certain need has always been satisfied are best equipped to tolerate deprivation of that need. Those who have been deprived will react differently from those who have not. A young child who feels secure and loved at home will adjust to the hospital situation more readily than a child who has suffered past family rejection. Recognizing the hierarchy of needs, the nurse gives high priority to maintaining the patient's oxygen supply, nutrition, fluid and electrolyte balance, and excretory and motor functions. Highest priority will be given to life-threatening situations such as an obstructed airway, shock, and hemorrhage.

Safety needs include a desire for a safe, orderly, predictable world. Fear of disapproval, need of protection, need of routine, and fear of unfamiliar and strange things underlie the need for reassurance. After life-threatening situations have been overcome, and while administering to the physical needs of the patient, the nurse can address herself to the patient's safety needs. She can orient the patient to his room, the hospital unit, and hospital routines to reduce the patient's fear of the unknown. Use of side rails, assistance to patients who have difficulty ambulating, checking identification bands before administering medication, and the use of sterile techniques are measures that protect the patient.

Love needs emerge as the physical and safety needs are met. There is a need to give and receive love and for a sense of belonging. Involvement of the patient with his family and other patients on the ward may be important during this phase.

Self-esteem is based on a capacity for achievement and for respect from others. Self-esteem may include desires for strength, achievement, adequacy, confidence, independence, freedom, reputation, prestige, recognition, attention, importance, and appreciation. Satisfaction of these desires contributes to feelings of self-confidence, worth, and the capability of being useful and necessary. The nurse can help by indicating that the patient is worthy of attention by calling the patient by name instead of depersonalizing him with a room number or diagnosis, by having the patient participate in the planning of his own care, and by recognizing and acknowledging his progress.

Self-actualization is not well understood and seems to be an exception for most people in our society. Its main impetus is the desire to fully realize one's potential. Since self-actualization has more preconditions than lower needs, it emerges on satisfaction of the other needs. Self-actualization is more prevalent among basically satisfied people. Living at a high need level means greater biological efficiency, greater longevity, and less disease. Higher need gratification produces more desirable results such as happiness, serenity, and richness of life. Pursuit and gratification of higher needs represent a general trend toward health. The higher the need, the greater the degree of love-identification (affection for more people), with resulting desirable civic and social consequences and stronger individualism.[2]

PATIENT'S ROLE IN PLANNING

The patient should be included in the planning of his nursing care. He is the most important single source of information for the assessment phase. How helpful he is for setting priorities and planning care depends on his physical and mental state of health, his understanding of the current situation, and past abilities for problem solving. The nurse must assume responsibility for planning care and setting priorities for the acutely ill patient until his physiological and safety needs have been satisfied. An increase in the patient's need for love and self-esteem indicates he is better able to participate in the planning of his care.

At this point, there is an increasingly apparent need for the nurse to educate the patient about his condition and limitations to supply him with a foundation on which to base decisions. The nurse may teach the patient how to do problem solving by showing him the process. Together they identify and define the problem, recognize and assemble relevant facts, recall known information, identify needs for more information and locate its sources, and finally, organize, analyze, and interpret the information. They also assess patient and family resources, develop mutually acceptable goals, and agree on actions and alternative solutions, taking into consideration modifications in the patient's physical and cultural setting, the patient's personality and values, and his and his family's expectations. The plan is then put into action with the patient's cooperation. Patients are more likely to cooperate in their care if they understand the situation and have helped plan their regimen. They should also help evaluate the results. This helps meet their love and esteem needs and does not allow their problem solving skills to degenerate through lack of use.[3]

NURSING CARE PLANS

The nursing care plan states problems, objectives, actions, and responses. Vague and general statements are relatively useless, so the more specific and concise the statement of the problem, the easier it is to define the objective and to describe the nursing action. Present and potential problems should be listed. Problems with which the patient is coping well, and for which no nursing intervention is necessary, need not be listed on the nursing care plan.

Long- and short-term objectives should be defined and stated concisely. Each objective should contain a performer (the patient), a performance, and standards. It should identify the terminal behavior that will be accepted as evidence that the patient has met the objective. It should define important conditions under which the behavior is expected to occur and specify an acceptable performance level. Objectives should be realistic and attainable, supporting the patient's needs and mutually acceptable goals.[4]

A common error in writing objectives is to make them too general. To remedy this, one goal may be divided into several component objectives. Such words as "know," "understand," and "appreciate" are open to interpretation and should be avoided. Words less subject to interpretation such as "identify," "list," and "compare" should be used instead. The objective should describe patient rather than personnel behavior.[5]

Personnel behavior is the nursing approach that is determined by the objective. The prescribing of nursing approaches makes up the nursing order. One nursing interaction may meet several objectives simultaneously, whereas several nursing actions may be necessary to accomplish one goal. Nursing actions can be evaluated by assessing the patient's response. The objective is met when the patient's behavior is the same as the terminal behavior described in the objective.[6]

Characteristics of nursing care plans. The nursing care plan is developed for a specific patient. It should not be so general that it could be applied to almost anyone with the same medical diagnosis. Individuals react differently to illness, and the care plan should reflect this individuality through nursing orders that take into account individual differences.

The care plan identifies present and potential problems. Long- and short-term objectives are developed to meet mutually acceptable goals. The plan takes into account the psychosocial needs of the patient and the interrelatedness of those needs to the physiological needs. It reflects patient and family participation and coordination with the overall health care.

The care plan indicates the patient's location on the hierarchy of needs continuum. It should be current and flexible. Consequently, the care plan is written in pencil so it can be changed as the patient's needs change. The nursing care plan should be realistic; the objectives should be attainable. Unrealistic goals contribute to morale problems.

Nursing care plans prescribe nursing actions. Those actions are based on scientific principles and should be therapeutically effective. They must be specific. What directions does "force fluids" give a nurse? How much of which kinds of fluids? When? How? What is allowed on the patient's diet? What are his likes and dislikes? When does he prefer which types of fluids?[7]

Research findings about the use of nursing care plans. Studies of nursing care plans indicate that the plan is used primarily as a place for the notation of functional duties relative to the physician's therapeutic plan. The plans do not reflect the patient as a total person. Comprehensive nursing care planning is not evident. Plans usually do not mention medication precautions, fluid intake requirements, dietary adaptations, environmental adaptations, protective measures, rehabilitation, teaching, referrals, or psychological support. Patients' hygienic needs are mentioned, but notations are usually brief and without apparent rationale. In general, low priority is given to nursing care planning within the general scheme of patient care activities.[8]

NURSING CARE CONFERENCES

The primary purpose of the nursing care conference is the development and revision of nursing care plans. It is an opportunity to identify and solve problems. Sharing information increases precision in the identification of problems, especially for patients with particularly challenging problems. It provides an opportunity for the staff to learn specialized nursing care and an orientation to infrequently used equipment or procedures. The textbook picture of the patient's condition can be compared with the actual situation, and standard care routines can be reviewed.

Team conferences may update the nursing care plans for the entire case load. Critical incidents can be analyzed in an effort to prevent them from recurring. Staff educational needs may be identified and worked through. Examples of excellent care may be reviewed to identify the contributing elements. Positive reinforcement should help the staff incorporate the identified factors into routine care procedures. Team conferences can prevent and help resolve interpersonal problems by providing an opportunity to discuss and work through those problems. Consequently team spirit can be promoted.[9]

Care planning conferences should be limited in time and scope. Fifteen to thirty minutes is ordinarily the optimum time limit to discuss one patient's care thoroughly or to have a limited discussion about the care of a few patients.[10] The staff should be informed in advance of the time, place, purpose, and length of the planned conference. It is best to choose a time that least interferes with other activities. Arrangements should be made for coverage of the unit during the conference. It is important that team members attending the conference be relieved of patient care responsibilities if the meeting is to proceed without interruptions. The other team on the unit or the head nurse may cover. If there is only one team on the unit, half may attend the conference first and the other half later, or one person can be assigned to cover the unit while the others attend the conference. By planning their other work around the conference, the staff can attend well prepared and ready to focus on the purpose.

If a nursing care conference is held at the same time every day, it will probably be accepted as part of the daily routine. Interest may be stimulated if the team decides whom they want to discuss. At the end of a conference the team can choose whom they want to discuss the next day. Posting time, place, and name of the patient(s) to be discussed encourages staff preparation.

Acceptance of the premise that the total group has more information about a subject than any one member will increase the staff's appreciation of group productivity. Consensus or majority rule for planning of nursing approaches increases the commitment to those decisions. It is important to assess the team's interest and needs and to identify and define the problems early in the conference, since identification of the problem necessarily precedes planning intervention. The team members' readiness and needs influence their learning rate, and their participation in setting goals helps make learning activities more meaningful and useful to them. Analyzing nursing care given in relationship to goals helps team members validate their behavior and plan and invent ways to improve patient care. When the members of the team do not understand reasons for care, they can be informed to improve their knowledge and understanding. Making the relationship between learning activities and goals more obvious increases motivation for learning. Learning in a real instead of a contrived situation also facilitates learning and retention.[11]

The team leader has special responsibilities for team conferences. She must learn as much as possible about the patient and his condition through observation, interviewing, and reviewing records. A review of the disease and reasons for medications and treatments is helpful as is a written list of points for discussion.

Another responsibility of the team leader is preparation of the meeting area. Are the temperature and ventilation controlled? Are the chairs arranged? If smoking is allowed, are ashtrays available? Sometimes group process is improved by serving refreshments. Have arrangements for those items been completed?

Start the conference on time. Late arrivers are more motivated to be prompt if they feel they have missed something. The leader may begin the conference by introducing the chosen topic. Either she or a team member gives a brief review of the patient's condition. The team leader may stimulate the conversation with key questions. Does the patient have any complaints? What are his preferences?

The team leader should make sure that the discussion is relevant to the chosen topic and should encourage everyone to participate. The person who rarely participates because of fear of speaking in front of a group may be asked to collect specific data before the meeting and present it. Such contributions should be recognized for positive reinforcement.

The team leader may try to get information first from the more reticent team members, and later ask for additional information from active participants. Ask questions that can be answered yes or no to the person who tends to ramble. A verbose person may have to be interrupted, and future indications of wanting to contribute ignored. With an active group the team leader needs to keep the discussion moving from point to point. Increasingly difficult questions may be used to promote a thorough discussion.

When antagonism exists among team members, it is important to discover the cause. If caused by misunderstanding or lack of information, it should be corrected immediately. A private conference may be necessary if one person appears responsible for the group's antagonism.

Although the primary purpose of nursing care conferences is to develop and revise nursing care plans, they also offer the team leader opportunities for teaching, especially material related to the improvement of nursing care. She should record problems and approaches on the nursing care plan as the conference progresses and evaluate and summarize the major points during the last few minutes of the conference. Information from the nursing care plan is then available to all. The leader serves as a role model by showing the staff how to use the plans, referring to them when making out assignments, giving and receiving reports, and administering nursing care.[12]

MULTIDISCIPLINARY TEAM CONFERENCES

It is not uncommon for nurses, physicians, social workers, dietitians, physical therapists, and other health personnel or individuals from related disciplines such as teaching to meet together to exchange information about a patient. The nurse relies upon the nursing care plan to make valuable contributions at the conference and uses new information gained there to revise it. A multidisciplinary telephone conference may be more practical in a community health setting where it is difficult, time consuming, and expensive to bring together professionals from several locations to discuss a patient.[13]

NOTES

1. Little, D. E., and Carnevali, D. L.: Nursing care planning, Philadelphia, 1969, J. B. Lippincott Co., pp. 47-53; Mayers, M. G.: A systematic approach to the nursing care plan, New York, 1972, Appleton-Century-Crofts, pp. 14-15, 28-33.
2. Maslow, A. H.: "Higher" and "lower" needs, J. Psychol. 25:433-436, 1948; Maslow, A. H.: A theory of human motivation, Psychol. Rev. 5:370-396, 1943.
3. Collins, R. D.: Problem solving: a tool for patients, too, Am. J. Nurs. 68(7):1483-1485, 1968; Little and Carnevali, pp. 54-55.

4. Mager, R. F.: Preparing behavioral objectives, Belmont, Calif., 1962, Fearon Publishers, Inc.
5. Smith, D. M.: Writing objectives as a nursing practice skill, Am. J. Nurs. **71**(2):319-320, 1971.
6. Little and Carnevali, pp. 57-64.
7. Lambertsen, E. C.: Nursing care plan should reflect present and future patient needs, Mod. Hosp. **103**:128, Oct., 1964; Wagner, B. M.: Care plans: right, reasonable, and reachable, Am. J. Nurs. **69**(5):986-990, 1969.
8. Ciuca, R. L.: Over the years with the nursing care plan, Nurs. Outlook **20**(11):706-711, 1972; Kelly, N. C.: Nursing care plans, Nurs. Outlook **14**(5):61-64, 1966.
9. Lockerby, F. K.: Communication for nurses, St. Louis, 1968, The C. V. Mosby Co., p. 65; Mayers, pp. 260-262; Swansburg, R. C.: Team nursing: a programmed learning experience, Unit I, Philosophy of team nursing, New York, 1968, G. P. Putnam's Sons, pp. 41, 47.
10. Newcomb, D. P., and Swansburg, R. C.: The team plan, New York, 1971, G. P. Putnam's Sons, p. 131.
11. Douglass, L. M., and Bevis, E. O.: Leadership in action: principles and application to staff situations, St. Louis, 1974, The C. V. Mosby Co., pp. 58-108.
12. Kron, T.: The management of patient care, Philadelphia, 1971, W. B. Saunders Co., pp. 113-124.
13. Mayers, pp. 262-263.

Selected readings

Barbara Butler, Mary Jane Duke, and Toni Stovel present a case study and care plan. In her study of nursing care plans, Nancy Cardinal Kelly found that most of the information on care plans concerns nursing functions as they relate to physicians' orders. She identifies information usually omitted from plans. Ms. Kelly outlines a master plan and lists appropriate observations under each major topic heading.

Dolores Little and Doris Carnevali discuss barriers to written plans, influences of the environment, and tools and techniques to assist care planning. They suggest ways in which nursing care plans can be used and offer guidelines for implementing those plans. Barbara J. Stevens further elaborates on "Why Won't Nurses Write Nursing Care Plans?" She lists reasons for using care plans and ways to overcome the obstacles that interfere with the writing and implementing of plans. Robert L. Hanson maintains that nursing histories and care plans should be retained and shared, rather than thrown away. He reports on one study that indicates over half the entries on care plans from previous hospitalizations were relevant to the current hospitalization. Another study indicates that use of nursing histories and care plans as part of the referral system supplies more information than regular referral forms.

ANOREXIA NERVOSA: A NURSING APPROACH
Barbara Butler, Mary Jane Duke, and Toni Stovel

Anorexia nervosa is defined as the condition of "self-inflicted starvation, without recognizable organic disease and in the midst of ample food."[1] The seriousness of the illness is indicated by a mortality rate of approximately fifteen percent.

Reprinted with permission from The Canadian Nurse **73**(6):22-24, 1977.

It is a complex problem and there is some dispute regarding the etiology of the illness. It occurs most frequently in single females in their adolescent or young adult years. Generally, the patients are of average or above average intelligence; often, they have a history of obesity. Although the literature is not unanimous in documenting this, those diagnosed as suffering from anorexia nervosa are described as having been quiet, obedient children, often from financially or socially successful families.

SYMPTOMS

Anorexia nervosa is characterized by some or all of the following symptoms:
- amenorrhea
- disturbance in body image and body concept of delusional proportions
- perverse eating habits, including:
  1. starvation diets with compulsive overeating;
  2. gorging followed by self-induced vomiting;
  3. hoarding of food;
  4. excessive use of laxatives and enemas.
- difficulty in interpreting body cues, such as:
  1. inability to recognize hunger;
  2. hyperactivity and denial of fatigue;
  3. failure of sexual functioning.
- a low basal metabolic rate
- constipation
- a sense of ineffectiveness, that is, a lack of self-awareness. They see themselves as always responding to others' demands rather than to their own desires.

Along with the generally recognized symptoms, we have noted several common behavioral characteristics in patients having anorexia nervosa. One of these is a child-like quality and another is extreme anxiety related to gaining weight. The patient attempts to deal with this great fear of weight gain and to gain control by any means possible, a behavior described as "manipulation."

Manipulation has been defined as a "process by which one individual influences another to function in accord with his needs without regard for the other's needs or goals."[2] It can be seen that manipulation is an interpersonal phenomenon. Within the nurse-patient relationship, the nurse strives to limit manipulative behavior and at the same time assists the patient to learn more mature methods of relating to others in order to satisfy his needs. The use of cooperation, collaboration and compromise are seen as more effective interpersonal methods for need gratification.

CASE STUDY: MARGIE

Margie, a twenty-one year old, was first diagnosed as having anorexia nervosa in England when she was sixteen years of age. At that time, she discovered that her unmarried sister, two years older, was pregnant. Margie was quite disgusted with the whole matter and was extremely fearful that she, too, might become pregnant. She associated pregnancy with a feeling of fullness in her stomach. It was at this time that she developed irregular menstrual cycles, began dieting, and lost 7.7 kg (17 lbs).

Margie's parents were both successful in their chosen careers. Their marriage, however, had dissolved when Margie was a young girl. Margie had a history of three previous hospital admissions and intermittent psychiatric treatment on an outpatient basis. In addition she had been admitted twice to medical wards for treatment of pneumonia.

More recently, Margie had had one previous admission to our hospital and although she had gained 4.5 kg (10 lbs) her stay was described as unsuccessful. She would sneak food from other patients' trays and hide it in her room under her pillow, between her clothes, and in drawers. This was a constant problem and her room often reeked of stale food. She would harrass the dietary staff for extra food, beg candy from other patients, then gorge herself and induce vomiting several minutes later. Margie was in constant conflict with her need for hunger satisfaction and having to deal with feelings of guilt and fullness. This led to many outbursts and tantrums which proceeded to increase her self-dislike. Eventually it became clear that her stay in hospital was no longer producing worthwhile change, and discharge was recommended.

We readmitted Margie from a medical ward in another hospital where she had been a patient for two-and-one-half weeks for treatment of malnutrition. Her physical status was considered to be precarious; her resistance to infectious diseases was low. In fact during that admission, she had lost another pound so that she now weighed 33.27 kg (73¼ lbs) in spite of her height of 170 cms (5'8"). She appeared gaunt and frail. Her sunken eyes and pallor gave her a ghost-like appearance. She was unsteady on her feet, and unable to speak more than a few words at a time because of her exhaustion. On closer observation, she showed further signs of malnutrition: anemia, poor skin turgor, little muscle tone and lack of subcutaneous fat.

The nursing staff on the psychiatric unit felt well-prepared for Margie's admission. Articles on anorexia nervosa and manipulation were made available. The dietician, occupational therapist, social worker and psychiatric resident were involved to help establish staff agreement on nursing management and thus consistency in her care. We met to formulate the treatment plan that covered all present and anticipated problems. Explicit and detailed pre-planning left little room for patient manipulation. (See Kardex outlining Margie's initial care plan, p. 99.)

Because of Margie's physical instability and previous management difficulties, she was initially put on bedrest in pyjamas; her clothes and possessions were locked up; her visitors and recreational activities were limited. These activities and privileges were slowly increased as her health status improved. It was agreed that the goal of this admission was to attain physical stability and health through the establishment of better eating habits. No attempts were made to explore with Margie the underlying reasons for her behavior through intensive psychotherapy. Those would be achieved later on an outpatient follow-up basis with her psychiatrist.

Weekly contract meetings were established soon after her admission. Each Monday morning, Margie, her primary nurse and the psychiatric resident met to discuss and agree on care plan revisions. Prior to the meeting, the resident and the nurse together reviewed any possible plan changes which were then discussed at the meeting. These meetings succeeded in decreasing staff confusion about Margie's manipulative behavior and also encouraged consistency of care with an open and honest relationship between staff and patient.

We encouraged Margie to become involved in these meetings by allowing her a choice within the boundaries we had set for her. For example, Margie could suggest menu changes or help us decide changes in activity level. We found that when Margie took responsibility

NURSING KARDEX—INITIAL CARE PLAN

Short term goal — Weekly weight gain of 0.91 kg (2 lbs)

Long term goal — Physical stability and health through re-establishing better eating habits.

Problem | **Plan**

Physical instability
— record intake and output
— take vital signs and temperature prior to giving medications
— bedrest, in pyjamas
— meals in room

Anxiety
— Chlorpromazine 50 mg QID and increased to 175 mg QID
— consistent staff visits q 15 minutes
— in pyjamas with clothes locked up

Obsession with food and fear of weight gain
- hoarding
- gorging
- vomiting
- weight loss
- abuse of laxatives

— 0800-0845 breakfast
— 1000-1030 snack
— 1200-1245 lunch
— 1500-1530 snack
— 1700-1745 dinner
— 2100-2130 snack
— consistent staff members to sit with patient during meals and snacks and for one hour following
— not to leave room—use call bell if necessary
— no conversation during meals and snacks with social conversation following
— no psychotherapy
— allow patient to eat at own pace but at end of allotted time remove tray from room and calculate number of calories not eaten (keep caloric values in chart for easy calculation)
— equivalent oral Sustagen supplement given with HS snacks
  a) for total daily calories missed when exceeding 400 calories
  b) for emesis—supplement per volume
— direct conversation away from food
— increase roughage in diet
— Metamucil 30 cc BID
— weigh once a week

Manipulation and resistance to treatment
— weekly contract meetings - Monday a.m.
— involve patient in own care plan
— be firm and consistent in manner
— follow care plan explicitly
— patient to have no direct contact with dietician

Dependency
- on mother
- on material possessions

— mother 1/2 hour visit per day (no other visitors)
— one phone call per day
— personal articles limited—no further articles brought in unless exchanged for those in present possession

Boredom
— provide limited occupational therapy supplies
— provide consistent volunteer member for companionship other than nurses
— increase privileges slowly so that we have something to offer patient at each contract meeting.

for her care plan she was more willing to follow it. This increased her motivation, self-esteem and sense of trust towards staff and, in turn, the staff's anxiety lessened as progress was made. All care plan changes were thoroughly noted in Margie's chart and there were no further changes made until the next meeting.

Margie's conversation centered around food, diets, and her body image. She was constantly worried that she was "fat": "My stomach is huge, I'm fat"; "Do I look fat?" This misconception of body image was of delusional proportions and was dealt with by redirecting conversation to other areas of interest such as sewing, fashions and poetry. As can be seen by the Kardex, there was constant supervision during and following meals. This was done to prevent hoarding of food and to control vomiting.

We felt the amount of time given to Margie was necessary, at first, due to her lack of physical stability and her unpredictable behavior, sometimes being a charming and sweet girl but just as often a screaming and demanding child. Her manipulative tactics were evident in statements such as "I'm hopeless, I'm ugly and horrible, nobody loves me," or "You're nicer than the other nurses." It was often frustrating for the nursing staff to deal with her constant manipulation and demanding behavior. The amount of time spent with Margie created a feeling of isolation for those working closely with her and was a general energy drain for all staff members. We were fortunate to be able to work through frustrations by sharing our feelings with one another and, of course, a sense of humor helped.

As her physical status stabilized, Margie's activity was slowly increased. From bedrest, she was allowed to sit up in her chair for 30 minutes twice a day, then go for supervised walks in the hallway, then spend a half hour in the patients' lounge and so on. At the same time, she was gradually given back some of her possessions—clothes, jewelry, embroidery, sewing. All these privileges were gained back slowly and only granted at the weekly contract meetings.

Margie's obsession with food never really decreased but she did gain confidence in herself and her diet. As this trust built up, staff slowly decreased time spent with her following meals and finally she was able to eat on her own. Margie was allowed more control over her own care plan changes and although there were occasional setbacks in the form of hiding food from her tray, and vomiting once while on a weekend pass, she managed to control this behavior and it soon disappeared.

On discharge, Margie weighed 40.9 kg (90 lbs) the goal she had set for herself on admission. She was still very thin but she had gained physical stability and was well motivated to continue her diet. It was a fulfilling experience for the staff to observe Margie slowly improve, to gain some independence and begin to establish some healthy relationships. It has been two years since this admission and there have been three admissions since, but each time there is a more healthy response. Margie's weight today is 46.8 kg (103 lbs); she has a part-time job in a daycare center and is beginning to develop a close relationship with a young man.

CONCLUSION

Patients with anorexia nervosa pose difficult and challenging problems for members of the health care treatment team. For nurses, the behavior patterns of these patients are often a source of frustration, bewilderment and anxiety. The establishment of nurse-patient contracts as a mechanism for limiting the patient's manipulative behavior and at the same time, involving her in the treatment program are seen as effective nursing interventions.

REFERENCES

1. Bruch, Hilde. Anorexia nervosa and its differential diagnosis. *J. Nerv. Ment. Dis.* 141:555, Nov. 1965.
2. Kumler, Fern R. An interpersonal interpretation of manipulation. *In* Burd, Shirley F. *Psychiatric nursing.* New York, Macmillan, 1963. p. 116.

BIBLIOGRAPHY

Bruch, Hilde. Anorexia nervosa and its differential diagnosis. *J. Nerv. Ment. Dis.* 141:555-556, Nov. 1965.

Schmidt, Mary. Modifying eating behaviour in anorexia nervosa, by . . . and Beverley A. B. Duncan. *Amer. J. Nurs.* 74:9:1646-1648, Sep. 1974.

NURSING CARE PLANS

Nancy Cardinal Kelly

A giant step toward solving many of the communication problems in nursing would be the development of a method for writing a truly comprehensive nursing care plan. Nurses have always planned patient care, but today, when a hospitalized patient is frequently transferred through a series of specialized departments in the course of his treatment and his daily care is divided between both professional and auxiliary nursing personnel, continuity of care is possible only when a patient's needs are first analyzed and then written in detail on a nursing care plan.

A well-written plan provides a central source of information about the patient and a description of his nursing needs. The nurse requires such a description to give auxiliary workers specific instructions and evaluate the quality of nursing care the patient is receiving. A nursing care plan has inestimable usefulness to the nursing staff for patient-centered conferences, change-of-tour reports, and nursing rounds with the doctor. A nursing care plan does not ensure optimal patient care, but it will never be attained without a plan.

NURSING CARE PLANS INADEQUATE

Although the prerequisites for good planning have been developed and defined, nursing care plans are inadequate in most hospitals. The best available plans contain the doctor's orders and a few notations about diet, hygiene, and whatever allergic reaction the patient may have. The worst ones look like scratch pads—a singular mixture of out-of-date instructions, blank expanses, scratched out medication orders, and amateur art. Why has the theory of comprehensive nursing care, a concept which has been taught to students for years, been reduced to doodle-pad entries? Perhaps we have been preaching it, not really teaching it. Whatever the cause, there have been few efforts made to provide effective guidelines for the development of a comprehensive plan of care.

During the nurse's transition from student to beginning practitioner, she receives little explanation of the difference between a student nursing care plan, designed to elicit the principles basic to nursing action, and the nursing care plan, actually a nursing order form, which she is expected to use in nursing practice.

Reprinted from Nursing Outlook 14(5):61-64, 1966. Copyright The American Journal of Nursing Company.

In many institutions, the stationery used for planning nursing care, usually a Kardex or similar record form, includes few headings which suggest the kinds of information necessary for planning care. Some hospitals provide each ward unit with a sample nursing care plan, one designed to fit the requirements of an imaginary patient. But it is difficult to adapt a model describing one patient's plan of care to the needs of every patient.

Nurses are afraid of making mistakes, because they have never gotten out from under the spell of their instructors' repeated precautions on preventing error. Perhaps this is one reason why, when it comes to problem-solving techniques used in planning patient care, the columns on some nursing care plans, reserved for "problem" and "approach," are left singularly innocent of notations. Nurses may be so afraid of making errors of judgment in solving patient problems that they make no judgments at all.

Patient-centered conferences seem to shift between two extremes: time-consuming lessons in pathology and brief statements to the effect that the majority of the patients need "routine care." The expression "routine care" is applicable only to the care of equipment; it can have no other connotation when used to describe the type of nursing care required by a patient. Pathology does influence the patients' needs, but it is more closely related to *why* a patient must be given certain care than to *how* his needs will be met. When the nurse recommends "routine care" for a patient, she assumes that auxiliary personnel are competent to judge the individual needs of this patient. In other words, she is delegating to unqualified persons one of her most important functions.

Since the day of the "confusion of tongues" when our ancestors stopped work on the tower of Babel, innumerable ideas have been advanced for the improvement of communications. This ancient concern is still with us, so it is not surprising that nurses still have difficulties with their communication system.

An unstructured form for nursing care plans does not provide the nurse with any real guidance. Most types of purposeful communication require an outline so that necessary information may be obtained and irrelevant material excluded. Interviewers use an outline; instructors follow lesson plans; physicians record patient histories or physical examinations according to a standard pattern.

The nurse lacks a standard pattern for developing a nursing care plan. A more structured form with headings would outline the components of comprehensive care and suggest areas for nursing action. For example, the headings might read: "Physicians Orders," "Protective Measures," "Physical Care," "Patient Preferences," "Rehabilitation," "Recreation," "Patient and Family Teaching," "Psychological Problems," "Spiritual Care," "Referrals."

Such headings, besides being a good teaching tool, would place certain demands on the nurse, requiring her to give consideration to each of these subdivisions. To save her writing time and increase the efficiency of the form, a checkoff system might well be used for such routine nursing procedures as: Type of bath: bed, tub, shower, other; Assistance needed: out of bed, dressing, to bathroom. A combination of related forms, a combined nursing care plan and nursing notes, or a combination of nursing care plan and an assignment card might save time, reduce error, and avoid duplication of effort.

A STUDY IS DEVELOPED

When I first came to these conclusions, I decided that I needed more information from my coworkers to provide a more stable peg on which to hang any authoritative recommendations for improvement. In the spring of 1964, I made a study of the types of records nurses were currently using to plan nursing care, the information being recorded on the plan, and the respondents' opinions on whether revisions or changes in the information recorded on the plan were needed for better planning.

A preliminary survey of the stationery in ten hospitals was made to find out what types of forms were being used to plan patient care and what printed headings appeared on them. Since the completion of the study a review of plan cards from an additional ten hospitals supports the original findings.

The typical forms, usually Kardex, had these printed headings: the patient's social status, diagnosis, medicines, treatments, diet, bath, and activities permitted. Of the four plans which used checkoff systems, three were restricted to the type of bath and activities permitted; one provided for the type of spiritual care needed, the degree of isolation required, and a few other topics which evidently posed problems for this particular institution. Several forms included the heading "Nursing Objectives" and provided space for the nurse to record them. Some plans had the words "Problem" and "Approach" printed over "Reserved" columns. None of the forms included headings which referred to such fundamental areas of nursing care as rehabilitation plans, dietary preferences, patient teaching, referrals, or psychological factors, nor did they indicate any medication problem areas, with the exception of one card which had the printed heading "Anticoagulant Therapy."

A questionnaire was developed and distributed to nurses practicing in four general hospitals in New York City. Two of them had over 1,000 beds and two had over 200 beds. The participants were a knowledgable group, most of them head nurses, supervisors, or instructors. The questionnaire contained statements concerning nursing functions related to: the physician's therapeutic plan; the physical care of the patient, including the prevention of accidents or disease complications; the facilitation of the patient's adjustment to living, with whatever patient teaching or referrals his rehabilitation might require; psychological support; and spiritual care. Respondents were asked their opinion on the advisability of making changes in the form used for planning. Suggestions and comments were requested also.

A great majority of the respondents wanted sufficient information written on the plan to constitute a truly comprehensive plan of patient care, and most of them reported that current planning was inadequate. But there were some surprising differences in present usage and opinions about change.

ANSWERS TO THE QUESTIONNAIRE

According to the answers, nursing objectives were seldom stated on the nursing care plan, and a slight majority believed they should be omitted. I agree with this opinion, for I question the need for nursing objectives on a plan which is actually a nursing order sheet. By their very nature, these objectives tend to be general statements. If an objective is considered necessary, why not develop it and print it on the plan? For example: Prevent complications, rehabilitate, teach, support, assist with cure, and comfort the hopelessly ill. This seems to take care of all contingencies and would be a constant reminder of the primary elements in good patient care.

The study indicated that there was more information available in nursing care plans about nursing activities related to the physician's therapeutic plan than about nursing functions in other areas. This confirms Smith's opinion that the doctor's orders receive more attention from nurses than purely nursing measures do.[1]

Medication precautions were seldom mentioned on plans, and opinion was divided as to the usefulness of a list of ordered medicines on a patient's care plan. Several nurses explained their reasons for thinking so: (1) medicines are charted on several other forms, and the frequent changes in medication orders necessitate constant revision; (2) frequent recopying can result in errors; (3) when nurses are in doubt about a medication, they consult the doctor's order sheet; and (4) the space needed to list medicines would serve a better purpose if it were used for an analysis of patient problems.

Plans did include the patient's hygienic needs, but little attention was given to fluid intake requirement or any dietary or environmental adaptations necessary for comfort. Few plans listed protective measures, except for some written instructions on the prevention of respiratory complications. Very few respondents admitted to the use of plans made for rehabilitation, patient or family teaching, referrals, or psychological support.

There seemed to be a misunderstanding on the part of some nurses about the psychological implications of certain behavioral reactions to illness. Some of the respondents who wished to exclude written plans for nursing action in response to sleeplessness, crying, and hostility, wanted to include psychological support.

The results of the study seemed to demonstrate that there was a relationship between the headings printed on the forms and the type of information which nurses record. The majority of the nurses who participated in the study approved of the following revisions of the forms: (1) the addition of printed headings with sufficient space for the nurse to record plans for patient preferences, safety precautions, rehabilitative activities, patient teaching, and psychological factors; (2) a printed checkoff system to indicate specific patient needs, such as assistance with feeding, type of bath, and ambulation privileges; and (3) the development of a combined nursing care plan and assignment sheet.

Some nurses disapproved of the addition of any of the printed headings offered for their consideration. One believed that headings "would destroy individuality and make the development of the nursing care plan mechanical rather than creative." This is a valid criticism. Loss of creativity is something to be feared, but I think a standard pattern would merely remind the nurse of the comprehensive nature of the plan and help her to organize her information, and in so doing, give better patient care.

The real threat to creativity will come with the use of electronics equipment (those wonderful computers!) which will take over the clerical workload now such a burden to nurses. A computer can solve routine or middle-management problems, but it is only a communication tool, not a brain, and is dependent on the information programed into it in order to supply the correct answers. It can attack a problem with infinite variations and solve it, but nurses must supply the specifications needed to meet all contingencies. Interestingly, the computer's use in nursing service at the present time is confined to nursing procedures related to the physician's therapeutic plan—the area in which nursing activities are already well organized. According to DeMarco, many other applications of the data processing equipment to nursing functions are being contemplated. For example, "nursing care plans which can be printed out at the beginning of each shift and given to team members so they will know exactly what care a patient requires and can plan the best approach to his care."[2]

Surely nurses, in institutions where computers are used, are busy accumulating data on nursing measures which will meet the patient's needs and which can be programed into the machine. The machine will turn out hackneyed or individualized plans, depending on the nurse's ability to determine the components of a good nursing care plan.

A SAMPLE MASTER PLAN

Whether for computer use or simply for better care in general, the first thing to be done would be the development of a master plan which will represent an analysis of patient care needs. Then, the plan should be tested in a working situation, so that adaptations can be made to meet the requirements of specialized services. The space available on the individual plan card (Kardex) is limited, with room for only general headings. If the master plan provides a further elaboration of nursing measures, it can be used as a supplementary guide to developing individual plans of care. It can also furnish a checklist or nursing audit sheet with which the head nurse, instructor, or supervisor can evaluate the quality of patient care and test it against a nursing care standard "to insure that certain fundamental things are done for each patient."[3]

The types of plans discussed in this article are merely suggestions presented for consideration. They cover the fundamentals of patient care.

Nursing plans related to the physician's orders
    1. administration of medicines
    2. medication precautions
    3. diet requirements and preferences
    4. measurement of fluid intake and output
    5. treatments
    6. determination of vital signs, and weight
    7. physical and psychological preparation for diagnostic tests and surgery
    8. reinforcement of physician's instructions
Nursing plans related to hygienic care
    9. type of bath required: bed, tub, shower, and supervision for partial or complete selfcare
   10. skin lubrication, rather than too frequent bathing for the aged and for patients with long-term illness
   11. frequent partial and complete bath for incontinent patients
   12. type of care needed for mouth, back, feet, skin, nails, and hair
   13. arrangements for shaving men patients
Nursing plans related to environmental adjustments
   14. control of heat, light, ventilation, noise
   15. safeguarding patient's property
   16. consideration of patient's convenience in arrangement of furniture and equipment
Nursing plans related to the assistance needed by the patient
   17. preparation of patients for meals, with special attention to dentures
   18. prompt feeding of patients to keep food warm or cold as indicated
   19. ambulation: dangling, bed to chair, bathroom, walking
   20. dressing patient
   21. means for effective communication with the aphasic patient; with one having speech difficulties
Nursing plans related to safety precautions
   22. assessment of levels of consciousness and degree of mental responsibility
   23. warnings about sensory and bodily defects
   24. provision for call bells or lights
   25. safe bedside unit, equipment in working order, with bedrails in place when necessary

26. constant attendance, and safety belts on stretcher and wheel chair during transportation
27. safe administration of heat, cold, and flammable gases

Nursing plans related to the prevention of complications

28. maintenance of a patent airway, by positioning, intubation, suctioning
29. provision for good body alignment, by positioning, the use of supportive devices, such as pillows, bed board, foot board, appropriate mattress, bed
30. prevention of contractures, decubitus ulcers, circulatory disturbances, hypostatic pneumonia, by arrangements for moving and turning patient
31. prevention of respiratory complications, by deep breathing and coughing exercises
32. avoidance of circulatory constriction due to mechanical appliances
33. warning against massage of extremities
34. prevention of fluid and electrolyte imbalance, by estimating food consumption and measuring fluid intake and output
35. responsibility for observing administration of parenteral fluids to avoid infiltration into tissues
36. prevention and detection of clogging in drainage tubes
37. prevention of cross infections
38. degree of isolation necessary
39. protection from excessive irradiation
40. prompt relief of pain to avoid deleterious physiological reactions to pain

Nursing plans related to problems of elimination

41. provision for regular opportunities for defecation and micturition, privacy, and thorough cleansing of soiled skin
42. responsibility for observing abdominal distention when patient is incontinent of urine or feces, and when he is suffering from urinary frequency, diarrhea, or constipation
43. provision for offering bedpan frequently whenever diuretics are administered
44. appropriate fluids and diet
45. method for reporting each defecation
46. for patients with retention catheters: aseptic techniques; frequent changes of tubing and collection receptacle; prevention of kinks and pulling on catheter and avoidance of raising the tubing or receptacle higher than the bladder; arrangements for changing catheter or irrigating it as frequently as ordered

Nursing plans related to rehabilitation

47. positioning to maintain correct body alignment
48. passive or active exercises as ordered
49. consultation with physical and occupational therapist to plan supplementary exercises and activities nurses should follow to facilitate rehabilitation
50. consultation with speech therapist and use of simple, nonspecialized techniques to assist in rehabilitation of patient with speech difficulties
51. provision for recreation and companionship

Nursing plans related to patient and family teaching

52. teaching program which considers: intellectual status and economic resources of both patient and his family; family's attitude; patient's degree of disability and activity still open to him
53. general health teaching such as hygiene, permitted activities, rest, sleep, diet, elimination
54. special instruction for activities of daily living, exercises, use of prosthetic devices
55. self or family administration of medicines, treatments, and surgical dressing
56. information about my symptoms which require attention

57. allocation of sufficient time to repeat instruction and reinforce learning
58. detailed explanations of physician's instructions
59. provision for written instructions

Nursing plans related to psychological support

60. detection of psychological problems, such as feelings of isolation, boredom, discouragement, depression, hopelessness, apathy, dependency, hyperactivity, tension, anxiety, fear, distrustfulness, demanding behavior, hostility, anger
61. evaluation of physiological reactions which might indicate anxiety: pallor, cold clammy skin, nausea, vomiting, increased pulse and respiration rates
62. assessment of other reactions, such as restlessness, insomnia, lack of appetite, pain
63. listening to patient and noticing which subjects are constantly repeated or avoided; which response from nurse improves his morale
64. nurse's response to psychological problems: has respect for the person; withholds derogatory judgments; gives comfort and encouragement; inspires trust; is compassionate; recognizes the patient's need for independence; withholds advice outside her field of competence
65. arrangements for patient's active participation in plan of therapy
66. fostering a permissive attitude toward visitors
67. guarding all patients, including the supposedly unconscious, from hearing reports of alarming symptoms and discouraging prognosis
68. explanation of even the most innocuous medical terms which might cause apprehension
69. a full explanation of all procedures
70. relief of pain which requires psychological support as well as comforting and medical relief
71. aid for the stoic as well as the patient who frankly admits to having pain

Nursing plans related to spiritual care

72. type of spiritual support needed from clergyman, family, nurse

Nursing plans related to referrals

73. assessment of patient needs
74. consultation with resource personnel
75. reminder to physician of services available to his patient
76. working knowledge of community agencies

Specialists and groups will have to analyze patient needs before planning problems can be solved. One plan has a detachable assignment card, forming a combined plan and assignment. Either a more structured form (Kardex) with printed headings outlining the components of comprehensive nursing care, or a detailed master plan can be used as a teaching tool and as a review of nursing practice; used in combination, they can provide the all-important guidelines which are urgently needed to develop a comprehensive plan of patient care.

REFERENCES

1. Smith, Dorothy M. Myth and method in nursing practice. *Amer.J.Nurs.* 64:68-72, Feb. 1964.
2. DeMarco, J. P. Automating nursing's paper work. *Amer.J.Nurs.* 65:77, Sept. 1965.
3. Slee, V. N. The medical audit. *Hosp.Progr.* 46:106-109, Jan. 1965.

NURSING CARE PLANS: LET'S BE PRACTICAL ABOUT THEM

Dolores Little and Doris Carnevali

The idea of written plans for nursing care is not new. For years we have had plans that run the gamut from stereotyped routine orders for certain groups of patients to the highly individualized academic exercises of nursing students and the in-depth planning of clinical nursing specialists. Nurses in psychiatric and public health settings also have used written plans of care as a *modus operandi* for some time.

Why the sudden impetus to provide written plans of care for greater numbers of patients? Nurses are becoming aware of a broader spectrum of patient problems and have been developing increased skills in perceiving and coping with them. They are also aware of their responsibility for coordinating the efforts of many more people who participate in patient care. Yet, despite this magnification of patient care responsibilities, the nurse's time with patients has become an increasingly elusive commodity. All of these developments support the idea that nursing care must be more systematically planned to provide for individualization of patient care, for economy in the use of time with patients, and for coordination of all of the efforts on the patient's behalf.

Nursing care plans that are written seem to offer a method of achieving these goals. Within the guidelines of a plan of care, definite areas of information-gathering and nursing actions may be assigned; there is less likely to be duplication or omissions in either the assessment of a patient's needs or the nursing actions taken to meet these needs; and the staff members can use their interactions with the patient more profitably.

BARRIERS TO WRITTEN PLANS

As desirable and justifiable as written nursing care plans may seem, one must still cope with the thorny problem of introducing their use on the busy clinical unit. One of the barriers to their initiation may lie within the nurse herself. Unless she feels responsible for making a plan of care for her patients and putting it in written form so that it can be communicated to others who are also charged with patient care, the plan may not materialize. Then too, since there are few work settings where written plans of care are a routine, there are few models to follow, either in the plans of care themselves or in other nurses who are creating and implementing them.

Even the concept of a written plan of care that the nurse developed as a student may form a barrier to utilization of such a method when, as a graduate, she is faced with more extensive responsibilities. Do nurses find it impossible to formulate simple or partial nursing care plans because they conceive of them as being complete recipes for meeting the patient's nursing problems—the physical, emotional, intellectual, social, economic, and so on? Do they equate simple plans of care with "simple" nurses? Or do they feel that a degree is a prerequisite for planning patient care? In the world of reality there must be some point on the continuum between no plans of care and totally planned care—a point where a compromise can be reached that will serve both the patient and the nurse well.

A second barrier may be the difficulty of easing written care plans into our present

Reprinted from Nursing Forum 6(1):61-76, 1967.

pattern of ward assignment and staffing and our hope that a better pattern will soon emerge. It is true that in hospitals consideration is being given to organizational changes directed toward moving the nurse "back to the patient's bedside," where there is more opportunity for her to assess the patient's needs as well as his response to nursing actions—conditions which should facilitate planning nursing care realistically. If these changes have not been achieved to any great extent, does this mean that we must await further developments before attempting written care plans? A more positive approach would be to examine the potential means for planning care even on a limited basis in the present situation and, from this point of departure, to work to make conditions more conducive to expansion of this way of nursing.

INFLUENCE OF THE ENVIRONMENT

There can be no question that conditions in the work environment will have their effect on the character and extensiveness of planned nursing care. There are certain conditions that can facilitate and enhance the nurse's effectiveness in planning care and bring about economy of the time in which it is accomplished. Support from strategic figures in the setting will help to set role expectations that include planned care for patients, whether the nurse functions as a team leader or as a medicine-and-treatment nurse in a functional type of assignment. The nurse's way of life begins to change as expectations of her and her self-expectations shift.

Then, the whole nursing staff can enhance the quality of nursing care plans, while economizing in time expenditure, by the development of a philosophy of nursing care for the agency or institution—one that states goals and boundaries. This statement forms a framework within which each of the smaller units may develop its own more specialized set of objectives that are appropriate to the patients it serves. Thus, when the individual staff nurse plans her care, she is charged, not with the global problem of philosophy and goal formulation, but with adapting and individualizing the more general objectives to the particular needs of her patients. It can readily be seen that the objectives appropriate to the postpartum unit might not be particularly serviceable on the preventive medicine and rehabilitation unit. Those formulated by nurses on a surgical unit would vary from the objectives on a unit where nurses are involved with the care of terminally ill patients. Yet, for each of these units sets of objectives can be created which will fit within the total objectives of the institution.

In the same fashion the nurse adapts the unit objectives to the development of objectives for her individual patients. For example, in a recent study* in which nurse specialists were charged with the responsibility for planning, giving, and directing the care of a group of chronically ill patients, they first determined the over-all objectives for nursing care on the whole unit. One of these objectives was to encourage independence in the patients, who, as a group, have over the years, been characterized in the literature as being passive and dependent. For the nurse who was caring for the Mexican man who spoke no English, the pursuit of this objective meant that when he was placed on self-medication, labels were written in Spanish, the record forms he was to keep were translated from English to Spanish, and a fellow patient who was fluent in Spanish was used to assist in communicating with him. For a patient with cardiac insufficiency, the over-all objective was adapted to

---

*United States Public Health Service Grant No. HU 00094-02, "Nurse Specialist Effect on Tuberculosis."

discovering actions that would support his observed need for independence without compromising his physical condition.

And so it went from patient to patient. The goal for all of them was increased independence, but it was modified according to the needs and potential of each one. The economy of time and effectiveness of nursing care was not limited to the activities of the professional nurses. A ward climate developed in which all nursing personnel became involved in perceiving needs related to this objective, in devising means for achieving the objective, and in assessing patient response.

Support for a more experimental approach to nursing care is also a consideration in the preparation of nursing care plans. If nurses are to make judgments and prescribe nursing care, there has to be acceptance of their right to deviate from traditional routines and even, perhaps, to make a mistake. Nurses now have the responsibility to plan care; they also need, but may not want, the authority to do so.

BASIC COMPONENTS OF WRITTEN NURSING CARE PLANS

Any nursing care given in a purposeful fashion follows a pattern, whether the plans for it are written or quickly thought through at the bedside. The four essential components are:

1. *Observation and assessment of the patient to rule in or rule out present or potential nursing care problems.* In the written care plan the observation is followed by a written statement of the problems that have priority and that are to be dealt with in current nursing approaches.

2. *For each problem perceived there are patient goals or objectives.* In the written care plan these goals are not allowed to remain implicit but are explicitly stated in terms of the patient response which will indicate that they have been achieved.

3. *For each problem, and perhaps each goal, there are nursing actions to be undertaken as a means of accomplishing the goal and relieving the problem.* In the written care plan these actions are stated in such a way that they can be understood by all nursing personnel and, if the nursing care during a tour of duty is shared, can be assigned according to the knowledge and skill of the participating staff members.

4. *For each problem there are patient responses that must be assessed, in order that the nursing care may be evaluated and readjusted as a result of a more discriminating approach.* In the written care plan the cues of patient response that are helpful in making and interpreting one's observations are written and made available, so that personnel may gain skill in making and reporting back on pertinent data.

These four basic components are skills and behaviors which nurses use routinely in their practice of nursing, with or without awareness.

THE MEDICINE-AND-TREATMENT NURSE

A nurse on a ward assignment usually functions, with or without team members, in providing nursing care to a case load of a given number of patients, or she has the functional assignment of administering medicines and treatments to many patients. How can this second nurse, who is primarily concerned with assisting the physician and carrying out his therapeutic plan, put into operation the written nursing care plan idea? Anyone intimately involved with nursing activities of the medicine-and-treatment nurse on one of today's hospital wards feels that she is engaged in perpetual motion. The number of complex treatments she is called upon to know and administer and the rate at which innovations are introduced seem overwhelming. Often the exigencies of the situation cause the nurse to feel that she has accomplished miracles merely by getting the tasks completed on schedule, and the treatment, rather than the recipient of the treatment, tends to become the focus of her concern. One way of refocusing the nurse's attention on the patient may be through the nursing care plan route.

The medicine-and-treatment nurse is dealing primarily with the therapeutic aspect of the patient's care. Therefore, one logical point of departure for her is to deal simultaneously with nursing care problems related to the therapeutic regimen and the adaptation and individualization that may be possible in this area. In the case of medications, she might consider the questions: Is there a special way *this* patient likes to take his medication? Would a special approach ensure his acceptance of medication? If he is going home with a medication, what does he need to know? When should the teaching begin? What feedback of the learning process is needed? In what way does his family need to be involved? When dressings or treatments are required, techniques specially adapted to the individual patient always seem to be needed. Also, patients who are going to be carrying out treatments at home are in need of learning experiences that are provided with some continuity prior to discharge.

Another approach to the development of written care plans which might be adapted by the medicine-and-treatment nurse is the selection of a common care problem for study. Often in morning report or in her rounds of patients she becomes aware of recurring problems. On such occasions she might indicate a specific nursing problem and the patients in whom it is manifested, then in subsequent patient contacts gather more information about the commonalities and differences of the problem as it occurs in these patients. From these data and her knowledge of the basis of the problem she could begin to derive goals and the nursing actions to be prescribed. Some actions she might undertake herself; others she might share with other nursing personnel who also care for the patients. Conferences on findings and patient feedback often will generate alternative nursing actions to be tried or bring to light new problems to be solved. Thus plans of care grow, together with the habit pattern of being on the lookout for nursing problems and their commonalities and variations. Also, from a systematic collection of the responses of patients to particular nursing actions can emerge a more discriminating approach to selecting nursing interventions.

One common nursing problem that the nurses on the evening and night tours of duty may frequently face is the patient's inability to sleep. Too often the p.r.n. sedative is the only nursing action taken, and the only evaluation made is that of the number of times the patient's light is turned on subsequently. Why not try to find out the previous sleep patterns of the patient with sleeping difficulties? What are the factors in the current situation that are keeping him from sleeping? What are the possible nursing actions that suggest themselves from the information that is received? Could they be tried and evaluated? Could knowledge of successes and failures in nursing actions and predicted patient responses be shared with nursing colleagues on one's own ward and on other wards? Why not have inservice conferences that emerge from the patient problems on the wards, with eventually a cross-disciplinary approach if this is appropriate, instead of lectures and films from other disciplines about general topics of interest to nurses?

THE TEAM LEADER

The nurse in a team-leadership position is charged with the responsibility of planning care for a group of patients and of working through her colleagues and other nursing personnel for its implementation. The merit of written goals of care and nursing objectives in this type of assignment seems obvious, yet the magnitude of the activities and the complexities of this demanding role seem to make the necessary impossible. The same pattern of small beginnings suggested for the medicine-and-treatment nurse is applicable here: start with one patient whose problems seem to have priority, or with one common nursing care problem for a group of patients, as a basis for written plans of care.

Another logical point of departure for the team leader is the selection of a newly admitted patient for an initial experience with written plans of care. Actually, the "thinking aspects" of planned nursing care begin prior to the nurse's first contact with the patient. Take, as an example, a teenage boy who is being assigned to a ward for diagnostic studies; the tentative diagnosis is "possible ulcerative colitis." The nurse can immediately begin to plan the nature of her first contact with the patient, the priorities of the information needed, and the possible nursing actions that will be most appropriate to the patient's first needs. Several bits of information form the basis for the nurse to call forth knowledge that can be used to identify potential nursing problems to be ruled in or ruled out. The cues are: adolescent, boy, and possible ulcerative colitis. The nurse recalls that, to an adolescent, mother and father figures may trigger rebellion and that members of this age group are easily bored and restless. The modesty of an adolescent boy may pose particular problems with a predominantly female staff and the symptoms of ulcerative colitis. The diagnosis itself calls to mind certain potential behavioral patterns: withdrawal, meticulousness, the need for routines, and the need for details of information.

When the potential problems have been delineated, the first and subsequent nursing contacts can be used to validate each problem as relevant or irrelevant to this patient's response. The problems or patient characteristics which are verified form the framework within which the nurse will fit the physician's plan of diagnostic tests and treatments and from which she will prescribe the nursing care. Having done this much thinking and preliminary planning, the team leader may offer suggestions to the aide who is to carry out the admission procedure regarding approach and the cues to which the aide should be alert. In this way, planned nursing care is individualized but is woven through, not around, the established ward routines.

For herself, the nurse may set several goals in her initial contact with the patient: establishing a nonmaternal tone for the relationship, offering the patient any details of information he seems to want, and noting any cues to his response to hospitalization or illness. Early observations may suggest more questions than answers. However, with members of the team and nursing personnel on other tours of duty sharing the awareness of the problems and approaches currently being used and evaluated, the promise of observations from many perspectives offers the potential of a continuing flow of information. Some of the problems first predicted may be ruled out, and others that were not foreseen may be discovered. Similarly, nursing actions are tried and are retained or discarded. Each addition or revision, as well as each evaluation of patient response, helps to make the plan more complete, yet of itself may require little additional effort from each person involved.

THE NURSE IN A SPECIALIZED AREA

Written plans of nursing care need not be limited to nurse specialists or staff personnel. One group of nurses who could implement written plans of nursing care immediately are the private duty nurses. These nurses are in an enviable position, because their nursing activities are usually focused on the problems of one or a few patients, and they do not have many of the distractions of indirect care or administrative procedures. The close evaluation of patients that is common practice among these nurses, if recorded in nursing care plans describing patient response to nursing actions, could make a tremendous contribution to nursing's body of knowledge. In addition, this careful documentation of actions and responses would permit evaluation of patient condition from shift to shift and from day to day and thus not only would assure more continuity from one nurse to another but would provide for smoother transition if the patient's care were resumed by the ward staff.

Plans such as these could also serve as models, so that when other patients with similar conditions are admitted there would be more background on both potential problems and potentially effective nursing interventions. Thus, blocks of knowledge about commonality of problems, effective nursing actions, and characteristics of patient response can evolve.

Those who have planned continuing education programs are well aware that private duty nurses are interested in upgrading their practice. The development of nursing care plans and the sharing of them with ward staff would permit an evaluation of the nurse's skill in perceiving nursing problems and selecting appropriate nursing actions. In short, written plans by private duty nurses could prove to be a vital, patient-centered learning experience for both groups.

Other groups of nurses who work intensively with patients could develop and implement nursing care plans for patients which would help them to nurse more effectively and which, if shared with their colleagues, would contribute to the body of nursing knowledge. Nurses in operating rooms, in recovery rooms, and in intensive care units, both medical and surgical, could make major contributions by building files of written nursing care plans.

EXTRA-INSTITUTIONAL USE

Although this article has been concerned primarily with institutional nurses, mention should be made of another group of nurses who see patients over a longer period of time and who therefore have much case material to offer and much to gain by initiating written plans of care. These are the office and clinic nurses. Patterns of response to illness and therapy over the years could be recorded in the same way as the patient's medical record is kept. A transfer of information from office nurse to hospital nurse and back could mean less interrogation of the patient and more individualization of care. The presence of copying machines in many offices and institutions makes sharing of this information much less difficult than it would have been even a few years ago.

Nor should the use of the data on the hospital nurse's written plans be limited to hospital personnel. The increase in the utilization of convalescent centers, nursing homes, and public health agencies, as well as the patient's family, for posthospitalization care emphasizes the need for a written form of communication regarding the nature of the experiences the patient has encountered, physiologically and psychologically, and his response, his current level of recovery and independence, and any continuing problems of treatment or adjustment that will influence his care. A potentially important referral that is frequently not made is the one from the hospital nursing department to the occupational health nurse for the patient with continuing problems who is returning to an occupational setting. Such a referral would provide this nurse with a better basis for making nursing judgments in her subsequent contacts with the patient. In other words, nursing care plans offer not only content and learning opportunities to those who prepare them but background to those who care for the patient subsequently.

TOOLS AND TECHNIQUES

Three kinds of tools can assist, or perhaps even make possible, the development of a system of written plans of care: the nursing history form, a form for plans of care, and dictating equipment and clerical assistance.

An easy-to-use nursing history form is important if the nursing care plan is to be based on assessment of the patient. The items included should be practical and the form simple, so that the information can be readily collected and recorded and used in care plans. The idea that all kinds of information should be collected as a basis for elaborate planning can result in an early demise of an experiment in written care plans.

The specific form for written nursing care plans should also be simple and practical. The equipment in present use range from 5 by 7 Kardex systems to three-ring notebooks. All of the forms seem to include columns for the statement of nursing care problems, objectives of care, and suggested nursing actions. One ramification of the Kardex plan is the duplication of the current cards each day by the ward clerk, so that each nurse has her own copies at the time of morning report. She then has them available for notation and such revision as seems warranted during her tour of duty.

One mechanical device that has been found to facilitate the implementation of written plans of care is the dictating machine or the pocket recorder, with clerical help available for transcription, similar to the assistance available to physicians. Nurses can dictate histories, plans of care, and day-to-day observations of patient responses when they have a few moments and the information is still fresh. These dictated notes have been found to be invaluable in the subsequent evaluation of the patient's responses to nursing actions or to the illness itself; they form the basis for retaining or revising the plan of care. One important factor, of course, is the necessity for keeping the transcriptions current.

The use of dictating equipment conserves the nurse's time, and the dictated notes have been found to present a vivid picture of the patient, his nursing care needs, and, over a period of time, his progress. In settings where this technique for obtaining nursing records has been used, physicians and paramedical personnel have also found recorded data helpful to them. Thus, continuity of the patient's care was extended beyond that provided by the nursing personnel.

GUIDELINES FOR IMPLEMENTING NURSING CARE PLANS

A statement of one set of guidelines for developing a system of written nursing care plans may summarize the ideas presented in this article:

1. There should be developed within an institution realistic over-all objectives of nursing care which take into consideration the average length of stay, the nature of the presenting problems, the potential of the staff to cope with these problems, the availability of staff and paramedical services, and the role of the nurse in this setting.

2. Each ward needs to customize the larger institutional objectives to the specific problems of and objectives for the group of patients on the ward.

3. Nurses have the responsibility and qualifications to initiate and operationalize nursing care plans. This is their unique function. Nursing actions may be delegated—the planning should not.

4. Nursing care plans, whether simple or complex, offer the potential of more individualized, more coordinated care and, in addition, provide valuable means of growth to the staff.

5. The processes of identifying potential problems from previous knowledge and presenting cues, of being aware of the nature of patient response, of selecting from among alternative nursing actions, of seeking clues to patient response to these actions, and of capturing these ideas in the words of a nursing care plan can be learned and can become a habit—a way of life.

One final point should be emphasized. Just as nurses vary in the abilities and personalities they bring to nursing and in the nature of their preparation, so nursing care plans will vary. When a system of written nursing care plans is introduced in an institution or agency, some nurses may feel uncomfortable about their ability to "measure up." Improvement in the task, rather than abandonment of it, should be the motto of these nurses. If only the nurses who are best in their field were to practice nursing, many patients would go begging for nursing care. If only nurses who feel confident about trying their hand at written plans of care participate in this facet of nursing care, the benefits that can accrue to both patients and nurses and to the nursing profession as a whole will be a long time coming.

WHY WON'T NURSES WRITE NURSING CARE PLANS?

Barbara J. Stevens

Most nursing administrators agree that written nursing care plans are necessary for implementing quality nursing care. Yet, in spite of administrative support and encouragement, many nurses fail to write care plans. When written, care plans are often found to be outdated or incomplete, indicating only a token acceptance of the concept of care planning. Why is there such resistance to writing care plans?

So many credible reasons can be given for use of the nursing care plan that the failure to write plans is sometimes puzzling. The following reasons are the most common lines of support for the care plan: (1) Nursing as a profession must be willing to identify its own content, above and beyond the carrying out of medical orders. (2) Consensus of nursing approach requires a written plan of care. (3) Continuity of nursing approach (over three shifts) requires a written plan of care. (4) Formulation of a written plan will help the nurse to clarify and solidify her nursing goals. (5) It is necessary to clearly identify components of nursing care in order to have a check against care omissions. (6) Nonprofessional personnel need to have clearly established and well communicated nursing directives.

These and many additional reasons can be given for the use of written nursing care plans, yet the foot-dragging continues. Some administrators have resorted to compulsory care plan requirements. For example, a director may require that all care plans be written before the charge nurse leaves at the end of her shift. Such a plan, while useful as a training mechanism, does not guarantee the quality of those care plans; nor does it get at the underlying resistance to writing care plans.

Many explanations have been offered for this resistance. The staff nurse usually offers the excuse of time. "If I spent my time on writing care plans, I wouldn't have time to do the

Reprinted from Journal of Nursing Administration 2:6-7, 91-92, Nov.-Dec., 1972.

care!" Another, although weak, explanation is that the written care plan serves no real purpose. "We do all the needed nursing whether or not we bother to write it."

Nurse administrators usually have a different set of explanations for the failure. Some claim that nurses lack the ability to identify the content of independent nursing functions. Others claim that nurses have difficulty in making nursing judgments. Still others state that nurses lack the skills of patient assessment necessary to obtain the input on which the care plan is developed.

All these factors may be relevant in selected instances; however, they overlook some important issues in the care plan failure, conceptual as well as operational issues.

THE CONCEPTUAL PROBLEMS

One conceptual problem has its base in the nursing educational system. The nurse is frequently educated to think that there is a "right" answer for every nursing problem. During the years of her education, she is exposed to instructors who judge her class and clinical assertions as either right or wrong, good or bad. This same nurse is taught that she is a scientist and must plan her clinical care on scientific principles. Thus the nurse comes to expect that if she makes the "correct" decision, she can expect the "correct" outcome.

After graduation she soon discovers that clinical practice is not so simple. She plans a good teaching program for Mrs. A, but Mrs. A still fails to learn. She has a great plan for decreasing the anxiety level of Miss X, but Miss X remains as anxious as ever. Since her previous education has convinced the nurse that the correct decision produces the correct outcome, she soon comes to question her own planning ability. When she loses faith in her own planning ability, the last thing she wants to do is to commit her plans to paper, where everyone can see her possible shortcomings.

Thus the uncertainty of patient outcomes is one primary reason that the nurse dislikes to commit her plans to any recorded system. The nurse tends to judge herself on patient outcomes rather than on the inherent worth of the proposed plan of care itself. This is not to assert that patient outcomes are not important, for indeed they are the whole aim of nursing. Indeed, when patterns in patient outcomes can be identified, the patterns help to delineate nursing care approaches that have high success or low success levels. (This interpretation concerns "probabilities" rather than rights and wrongs.)

Too often the nurse is taught to ignore the distinctive character of practical activity, which is *uncertainty*. Individual situations are unique and never duplicated. No complete assurance of outcome is possible. No matter how prudent, the nursing plan is not the sole determinant of the patient outcome. Overt action cannot avoid risk, and nursing involves more overt action than most other health careers by the mere fact that the nurse interacts with the patient for longer time periods and concerning a broader scope of needs. Certainly it is the aim of nursing planning to decrease variables that will negatively affect patient outcomes, but it is not possible to establish complete control of these variables.

Nursing, for example, involves more numerous acts of uncertain consequence than medicine. If the culture and sensitivity shows that an organism is sensitive to penicillin, the physician has little reason to doubt the outcome of this drug selection. If the nurse plans a strategy to encourage a disturbed new mother to accept her newborn, she has far less security in her selected strategy.

The more one has to deal with the behavioral and social sciences, the less predictable are the outcomes. A behavioral response can never be predicted in the same manner as can the result of a chemistry experiment. Even the nursing functions that rest upon more secure bases, such as the physical and biological sciences, may go wrong in the area of practical activity. The nurse may know where the sciatic nerve "ought" to be, but that does not assure that it will be there for this particular patient. The nurse may put on a dressing with perfect sterile technique, but that does not assure that the patient won't "readjust" the dressing and contaminate it after the nurse leaves.

The solution to this problem obviously requires an altered concept of nursing intervention. The nurse must learn that patient outcomes are ultimately uncertain. She must accept that nursing input, even though it is extremely influential, is in fact only one variable in any individual patient outcome. She needs to accept that a good plan may fail, but that the failure is not the only criteria by which to evaluate the nursing judgments that made the plan. She needs to accept, without a sense of personal failure, the need to readjust a plan that is not working after a reasonable test period. Thus the first conceptual problem can be resolved by a general understanding that the rightness or wrongness of the nursing plan cannot be determined totally by the patient outcome.

A closely related conceptual problem is that represented by the view that there is only one *right* plan. Nurses need to realize that many different plans might be evolved to meet the same nursing needs, and that, indeed, one plan might be just as likely to lead to the desired patient outcome as another plan. The nurse must not be expected to find *the* plan to meet each patient need; she should be expected only to find *a* plan. She must recognize that many different methods can lead to the same patient outcome. She must not feel responsible for finding the one plan that suits all her superiors; she is only responsible for determining a plan which seems to have a high success probability. Obviously, it is not only the staff nurse that must understand the multiplicity of potential methods. Until head nurses and supervisors recognize that differing approaches to problems are possible, it is unlikely that any staff nurse will want to commit her ideas on care to paper.

There is one more conceptual factor that causes nursing reticence about care plans. Care plans represent conclusions, but they usually fail to show the lines of reasoning behind those conclusions. In this case, care plans are just like physician's orders. When the physician orders that a leg be elevated, he does not include a long explanation of how he arrived at that decision. Care plans, too, are seldom constructed to show the reasoning behind the nursing order. This practice also conflicts with the nurse's educational orientation. As a student, she had to detail her reasoning and give supportive principles for each nursing judgment.

Thus the nurse often wishes she has a written form by which to substantiate her written care plan. This desire is more than just habit, however; certain kinds of nursing orders (strategies) may actually work better and be better enforced if the care supplier understands the aim of the strategy. For example, the nurse may have a valid reason for requiring that a patient do a difficult dressing change himself, but if her strategy is not immediately obvious to the rest of the staff, they may hesitate to follow the plan.

Thus, in establishing a system for recording nursing orders, one needs to consider the nurse's need to explain her judgments and strategies. If such option is not available, the nurse may hesitate to write nursing orders that have complex derivations.

THE OPERATIONAL PROBLEMS

If one analyzes the concept of the nursing care plan, it is apparent that the care plan is really a set of nursing orders. It will then be useful to contrast the treatment of nursing orders with the treatment of physician's orders. Many differences are immediately apparent. First, with the physician's orders, one physician has overriding responsibility and authority. Even when physicians work in teams, they have an established "pecking order." No intern sets out to countermand the attending physician's orders just because he would like to see the case managed in a different way.

Many head nurses, however, work on a principle by which any nurse on duty can "contribute" to the nursing care plan by simply writing down her desired order or by deleting orders that do not seem suitable to her. This egalitarian plan leads to a simple management problem: if it is everyone's job to write care plans, it is really no one's job. Unless some particular person is held responsible for each care plan, there is no way to insure that each care plan will be formulated. Thus the first operational problem is the need to center responsibility for each care plan in one individual.

Many head nurses have recognized the need to assign individual responsibility for nursing care plans. Too often, however, that principle is carried out by assigning the care plan as a daily function of the nurse caring for the patient or of the team leader. If either the bedside nurse or the team leader is responsible on a daily basis, this may lead to as many as four or five nurses producing nursing orders for a single patient, on a single shift, in a single week. The crux of this second problem is obvious: Many nursing plans involve a sustained effort over a period of time. Four or five different nursing approaches might all solve a particular patient need equally well. Daily alteration, however, from one approach to another, depending on the preference of the nurse on duty, is not at all as likely to solve the problem as a unified approach. How many times, for example, have two nurses frustrated each other over a decubitus because one nurse is trying to cure it by drying the decubitus with air and light, while the second nurse is trying to cure it from a different basis, by application of selected creams. This is perhaps an oversimplified example, but it makes the point that two approaches to a problem, both of which may be good in themselves, when combined, may be less effective than either one would be if used alone.

Suppose also that two nurses alternate care of Mr. C, and that each nurse identifies the same nursing need, the need for increasing the patient's independence. Nurse A sets about meeting this need by a little calculated neglect, forcing Mr. C to feed himself by her absence. The next day, Miss B takes over, but she has a different plan. She intends to promote independence by first winning Mr. C's confidence. Her plan for establishing rapport is to meet his dependent needs for a few days before beginning the move toward independence. Even though both nurses have the same goal in mind, Miss B's behavior will convince the patient that Miss A is cruel, and it will be more difficult for her to help him in the future. Thus the care plan needs to be under the direction of one nurse over a sustained period of time if nursing strategies are to be consistent. A strategy that changes every day is no strategy at all. Certainly, lines of communication should be developed to permit recommendations from other staff members, and procedures should be established for instituting emergency changes as needed. The head nurse or other selected authority should be responsible for evaluating plans and guiding the assigned nurses in their care plan formulations.

Another basic difference in the handling of nursing orders from the treatment of physician's orders is that many institutions record nursing care plan orders directly on a Kardex, changing that Kardex as the care plan is modified. This procedure leaves no permanent record of the nursing decisions that went into the patient's care. Thus material available for research is severely limited, and it may be difficult for a nurse to get a full picture of the patient's progressive care as a basis for future assessment, unless she has been following the case from its inception. Many nurse leaders are now recognizing the need for formal recording and retaining of nursing orders, either with the physician's orders or on a separate, but similar type of sheet.

While the conceptual and operational problems discussed in this paper may not be the only issues to arise in implementing a stable care plan system, they certainly are major factors to be considered. The following principles may be helpful to the nurse leader in meeting these obstacles:

1. Evaluate each care plan on its inherent worth as well as on patient outcomes.

2. Be supportive of nursing care plans that are thoughtfully and logically developed by the responsible nurses, even if you would personally have selected other strategies. (Adherence to the approved care plan should be required of all staff; the care plan cannot be treated as an optional guide).

3. Provide some means for the nurse to explain and communicate the reasoning behind her nursing care plans to other staff members.

4. Assign responsibility for a care plan to one particular nurse, over a sustained period of time.

5. Derive a system for staff input to the planning nurse.

6. Provide a system for review of care plans and of guidance to the planning nurses by a selected nurse expert.

If the staff nurse senses an attitude of acceptance for her planning, and if there is a clear system for the care planning tasks, then the nurse may be more receptive to the task of writing care plans.

THE NURSING HISTORY AND CARE PLAN: A THROW-AWAY?

Robert L. Hanson

You say that you put the nursing history and care plan in the round file after the patient is discharged? How odd that something on which nursing service and education puts such a high value suddenly has no value and is destroyed. Maybe you throw it away because it is blank, and maybe it is blank because the staff knows it will just be thrown away. Or maybe the information which has been recorded is considered to be just busy work to meet the expectations of nursing administration or the nursing instructor. But maybe, just maybe, you are discarding an extremely well thought out and assembled document which if retained and shared could serve to enhance the quality of the patient's nursing care in the future. Just possibly the nursing history and care plan is the continuity link between hospitalizations or between the hospital and an extended care facility or care by a public health nurse.

I would like to briefly share with you what is happening to nursing histories and care plans at Virginia Mason Hospital and how two studies involving nursing histories and care plans have added to our conviction that these should be retained and shared rather than round-filed.

Reprinted from Washington State Journal of Nursing **44**:21-23, Spring, 1972.

In the spring of 1970 some ambitious team leaders set out, on their own initiative, to revise the existing nursing history and care plan form. Spurred by their enthusiasm, and following a pilot study of the new form on Nursing Study Unit, the proposed nursing history and care plan was implemented for use throughout the institution in June of 1970. The nursing history was developed as an interview guide for obtaining and recording the patient's perceptions and expectations of hospitalization, his basic needs and the nurse's initial observations. In addition to the traditional columns for Date, Needs and Observations, and Approach, the care plan incorporates a column headed "C/P" for indicating whether the need is current or potential, and a column for evaluation. The evaluation column serves to record success or failure of an approach and its continuance or discontinuance and to indicate when a need no longer pertains.

Physically the form was constructed to fit in a standard five by eight inch Kardex tray, with a tab end which would allow for fastening the form into the permanent record. The form was also constructed so that two forms may be connected end-to-end to provide continuous columns in the care plan when more than one page is needed (and this is not an infrequent occurrence).

Basic to the rationale for some of the features described was the conviction that entries on the nursing history and care plan have historical value which may have future relevance to the patient's care. Thus, all entries on the nursing history and care plan are required to be made in ink.

A few months' experience using the new form gave further assurance that the nursing history and care plan has historical value, and a few nursing units began to file the nursing history and care plan upon the patient's discharge, to be used for reference should the patient be readmitted. Following Medical Records Committee approval, the nursing history and care plan became a part of the patient's permanent record on November 1, 1970, making it available to nursing upon readmission of the patient to any unit in the hospital. A little over two months later a procedure was implemented for providing a copy of the nursing history and care plan to agencies receiving our patients on referral.

It was in relation to the two practices, (1) retaining the nursing history and care plan as a permanent record and (2) sending a copy of the nursing history and care plan to referral agencies, that the two studies reported in the following were conducted.

I. A study to determine the relevance and utilization of information from a nursing care plan from a past hospitalization in planning the care during subsequent hospitalizations. The first study was conducted primarily to determine the validity of the conviction that the care plan had historical value and relevance to care in subsequent hospitalizations and would, therefore, be justified for retaining as a permanent record.

The study population included all patients admitted to Virginia Mason Hospital between January 25 and February 24, 1971, who had previously been a patient in the hospital and who had been discharged on or after November 1, 1970. Due to the number of patients who qualified, and the limitations on time for data collection, only 20 or 12.5 percent, of the population were included in the sample. The average patient had been discharged 4.55 weeks prior to readmission.

The method involved recording all entries for each patient in the Needs and Observation column from the care plan from the previous hospitalization on to a data collection sheet. In some cases quotes from the Approach and Evaluation columns were transcribed for clarification. All entries relating to the same need or observation were grouped together and treated as a single item. Each entry was then coded as falling into one of six categories: 1)

Anatomical, 2) Physiological, 3) Activity of Daily Living, 4) Behavioral-Emotional, 5) Sense or 6) Other, based on detailed definitions for each category. A total of 78 entries or groups of entries were classified. The frequency and distribution within these six categories in itself presented some interesting insight into nurses' care planning emphasis and behavior.

Following transcription of entries from the Needs and Observation column for a given patient, five avenues were open to seek information which would confirm or disconfirm relevance of each entry to the current hospitalization: 1) the nursing history for the current hospitalization, 2) the care plan for the current hospitalization, 3) the patient's current chart, 4) nursing personnel caring for the patient and 5) the patient himself.

For the purpose of this study, a patient's need, identified in the nursing care plan from a past hospitalization, was considered relevant to the current hospitalization if it pertained to the same anatomical part, physiological function, activity of daily living, behavioral-emotional characteristics, or sense as an identified need for the current hospitalization. It was recognized that the method introduced a potential for investigator bias in that relevance for each need was being sought. However, it was believed that recognition of this potential minimized the possible bias.

Collection of the data, particularly the portion involving patient interviews, was a fascinating experience in itself, and the resultant analysis of data led to a variety of conclusions. The most significant finding, however, for the purpose of this report was that 60.3 per cent of the entries on the care plans from previous hospitalizations were relevant to the current hospitalization. Acknowledging that the mean term between hospitalizations (4.55 weeks) for the study sample probably gave some favor toward a positive finding, we will repeat the study at a later date, including patients whose term between hospitalizations is longer. However, it is hypothesized from the experience and finding of the initial study that results will be only slightly different for a population with a longer term between hospitalizations. Even if a dramatic difference is found, the initial sample represents about 15 per cent of all admissions to our hospital which seems sufficient to justify retention of the nursing history and care plan.

II. Study to determine the value of the nursing history and care plan to agencies receiving patients on a public health nurse or interagency referral. Beginning on January 18, 1971, each referral sent to an extended care facility or public health nurse agency was accompanied by a copy of the patient's nursing history and care plan. (Postpartum referrals are not included in this discussion.) During the first two and one-half months, a questionnaire, designed to obtain the receiving agencies' responses to the nursing history and care plan, accompanied the referrals.

The questionnaire contained five multiple choice response questions and a sixth item which asked for any additional comments. The first two questions were directed toward determining whether the nursing history and care plan alone, and in conjunction with the completed referral form, provided more than adequate, adequate, or less than adequate information for initiating the care of the patient. The second pair of questions sought a comparison between the information provided on the nursing history and care plan alone, and in conjunction with the referral form, and the information usually received on a referral for the type of patient involved. The fifth question asked for the respondent's preference for receiving: 1) Referral form only, 2) Nursing History and Care Plan only, or 3) Referral and Nursing History and Care Plan together.

Seventy-nine questionnaires were sent with a return of 35, or 44.3 per cent. The returns represented responses from 18 different extended care facilities and 11 public health nurse agencies or districts. Responses from extended care facilities and public health nurse agencies were very similar and are reported here as a combined group.

Eighty per cent of the respondents indicated that the nursing history and care plan alone was "adequate" or "more than adequate" for initiating the care of the patient referred. When the nursing history and care plan was evaluated in conjunction with the referral form, there was an even higher positive response with 89 per cent indicating "adequate" or "more than adequate."

When compared to other referrals received for similar types of patients, the nursing history and care plan alone was indicated in 91 per cent of the responses as containing as much or more information than usually received. One hundred per cent indicated that the nursing history and care plan, in conjunction with the referral, provided as much or more information than is usually received for the type of patient referred.

The results of question five and the comments in response to item six provided us with the strongest reinforcement to continuing the practice of sending a copy of the nursing history and care plan with referrals. Ninety-one per cent of the respondents indicated preference for receiving the referral and nursing history and care plan together. The remaining nine per cent indicated preference for the referral only. Additional written comments were, for the most part, very positive with such statements as, "Definitely helpful to have care plan," and "We are very happy to see some sort of information being started from hospitals for continuity of care. Anything we can assist in keeping this going—please let me know."

CONCLUSIONS

Converting convictions into practice takes action. Beginning with the action of a few team leaders, we have seen over the past year the successful implementation of a new nursing history and care plan. We have achieved its incorporation into the patient's permanent record and demonstrated the relevance of the care plan to the care of a readmitted patient. A copy of the nursing history and care plan is being sent with interagency and public health nurse referrals and we have received strongly positive feedback from the recipients.

The obtaining of a nursing history and the initiating and maintaining of a good plan of care takes time, and a nurse's time is valuable. The closer the practical value of the nursing history and care plan is to the value of the time needed to obtain a nursing history and develop the care plan, the more likely we are to see nursing histories and care plans become a reality.

SUGGESTED READINGS for Chapter 3

BOOKS

Auld, M. E., and Birum, L. H., editors: The challenge of nursing, St. Louis, 1973, The C. V. Mosby Co. Unit III is a collection of articles related to nursing process.

Berni, R., and Readey, H.: Problem-oriented medical record implementation: allied health peer review, St. Louis, 1978, The C. V. Mosby Co. Describes problem-oriented records and discusses implementation and evaluation of the system.

Bower, F. L.: The process of planning nursing care, St. Louis, 1977, The C. V. Mosby Co. Discusses planning individualized nursing care, identifying nursing problems, selecting nursing actions, formulating evaluative criteria, and implementing nursing care plan.

Douglass, L. M., and Bevis, E. O.: Leadership in action: Principles and application to staff nursing situations, St. Louis, 1974, The C. V. Mosby Co. Presents principles of leadership, teaching and learning, group dynamics, delegation of authority, effective conference, and evaluation of personnel.

Duvall, E. M.: Family development, Philadelphia, 1967, J. B. Lippincott Co. Covers the family life cycle and family developmental tasks for expanding and contracting families.

Easton, R. E.: Problem-oriented medical record concepts, Englewood Cliffs, N.J., 1974, Appleton-Century-Crofts. Discusses problem list, data base, components of patient care notes, flow sheets, teaching, and nonproblem data.

Freeman, R. B.: Public health nursing practice, Philadelphia, 1963, W. B. Saunders Co. Discusses the pattern of public health nursing, services to individuals and families, supervisory and management responsibilities, services in clinics, schools, and occupational health programs, and professional responsibilities.

Freeman, R. B.: Community health nursing practice, Philadelphia, 1970, W. B. Saunders Co. Discusses the nature and process of community health nursing, agency structure, community structure, families, poverty, and the roles and functions of the community health nurse in various settings and programs.

Havighurst, R. J.: Developmental tasks and education, New York, 1952, David McKay Co., Inc. Discusses the characteristics of developmental tasks and developmental tasks in the various stages of a life cycle.

Johnson, M. M., Davis, M. L. C., and Bilitch, M. J.: Problem solving in nursing practice, Dubuque, Iowa, 1970, William C. Brown Co., Publishers. Presents an overview of problem solving and discusses patient problems vs. nursing problems, problem assessment, problem statement, and solving the problem.

Kron, T.: The management of patient care, Philadelphia, 1971, W. B. Saunders Co. Covers leadership, management, planning for patient care, conducting team conference, team nursing, use of care plan, and staff relationships.

Little, D. E., and Carnevali, D.: Nursing care planning, Philadelphia, 1969, J. B. Lippincott Co. Discusses current concepts and rationale for planning patient care, relationship of philosophy of patient care to nursing care plans, processes used in care planning, nursing history, nursing care plans, revisions of nursing care plans, nursing care plan forms, activating nursing care plan system, and teaching planning of nursing care.

Lockerby, F. K.: Communication for nurses, St. Louis, 1968, The C. V. Mosby Co. Covers communication, observing, listening, speaking, and writing.

Mager, R. F.: Preparing instructional objectives, Belmont, Calif., 1962, Fearon Publishers, Inc. Provides a programmed instruction for preparing objectives.

Mayers, M. G.: A systematic approach to the nursing care plan, New York, 1972, Appleton-Century-Crofts. Discusses systematic problem solving, the problem as basis for planning care, expected outcome as standard for evaluation, nursing action as strategy for solving problems, the patient's response as a test of good planning, nursing history, communicating patient care information, implementing nursing care planning, and current trends for improved patient care. Care planning in hospitals, institutions, community agencies, and nursing education are considered.

Neelon, F. A., and Ellis, G. J.: A syllabus of problem-oriented patient care, Boston, 1974, Little, Brown & Co. Discusses data base, problem formulation, progress notes, discharge summary, outpatient clinics, and teaching and learning. Gives many examples.

Newcomb, D. P., and Swansburg, R. C.: The team plan, New York, 1953, G. P. Putnam's Sons.

Describes a team plan, procedures for making a team plan work, and creativity through team leadership.

The problem-oriented system—a multidisciplinary approach, New York, 1974, National League for Nursing. Presents a collection of articles about the problem-oriented system.

Saxton, D. F., and Hyland, P. A.: Planning and implementing nursing intervention, St. Louis, 1975, The C. V. Mosby Co. Uses stress-adaptation and patient needs as the theoretical framework for nursing intervention. Presents numerous care plans.

Swansburg, R. C.: Team nursing: a programmed learning experience, Unit I, philosophy of team nursing, New York, 1968, G. P. Putnam's Sons. The first of four programmed learning units, this volume discusses philosophy of team nursing. Unit II covers differentiation of functions as a rationale for assignments. Team leadership is topic of Unit III. Unit IV discusses plan of care as goal of team nursing.

Travelbee, J.: Interpersonal aspects of nursing, Philadelphia, 1966, F. A. Davis Co. Discusses the nature of nursing, nurse-patient relationships, and nursing intervention. Explores the concepts human being, patient, nurse, illness, suffering, and communication.

Vaughan-Worbel, B. C., and Henderson, B.: The problem-oriented system in nursing: a workbook, St. Louis, 1976, The C. V. Mosby Co. Discusses the problem-oriented system and presents exercises for implementing and evaluating it.

Vitale, B. A., Schultz, N. V., and Nugent, M.: A problem solving approach to nursing care plans, St. Louis, 1978, The C. V. Mosby Co. A programmed text that shows how to develop a nursing care plan by using scientific problem solving.

Walter, J. B., Paradee, G. P., and Molbo, D. M.: Dynamics of problem-oriented approaches: patient care and documentation, Philadelphia, 1976, J. B. Lippincott Co. Discusses the problem-oriented system.

Weed, L. L.: Medical records, medical education, and patient care, Chicago, 1971, Year Book Medical Publishers, Inc. Discusses data base, problem plan, initial plan, progress notes, flow sheet, discharge summary, implications of the problem-oriented record, and computerization of the medical record.

Woolley, F. R., et al.: Problem-oriented nursing, New York, 1974, Springer Publishing Co. Discusses problem-oriented records and audits.

Yura, H., and Walsh, M. B., editors: The nursing process, Washington, D.C., 1967, The Catholic University of America Press. Discusses assessing patient needs, planning to meet those needs, implementing, and evaluating plan of care.

Yura, H., and Walsh, M. B.: The nursing process: assessing, planning, implementing, evaluating, New York, 1973, Appleton-Century-Crofts. Discusses components of nursing process.

PERIODICALS
Health team

Barham, V.: A patient oriented nursing system: an interdisciplinary project on the postsurgical service, Nurs. Digest 5(1):74-76, 1977. Describes the project.

Byres, P. J.: The role of the nurse in family-centered nursing care, Nurs. Clin. North Am. 7:27-38, March, 1972. Emphasizes the importance of a personal commitment to life experiences and a philosophy of nursing. Discusses roles of the nurse in family-centered nursing care.

Schlesinger, A. D.: Patients become part of health team, Hospitals 47:137-140, April 1, 1973. Discusses the importance of patient-directed health education programs for the hospitalized patient.

Tanner, L. A.: Family-oriented health care: is the interdisciplinary health team necessary? J. Psychiatr. Nurs. 9:18-22, May-June, 1971. Stresses the importance of prevention, emphasizing social and emotional aspects of health and illness using interdisciplinary teamwork for giving comprehensive family health care.

Nursing care plans

Anderson, B.: Nursing by trial and era—the standard misconception, Superv. Nurse 7(7):35-41, 1976. Discusses the nursing care planning process.

Bain, B., and Bailey, J.: How a communication tool led to the development of a nursing care plan, Nurs. Outlook 15(10):48-51, 1967. Describes a general nursing care plan for thymectomy patients.

Baldwin, S. M.: Made to measure, Nurs. Times 72(12):468-469, 1976. Stresses the importance of setting nursing objectives and planning care.

Boore, J.: The planning of nursing care, Nurs. Mirror 141(15):59-62, 1975. Discusses collection of data, assessment of needs, and planning of care for the patient with cancer. Presents a framework for the nursing history.

Calnan, M. F., and Hanron, J. B.: The team conference, Superv. Nurse **2**(4):83-87, 1971. Discusses team conference as method of problem solving.

Ciuca, R. L.: Over the years with the nursing care plan, Nurs. Outlook **20**(11):706-711, 1972. Describes how nursing care plans have moved through three phases: a means of communications, an assessment and diagnostic tool, and an incorporation of a multidisciplinary approach. Study found the nursing care plans to be incomplete or nonexistent in most of the patient care settings studied. Nursing care plans primarily noted functional duties without explanation or rationale and did not reflect comprehensive patient care planning.

Collins, R. D.: Problem solving: a tool for patients, too, Am. J. Nurs. **68**(7):1483-1485, 1968. Discusses teaching patients how to do problem solving.

Copp, L. A.: Improved patient care through evaluation. III. Your plan of nursing care, Bedside Nurse **5**(9):25-28, 1972. Discusses planning and delegating patient care.

Cornell, S. A., and Baush, F.: Systems approach to nursing care plans, Am. J. Nurs. **71**(7): 1376-1378, 1971. Describes computerized nursing care plans.

Deininger, J.: The nursing process: formulation . . . care plan, J. Pract. Nurs. **25**(11):27, 37, 1975. Discusses the purposes and objectives of the nursing care plan.

Dickie, C.: Care in the community, N.Z. Nurs. J. **65**:22-24, Nov., 1972. Presents the nursing care plan and progress notes for one family the author cared for in the community.

Dunlap, L., and Matteoli, R.: A team function: developing a nursing care plan in a psychiatric setting, J. Psychiatr. Nurs. **8**:19-23, Sept.-Oct., 1970. Staff developed a nursing care plan on a psychiatric patient as means of learning nursing process.

Fanning, V. L., Deloughery, G. L. W., and Gebbie, K.: Patient involvement in planning own care: staff and patient attitudes, J. Psychiatr. Nurs. **10**:5-8, Jan.-Feb., 1972. Study explored the staff and patient attitudes toward patients' involvement in planning their own care. Both staff and patients agreed that the patient should be involved in planning process from admission. Females, patients under 30, and patients with contact with the staff for a year or more desired more staff control. The more educated desired more patient involvement.

Grant, N.: The nursing care plan 2, Nurs. Times **71**(13):25-28, 1975. Indicates that the data collected for nursing care plans can be used to determine staffing needs.

Harris, B. L.: Who needs written care plans anyway? Am. J. Nurs. **69**(8):2136-2138, 1969. Identifies types of patients who need nursing care plans.

Hefferin, E. A., and Hunter, R. E.: Nursing assessment and care plan statements, Nurs. Res. **24**(5):360-366, 1975. Research report of scope, specificity, and interrelatedness of patient problems and nursing intervention statements on ninety nursing care plans in relation to the use of an observation checklist or a nursing history form. Found that care plans reflected less than half of the patient problems identified on nursing histories.

Henderson, V.: On nursing care plans and their history, Nurs. Outlook **21**(6):378-379, 1973. Discusses history of nursing care plans.

Krall, M. L.: Guidelines for writing mental health treatment plans, Am. J. Nurs. **76**(2):236-237, 1976. Minnesota state law mandates that treatment plans be stated in behavioral terms.

Lambertsen, E.: Nursing care plan should reflect present and future patient needs, Mod. Hosp. **103**:128, 1964. Lists seven nursing care standards for good nursing care plans.

Little, D., and Carnevali, D.: The nursing care planning system, Nurs. Outlook **19**(3):164-165, 1971. Stresses the importance of incorporating nursing care planning into job descriptions and evaluation forms.

Malloy, J. L.: Taking exceptions to problem-oriented nursing care, Am. J. Nurs. **76**(4):582-583, 1976. Suggests using behavioral objectives instead of stressing problems.

Mansfield, E.: Use of patient care plans by aides, Nurs. Outlook **15**(4):72-74, 1967. Discusses how aides were taught to use nursing care plans at state psychiatric hospital.

Maslow, A. H.: A theory of human motivation, Psychol. Rev. **5**:370-396, 1943. Presents a hierarchy of needs—physical, safety, love, esteem, and self-actualization.

Maslow, A. H.: "Higher" and "lower" needs, J. Psychol. **25**:433-436, 1968. Discusses the characteristics of higher and lower needs.

McCloskey, J. C.: The problem-oriented record vs. the nursing care plan: a proposal, Nurs. Outlook **23**(8):492-495, Aug., 1975. Proposes using SOAP with care plans.

McKechnie, A. M., and Miller, N. R.: The nursing care plan, N.Z. Nurs. J. **64**:10-12, Dec., 1971. Discusses development of care plans based on Maslow's hierarchy of needs and patient profiles.

Monaco, J. T., and Conway, B. L.: Motivation by whom and toward what? Am. J. Nurs. **69**(8): 1719-1722, 1969. By taking cues from patient's behavior, the nurse can institute approaches that will enable the patient to develop own motivation toward accomplishment of established goals.

Muhs, E. J., and Nebesky, M. T.: A psychiatric nursing care plan, Am. J. Nurs. **64**(4):120-122, 1964. Presents a nursing care plan form and a guide to facilitate its use.

Nursing care plan, N.Z. Nurs. J. **65**:12-13, Feb., 1972. Presents a patient profile and nursing care plan.

Palisin, H. E.: Nursing care plans are a snare and a delusion, Am. J. Nurs. **71**(1):63-66, 1971. Discusses the problems involved with nursing care plans.

Pankratz, D., and Pankratz, L.: The nursing care plan: theory and reality, Superv. Nurse **4**(4): 51-55, 1973. Authors believe the goal of a nursing care plan for each patient is unrealistic and recommend the use of "standard care routines."

Randall, M. T., and Tacke, B.: A comprehensive nursing care plan, Nurs. Outlook **9**(12):767-768, 1961. Describes a three-page nursing care plan.

Ryan, B. J.: Nursing care plans: a systems approach to developing criteria for planning and evaluation, J. Nurs. Adm. **3**:50-57, May-June, 1973. Applies the fundamentals of general systems theory to a nursing care plan system. Diagrams a conceptual model and flow chart and lists criteria for evaluation in table. (See pp. 249-258.)

Smith, D. M.: Writing objectives as a nursing practice skill, Am. J. Nurs. **71**(2):319-320, 1971. Discusses writing objectives in terms of expected patient behaviors.

Sweet, P. R., and Stark, I.: The circle care nursing plan, Am. J. Nurs. **70**(6):1300-1303, 1970. Describes a nursing information record that begins in the prenatal clinic, goes to delivery room, postpartum floor, public health nurse for home visiting, and back to clinic for patient's postpartum check.

Thurston, E.: Orthopedic case study of a patient with a total hip arthroplasty, The ONA J. **4**(2):42-45, 1977. Presents a care plan for a patient with a total hip arthroplasty.

Wagner, B. M.: The nursing care plan, Nurs. Outlook **9**(3):172-174, 1961. Discusses the purposes, patterns, and forms of nursing care plans.

Wagner, B. M.: Care plans: right, reasonable, and reachable, Am. J. Nurs. **69**(5):986-990, 1969. Discusses the four essential components of a care plan and the characteristics of a good nursing care plan.

Wood, M. M.: Guide to better care . . . a nursing plan, Am. J. Nurs. **61**(12):61-62, 1961. Stresses the importance of recording on a special form anything that might help nursing personnel understand the patient's needs.

Woodcock, E., McGehee, T., and Grubb, C.: The blackboard and care plan—nursing treatment tools, J. Psychiatr. Nurs. **10**:15-17, Nov.-Dec., 1972. Utilizes the blackboard as a vehicle whereby group members' therapeutic needs could be made more visible to the patient and group. Nursing care plan form is then used to permanently record each treatment plan.

Nursing care conferences

Randolph, B. M., and Bernau, K.: Dealing with resistance in the nursing care conference, Am. J. Nurs. **77**(12):1955-1958, 1977. Analyzes activities of the opening, working, and closing phases of a nursing care conference. Enumerates specific suggestions for dealing with resistance.

CHAPTER 4

IMPLEMENTATION

Implementation is the actual giving of nursing care. It is nursing therapy or nursing treatments, each of which is the giving of nursing care. It involves carrying out physicians' orders and following hospital policies as well as implementing nursing orders. The nursing orders are the nursing activities identified on the nursing care plan such as "turn patient every two hours" and "give passive exercises four times a day."

Implementation of the nursing care plan contributes to comprehensive care because the plan considers the biopsychosocial aspects of the client. The nursing care plan should be used in referral systems to promote continuity of care; otherwise gaps or duplications in care may develop. The client and his family should participate in care planning, since they are key sources of information, and their involvement in planning will increase the likelihood of their cooperation with implementation. Therapeutic communication is another particularly important aspect of care planning because it helps the client identify his problems, explore possible solutions, and solve the problems. The nurse has a responsibility to teach the client the information and skills he needs to know to implement the care plan.

COMPREHENSIVE NURSING CARE

Comprehensive nursing care is essentially the same as total patient care and utilizes the holistic and individualized approaches. Comprehensive care involves the patient's physical, psychological, emotional, spiritual, social, cultural, economic, and rehabilitative needs, as well as his unique reactions to those needs. Nursing care plans based on observation and communication can provide the comprehensiveness needed to respond to those needs and can best be implemented when a health team pools ideas to identify problems or modify approaches.

Discharge planning should be part of each patient's care. The patient's ability to care for himself, the kind of help he needs, and the best way to provide that help are all factors to be considered. In an ideal situation the nurse will teach the client to care for himself.[1]

Referrals

By using the nursing process the nurse can determine who will need referrals for continuing care after discharge from the hospital. The nurse bases her assessment of the patient's need for referral on several factors. The patient may, for example, need nursing treatments administered or the family may be instructed in how to do the procedures. The patient may require rehabilitation or retraining in activities of daily living. Nutritional counseling may be necessary. If the patient or his family is unable to handle the required care, if there are mental problems, or if other members of the family have failing health, outside help may be beneficial to the family. Arrangements for the use of special equipment in the home can shorten a patient's hospitalization.[2]

To collect data on which to base a nursing diagnosis, the nurse can interview the patient and his family. The other means of data collection previously discussed are also available. Following are important questions to answer: What is the state of the patient's mental and physical health? What are his principal impairments and how do they affect his ability to function independently? What are his problems? How do they affect his activities of daily living, occupation, recreational activities, interpersonal relations, and general adjustment? What is his financial situation? What are the family resources? What is his living environment like? Is there a need for referral? What type of referral?[3]

Sometimes referrals are made rashly without consideration of the consequences to the patient. They are not practical if the patient cannot get to the clinic to which he has been referred because he has no transportation. Occasionally they are made in a routine manner without consideration of the patient as a unique individual. Not all alcoholics, for example, will benefit from Alcoholics Anonymous. At times the patient is excluded from planning for his own future, but he should be able to evaluate referral possibilities and reject suggestions if he so desires.[4]

The primary objective of a referral system is to assist the client in achieving the highest level of wellness possible. A referral may be a written or verbal statement of the client's problems and of other relevant data. It is used to transfer information about a client from one health team to another. Referrals to a public health agency, social agency, rehabilitative center, nursing home, clinic, other hospitals, and other departments within a hospital are common. The referral is a request for continued care, and the information system used assists continuity of care.[5]

Continuity of care

Implementation of a nursing care plan facilitates continuity of care. The nursing care plan aids in the consistent flow of nursing care from one nurse to another, from one shift to another, from one ward to another, from one agency to another, and from one discipline to another. It also contributes to continuity of care by identifying long- and short-term goals, listing patients' preferences and expectations, and proposing approaches for care.[6]

In an effort to reduce cost of care, it is important to move patients from costly facilities to less expensive ones. This may involve moving a patient from one ward to another, for example, from intensive care to a regular care ward and then to a self-care unit. It may be beneficial to transfer patients to a long-term care institution or to their homes.[7] Discharge planning may be done during nursing care conferences, change-of-shift reports, or at special times set aside solely for that purpose.[8] Some hospitals and public health agencies appoint people to be responsible for the continuing care program.

Part of the responsibility for the continuing care program includes the development of referral forms, orientation of staff to the use of the forms, and review of the use of the forms. The hospital nurse responsible for continuing care makes rounds regularly and discusses with staff and physicians the home-care needs of patients. The nurse supervises patient teaching for home care, arranges interdepartmental conferences to coordinate care, and meets with the health department nurse to plan for continuity of care.

The community health nurse provides the hospital with information about the health department's services and orients her staff to the care and referral forms necessary for referred patients. The nurse may arrange for the staff to visit the hospital to learn new procedures and arrange other in-service programs.[9] Plans for continuity of care should be made with the client and his family if they are to be successful. Therapeutic communications between health care providers and the client help assure that the client's needs will be met.

Therapeutic communication

The nurses' use of therapeutic communication—purposeful communication that contributes to the patient's recovery—may encourage the patient's participation in the problem-solving process. Through such purposeful communication, the patient can be helped to identify, explore possible solutions to, and resolve his problems.

Nonverbal communication, a nondirective therapeutic technique, is as important as verbal communication for conveying acceptance. The nurse's posture, facial expressions, and tone of voice should all convey acceptance.

An expression of acceptance is effective when a patient gives a lengthy account without much associated affect: "I understand," "Uh huh," "Yes, go on," "I see," or a nod of the head indicate that the nurse is interested and is following the trend of thought. This technique is especially useful when a patient is discussing a subject that arouses shame or guilt. If he perceives that information is accepted without judgment, the patient is more likely to relax and express himself freely. Acceptance should not be confused with agreement or approval. Because expressions of agreement and approval subtly influence the patient, they are not therapeutic techniques. Praise can have the undesired effect of creating a competitive situation, whereas the purpose of acceptance is to encourage exploration and aid the patient in problem solving.

But what if the patient is not ready or willing to talk? Then the nurse may make herself available, show interest in the patient, and indicate a desire to understand. Although the nurse may have to set limits on the amount of time she can devote to one patient, the patient should not be made to feel he has to give anything in return for the nurse's attention. The situation becomes nontherapeutic when the patient must deny his own feelings and perform for the pleasure of the nurse before he can receive help.

The nurse can allow the patient to introduce a topic with such comments as "What would you like to talk about today?" or "Would you like to tell me what's bothering you?" Such comments indicate to the patient that he is to take the initiative. The nurse should avoid small talk and conversational pleasantries that make the conversation social instead of therapeutic.

Once the patient begins to talk, the nurse can encourage him to continue with responses like "Really?" or "What then?" The nurse's nonverbal behavior also indicates that she remains interested and is following the discussion. With this approach the direction of the conversation is the patient's responsibility and the nurse does not distract him from his trend of thought.

Reflection is a technique that directs questions, thoughts, and feelings back to the patient. When the patient asks the nurse what he should do, the nurse asks him what he thinks he, the patient, should do. This approach indicates that the patient has a worthy point of view and the ability to make decisions. As the patient comes to understand that others view him as competent, he may begin to view himself as capable. The nurse is helping the patient learn to accept himself.

Restatement of an important thought expressed by the patient, using words similar to the patient's, helps him know he has successfully communicated. If the nurse misinterprets the idea, the patient has another opportunity to express himself. The nurse can verbalize the implied meaning of what the patient has said to further clarify the conversation and help the patient see relationships and meanings. The nurse should restate only what is fairly obvious to avoid imposing personal interpretations.

At times it is necessary for the nurse to verbalize feelings that are indirectly expressed. The patient may make a comment like, "I'm dead," which literally is not true. The nurse must attempt to identify the feelings that caused the patient to express himself in such a manner. Does the patient feel that life is no longer worth living? Does he feel lifeless? It is the patient's indirectly expressed feelings rather than his literal statement that should be pursued.

The nurse also may verbalize what she perceives: "I see that you are biting your nails, wringing your hands, clenching your fist. . . ." By verbalizing her observations, the nurse can make the patient aware of his own behavior, increase perception of that behavior, and thus facilitate the discussion of the behavior and its underlying dynamics. The patient should be encouraged to express his perceptions, for if he can discuss his feelings, he may have less need to act out behavior.

Sometimes the nurse may encourage the patient to focus on a particular idea or explore more fully certain points or subjects. This technique is especially useful when the patient is discussing several topics superficially.

The nurse can seek clarification when she does not understand what was said: "I don't believe I understand what you mean"; "If I understand, you mean. . . ." This also helps the patient clarify to himself what he really meant to say. The nurse may clarify the meaning of a word by asking, "What does that word mean to you?" Understanding the sequential relationships of events in time and place may help to clarify cause and effect and offer new perspectives: "Did that happen before or after . . . ?" Encouraging comparisons aids in the identification of recurring themes: "Have you ever experienced anything like that before? Was it anything like . . . ?" Keep comparisons within the context of the patient's experiences. Introducing the nurse's experiences for comparison changes the focus of the conversation from the patient to the nurse, and the conversation loses its therapeutic value.

Occasionally the nurse does need to give information to the patient. The patient has a right to know the nurse's name, whether she is a registered nurse, the amount of time the nurse can spend with him, and the purposes for recording parts of their conversation. Questions indicate the patient's need for information; the nurse's answers give him knowledge on which to base decisions. Receiving factual information in response to questions can strengthen the patient's faith in the nurse and improve the patient-nurse relationship.

When the patient distorts reality, the nurse can make factual statements to help him regain his perspective: "This is a hospital"; "I am a nurse"; "I don't see anyone else in this room, but there is a floor lamp in that corner." To avoid an argumentative or belittling approach the nurse can calmly present her own perceptions for consideration. Doubt about the patient's perceptions may be expressed: "I find that hard to believe! Isn't that strange?" Statements such as these allow the patient to know that others do not share his perceptions and give him opportunities to reevaluate the situation.

Silence is often uncomfortable for both the nurse and the patient. Why is the patient silent? Is he having difficulty starting? Is he embarrassed? Is he wondering if he has already said too much or if he should continue talking? The nurse's expectant silence encourages the patient to talk. It gives him an opportunity to think, collect and organize his thoughts, consider his feelings, weigh alternatives, and decide what topic of importance should be discussed next. Thoughtful silence should not be interrupted.[10]

Nontherapeutic technique

Nontherapeutic techniques interfere with the patient's problem solving process. When a nurse feels uncomfortable with silence or a certain subject, or wants information about another topic, she all too frequently changes the subject. If the nurse takes the initiative from the patient by directing the conversation away from what the patient considers to be more important, the patient may become frustrated.

Refusing to discuss a subject is nontherapeutic. The patient may feel slighted and may avoid seeking further help for fear of rejection. The nurse needs to identify topics and behaviors with which she is uncomfortable and resolve the underlying problems so that her approach can remain therapeutic.

It is wise to avoid evaluative responses. Judging the patient's feelings implies that the nurse knows how the patient should feel and what he should do. Giving approval tends to limit the patient's flexibility to think, talk, and act. It reinforces the behavior that pleases the nurse. Agreement with the patient indicates that his opinion is similar to that of the nurse. It limits his flexibility to change his mind later. The nurse's responsibility is to help the patient collect the data from which to formulate an opinion and make a decision.

Disapproval indicates that the nurse has passed judgment on the patient and that he is expected to please the nurse. Consequently, the patient is less free to express his feelings or ask questions and is less able to understand and participate in his treatment. If his conduct is causing harm to others, it should be noted by the nurse in a statement about the effect of his behavior rather than by an evaluative comment. "You are disturbing Mr. Jones, so we will have to remove you from this room," rather than "We are going to have to do this because you are naughty."

Disagreeing with the patient may inhibit his behavior or make him defensive. If the patient feels he is in opposition to the nurse, he may feel compelled to defend himself. As he defends himself, his position becomes more intransigent. This is especially nontherapeutic in situations in which the patient has delusions.

Reassuring the patient implies that there is little cause for anxiety. "You're going to be just fine. Everything is all right. Don't worry about a thing." False reassurances are meaningless to the patient and indicate the nurse's misunderstanding and lack of empathy. They comfort only the nurse. The nurse also may use denial to avoid an uncomfortable discussion. When the nurse denies that a problem exists, the patient will have difficulty identifying, exploring, and resolving his problems.

Telling the patient what to do also interferes with the patient's exploration of his problems. It fosters a parent-child relationship and dependency. Advising the patient indicates how the nurse believes he should feel, think, and act.

Interpreting the patient's experience denies him the chance to achieve his own insights. He may need to resist or deny any explanation of the unconscious motives behind his behavior. The nurse also runs the risk of making an incorrect interpretation. The nurse's goal is to help the patient develop self-interpretation skills and insight. The staff member should avoid seeking explanations from the patient, who should be asked to describe but not to explain. Without adequate insight, he may feel the need to fabricate answers, and a psychotic patient may even need to expand his delusional system. "Why?" is an intimidating question.

It is unwise to challenge the patient to provide proof of his perception or test his degree of insight. Pointing out the lack of proof will not ensure that the patient will have an insight regarding his delusions. They serve a purpose and are not easily given up until the needs they meet are fulfilled in other ways. When challenged, the patient tends to become defensive, expand his misconception, and seek support for his ideas.

Probing should also be avoided. Persistent direct questioning is less likely to reveal important information than a more open-ended interviewing technique. By directing the conversation, the nurse may neglect what is of most concern to the patient and may ask irrelevant questions. The nurse must be especially careful about asking social questions when silence has become uncomfortable. Inquiries into the patient's personal life may start a conversation the nurse is not expecting or prepared to handle; for example, by asking if the patient is married, the nurse may learn about a recent divorce or death of a mate.

The nurse should not make socially stereotyped comments, give literal responses to figurative comments, or belittle expressed feelings. Social conversations are usually loaded with clichés and patterned replies, both of which are nontherapeutic because they lack meaning and do not contribute to insight. Figurative comments do contain meaning, but literal responses to such comments do not help the patient achieve insights. If the patient has difficulty expressing himself, he may use figurative comments. The nurse can encourage him to express his feelings and avoid doing anything that might humiliate him.[11]

Barriers to communication

Research into patient-perceived barriers to communication indicates that patients perceive that nurses are too busy and overworked; they consequently do not feel free to bother them for services or information. They feel an obligation not to divert the nurse's attention from more critical patients and are reluctant to ask questions or complain because they fear negative reactions. Finally the patient feels it is futile to try to get anything done. They choose not to ask nurses questions because they rarely receive satisfactory answers, and they do not believe that the nurse has the authority to give information.[12]

HEALTH TEACHING

Teaching is a type of communication that helps the student learn. Learning produces changes in an individual's responses to his environment, and these responses reflect the cumulative effect of his past.

Counseling and guidance are related to teaching. There is a continuum from teaching to counseling, and the nurse's actions are determined by who has the most knowledge about the situation and the degree of self-direction possible by the client and his family. If the client lacks information about the situation and is not very self-directed, teaching is more appropriate. As the client becomes more knowledgeable and more self-directive, counseling, which is the sharing of ideas, is more useful. The nurse's approach may need to fluctuate between teaching and counseling as the situations and topics change.[13]

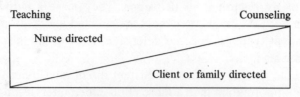

Teaching-counseling continuum

Settings for health education

Hospital. From Maslow's hierarchy of needs, one can assume that little learning can be accomplished during acute illness. During that time, all the patient's resources are focused on physical survival. As he begins to recover, he has considerable need for rest and sleep. The convalescent patient may be highly motivated to learn because he is anxious to go home and resume normal activities, but the patient facing the prospect of prolonged or permanent physical disability must resolve his conflicts about accepting his condition before he can concentrate on learning.

The family, as well as the patient, may not be too receptive to teaching during the acute illness phase. The nurse may have an opportunity during this period to establish a relationship with the family, although she should be aware that opportunities for contacts with the patient's family during hospitalization may be difficult. Teaching the patient's family about his condition and care should begin as soon as possible. If it is difficult to arrange to work with the family in the hospital, a referral may be sent to a public health nursing agency so that the family may be seen in their home.

The American Hospital Association is increasingly stressing the promotion, organization, implementation, and evaluation of health education by health institutions. Some hospitals have used the hospital facilities to house a community resource day or a "Hall of Health" for displays. Hospitals can offer health classes to community members, and some are providing preventive programs for their employees.[14]

Home. A major difference between teaching the client in an institution, such as the hospital, and teaching him in his home is that the nurse is a visitor in the client's home. In the hospital the patient is expected to conform to the hospital routines, but in the home the nurse is expected to adjust to the home situation. A home visit allows the nurse to make a more accurate assessment of family relationships, competencies, and facilities. Taught under these conditions, the client does not have to transfer knowledge from general instruction to his specific situation. The nurse can observe the care given by the family and look for additional educational and service needs. The family may be more willing to raise questions in a private situation and may gain confidence by the personal contact. However, teaching in the home does not allow the client to share experiences with others who have similar problems, and distractions, such as a crying baby or the need to put the wash into the dryer, may reduce teaching effectiveness. It is also an expensive method.[15]

Clinics and physicians' offices. The nurse's contact with clients in a clinic or physician's office is more intermittent than in a hospital. This intermittent contact makes it especially important for the nurse to do inclusive recordings about the clients so the records can be reviewed to determine what has already been taught. Preparation for teaching is facilitated by clinic appointment schedules and by having the client's charts ready for the appointment.

Group teaching may be used with clients who have similar problems. Because the nurse is likely to be busy while the physician is seeing patients, it may be necessary to schedule group teaching before or after clinic or office hours. If such scheduling increases the length of time the client has to spend at the clinic or office, it may be an inconvenience. On the other hand, teaching health care may improve the utilization of waiting time if more than one nurse is available.[16]

Schools and industry. Health records, required regular physical examinations, illness or injury reports, and attendance records help the nurse assess the health problems and learning needs of individuals and of various groups. Conferences with teachers or supervisors may be informative.

The nurse can teach health care as pupils or employees visit the health office or schedule classes or discussion groups for people with similar problems. Both schools and industry provide excellent opportunities to teach preventive health measures. Bulletin boards, handouts on various health topics, and health classes may be used to teach prevention.

The school nurse can take an active part in the development of a sequential curriculum for the health instruction program. The nurse is also a key person in the planning of in-service education for teachers and can serve as their consultant on content, materials, and activities for health education. Both the school nurse and the industrial nurse can help develop health resources within the institutions and serve as consultants to the community to encourage the development of resources. The nurse may develop adult health education classes and promote legislation and research relevant to school and industrial health. By making home visits, the nurse is able to assess the home situation, teach health care to encourage the implementation of health practices in the home, and encourage the use of community resources. The effectiveness of the health program in schools and industry largely depends on the interest and initiative of the nurse.[17]

Community. The nurse may wish to present health education to the general community in addition to groups with similar interests, such as expectant parents, mothers interested in breast-feeding, parents of retarded children, or cardiac patients. Group teaching provides an opportunity for people to share experiences and help each other. Practical, tested solutions can be discussed and problem solving practiced. Grievances, bitterness, and feelings of injustice may be expressed as people are learning to cope with a problem such as a chronic, debilitating condition. The disadvantages to teaching groups are that individual problems may get lost because a person is too shy or embarrassed to express them or because of the group's lack of interest in a specific problem. The discussion may be too generalized to be helpful, especially if there is considerable variation in the problems. For instance, a discussion about growth and development with parents of children ranging from 1 month to 20 years needs to be more generalized than a discussion about stimulation of preschool children, toilet training, how to handle temper tantrums, or how to cope with adolescence. Unfortunately, the people who need the service most are the least likely to take advantage of it. It is the highly motivated who respond to this relatively inexpensive method of health education.[18]

Some communities have provided health carnivals to do screening, offer demonstrations, and make health education available. Storefront health education centers provide health information, screening, and referrals on a regular basis. Health tape libraries are also used as a means of offering health education to the public over the telephone.[19]

Principles of learning

Principles are fundamental truths or laws based on man's past experience that help to explain known facts and guide actions.

Principle 1: conditioning is a process of learning. In classical conditioning one stimulus comes to substitute for another in evoking a response. A puff of air on the eye will automatically elicit an eyeblink response. If the air is accompanied several times by a tone, the tone alone will then elicit the eyeblink. If the sight of a bottle is followed by feeding, an infant will eventually respond with the sucking response at the sight of the bottle. However, if the sight of the bottle is not followed by feeding, the conditioned response will become extinct and the baby will no longer respond to the sight of a bottle with sucking. In classical conditioning the subject has no control over when the event will occur.

In operant conditioning the subject has more control over events. A specific response of the subject is necessary to obtain a reward. The antecedent (what happens before the behavior), the behavior, and the consequence (what happens as a result of the behavior) is the sequence of events that occur in behavior. The respondent behaviors of classical conditioning are usually automatically controlled by their antecedents. Because operant behaviors have an effect on their environment, they tend to be controlled by their consequences. Any consequence that strengthens (causes to occur more frequently) the behavior is called a reinforcer. A negative reinforcer causes the behavior to occur less frequently. Extinction, a process that eliminates or reduces the frequency of the behavior, is caused by withholding reinforcers. However, intermittent reinforcement increases resistance to extinction. Punishment causes the behavior to occur less frequently but increases avoidance behaviors. It does not teach new behaviors. Most operant behavior eventually comes under the effect of the antecedent stimuli. The teacher can use this knowledge of conditioning to reinforce learning experiences that are helpful to the client and help extinguish those that are detrimental.[20]

Principle 2: trial and error is a process of learning. Through this process, which consists of a series of random behavior, the learner is able to solve a problem. Solving the problem once does not guarantee having the ability to solve it a second time because the learner is usually unaware of the relationship between the problem and the solution. Success reinforces the response, and the random behavior is repeated. The teacher can help the learner save considerable time and energy by directing him toward a correct response. Giving the client facts he needs to know can help. Demonstration and return demonstration can be used. The nurse should expect the client to make some errors; ways to correct them can be calmly suggested. The nurse's approval and encouragement will help reinforce behaviors.

Principle 3: imitation is a process of learning. The imitative behavior may be conscious or unconscious. Many times we unconsciously imitate vocabulary, behaviors, or attitudes of people with whom we associate. At other times, such as during a return demonstration, we consciously attempt to imitate. The nurse needs always to demonstrate good health practices because the learner may imitate aspects of the nurse's behavior that were not planned as part of the learning experience.

Principle 4: perception affects learning. Perception is a conscious awareness of the environment that involves the reception of a stimulus by the sense organs, transfer of this impulse by the afferent nervous system to a sensory area in the brain, and the brain's interpretation of the impulse. Perception is affected by maturation and one's past: a teenager may seem very old to a young child but very young to an aging person. A person who has just moved away from the equator may desire a coat although his acquaintances are running on the beach in their swimming suits.

Errors in perception are common but have increased frequency for people with sensory problems. Therefore the nurse will need to be aware of perceptual difficulties for patients with impaired vision and hearing or nerve or brain pathology and to modify her teaching accordingly.

We tend to see and hear what we want to (selective perception), and our emotions affect our perceptions. The client is likely to feel anxious during his first hospital admission or first visit to a clinic. He may be upset about his diagnosis or prognosis and may need time to control his emotions before the nurse starts teaching. Offering explanations and allowing for questions may be helpful, but because of the impaired perceptions, the nurse should expect to repeat information.[21]

Principle 5: knowledge of concepts increases understanding. A fact is a particular piece of information about the world that may or may not involve the use of concepts. A concept is an abstract idea generalized from particular instances, whereas a principle is a fundamental law or truth that shows relationship between concepts. A concept should be analyzed to determine the relevant and irrelevant attributes. The relevant attributes are those which are critical to the definition of a specific concept; irrelevant attributes are characteristics that apply to other concepts as well as to the one being considered.

For teaching purposes the teacher can give examples and counterexamples of a concept and then have the student discover the concept through induction. It is also appropriate to define the concept and have the student give examples and counterexamples through the process of deduction. Induction or discovery learning is most appropriate for a complex concept. Errors in concept formation that commonly occur with both induction and deduction include overgeneralization, undergeneralization, and misconception.

Perception, or sensory impression, is the first phase of conceptualization: the person sees a small white tablet. The next phase is integration or the understanding of similarities, differences, and function relations: many medications are small white tablets; many are not. An inference is made generally during the generalization phase: a person may classify a small white tablet he has never seen before as a medication. In the final phase of abstraction, the person formulates an idea by mentally separating qualities or properties of a thing from particular instances: a small white tablet of that size and thickness with Bayer written twice on both sides is 5 grains of Bayer aspirin.

When organizing conceptual material, the nurse may list all the concepts to be learned. Specific concepts can be identified and principles containing a particular concept grouped together. This is an effective technique because the student needs to know the concepts involved before he learns the principle. The nurse may want to formulate a hierarchy of concepts to be learned. Within the hierarchy, a supraordinate concept is general whereas a subordinate concept is more specific. Medication is a general concept. Bayer aspirin is a more specific concept. A coordinate concept is on the same level of generality as the concept under discussion and may be used as a counterexample. Five grains of Bayer aspirin and 200 mg of meprobamate (Miltown) are coordinate concepts. Since people frequently make errors in concept development, the nurse has an important role in correcting misconceptions through reeducation.[22]

Principle 6: readiness is necessary for learning to occur. The student must have adequate physical and mental development to cope with a learning situation. Learning skills requires adequate neuromuscular development; mental readiness depends on intellectual development. The nurse obviously cannot teach a crawling baby how to walk with crutches because the baby does not have the physical or mental development required to learn that skill.

New learning should be based on previous knowledge and experience such as that which is documented in the nursing history and other health care records.

Knowledge of the occupation and level of education of the head of the household indicates the patient's socioeconomic class and suggests what health beliefs and practices to expect. Age indicates the approximate developmental level. The medical history may indicate past medical experiences, and old charts should reveal how the patient has reacted to past experiences. When planning for teaching, the nurse should determine what knowledge and experience is necessary to understand the subject and should determine if the learner has that knowledge. Before the nurse starts to teach the patient about his diabetic diet, she needs to determine what the patient knows about nutrition and how his condition affects utilization of food. Encouraging the patient to discuss his condition should help the nurse assess the patient's knowledge. If general questions do not elicit all the necessary information, the nurse may ask more specific questions. The nurse should begin teaching at the client's level of understanding.

Motivation can be enhanced by an organized presentation of data. Sequential organization of content from known to unknown, immediate to remote, concrete to abstract, and easy to difficult can facilitate learning. Many psychologists believe that motivation may be the most important single element in efficient learning. The student needs to know what he is to learn and needs to understand why that learning is desirable. Learning is most effective when the client feels the need to learn something, and the nurse may have to help the patient become aware of his need to learn.

Incentives help motivate learning and are especially useful for working with people who have little internal motivation. The nurse needs to determine what token will serve as an incentive for the client and may need to reward appropriate behavior until the client becomes more self-motivated. Motivation for promotion of health and prevention of disease is likely to be missing. When the student believes that the educational goals are useful to him, he has internal motivation that is self-directed and longer lasting than external motivation that has to be reinforced.

A good sense of humor on the teacher's part can help keep the student attentive by providing a break in the expected routine. The emotional climate also affects learning. A warm and accepting atmosphere can help focus the learner's attention on what he is to learn. Unfortunately, disruptive emotional overtones are frequently present in nursing situations. If the emotional climate is either extremely positive or negative, little learning can take place. A multitude of worries and fears accompany clients in their contacts with nurses. The patient may be uncomfortable or in pain and worried about the expense of health care. When hospitalized, he must adjust to a new situation, new routines, and removal from home. He may be concerned about family finances or child care. If the patient is ill at home, he will be disruptive to the family's normal routines. Because severe anxiety is incapacitating, the nurse should encourage the client to discuss his concerns and help him work through his anxiety before attempting to teach. A mild level of anxiety is motivating and may be utilized.[23]

Principle 7: reinforcement strengthens learning. Satisfaction reinforces learning. People tend to prefer to do what they enjoy, and a feeling of accomplishment or a satisfied curiosity tends to make us want to learn. Encouragement and approval from others are other forms of reinforcement. The establishment of a warm, pleasant, accepting atmosphere is also important. Allowing the client to progress at his own rate from easier to more difficult learning tasks will help ensure success. Signs of discouragement are indications that the nurse should slow down, review content, introduce a learning task in which the patient can expect to be successful, and praise the patient's accomplishments.[24]

Active participation is essential for learning. The more the teacher teaches the less the student may learn; consequently, discussions about a subject are probably more useful than monologue. Mohammed[25] found that 43% of the people tested were unable to profit from written health materials and many others were unable to benefit from materials as they are currently used. Consequently, the nurse should use written materials cautiously and may need to develop materials for her own use. By encouraging him to ask questions, the nurse can help activate the client's mental processes. By explaining what is being done and why, and by asking and encouraging questions, the nurse may get the client more involved. The nurse may allow the client to observe a demonstration and encourage him to return demonstrations as soon as possible, first under close supervision and later under less supervision. Because the strength of a learned response varies directly with the amount of reinforcement, the nurse should acknowledge the client's successes frequently. The longer the delay in reinforcement or the time interval between the response and the reinforcement, the poorer the learning performance. Consequently, the nurse should acknowledge the successful response immediately.

Learning that is not repeated becomes extinct. Different people need different amounts of repetition for effective learning, but everyone needs some. Most knowledge is forgotten shortly after the learning occurs. Consequently, repetition is especially important at first and then should be maintained intermittently to prevent extinction.[26]

The instructional system

The instructional system includes diagnosis of needs, formulation of objectives, selection and organization of content, selection and organization of learning experiences, and evaluation.

Before beginning formal teaching, the nurse should diagnose the client's needs. What does the client already know? What does he need to know? In determining the goals of the teaching situation, the staff member should formulate objectives. These objectives should state the terminal behavior, important conditions under which the behavior is expected, and the criteria of acceptable performance. For example, given a needle, syringe, vial, and cotton sponge (the circumstances or conditions), the client will withdraw 2 ml of solution into the syringe (terminal behavior) without contaminating the needle, syringe, or solution (criteria of acceptable behavior).[27]

Objectives can be classified into three domains: cognitive, affective, and psychomotor. The cognitive domain deals with the recall or recognition of knowledge and the development of intellectual abilities and skills. The affective domain describes changes in interest, attitudes, values, the development of appreciations, and adequate adjustment. The psychomotor domain emphasizes some muscular or motor skill, some manipulation of objects, or some act that requires neuromuscular coordination.[28]

Once objectives have been determined, content can be selected. The content should reflect contemporary scientific knowledge and include basic ideas, concepts, and modes of thought rather than factual detail. The content should have a balance of breadth and depth relative to the needs and capabilities of the learners. It should be adapted to the abilities of the learners and should be appropriate to the needs and interests of the students. To facilitate learning, the content should be organized sequentially. Movement should be from known to unknown, immediate to remote, concrete to abstract, and easy to difficult.[29]

Next the staff member must select and organize learning experiences. Lectures and reading assignments are fast, economical ways to acquire the knowledge and understanding required to meet objectives in the cognitive domain. Discussions, demonstration, and role playing tend to be effective methods for changing attitudes. Demonstration and role playing are also effective for developing skills. It is wise to have a variety of alternatives available because of the great number of variations in the way people learn. There are differences in aptitude, need, interest, and in other qualities. People respond differently to different learning experiences.[30] Various means and methods of teaching will be discussed later.

Evaluation may be used to determine to what extent the learner has accomplished the terminal behavior described in the objectives. Return demonstrations may be appropriate. Tests may be oral as well as written. The principal types of teacher-made test items are short answer, true-false, multiple choice, matching, and essay. Standardized tests are also available. Instead of relying on testing, the nurse may unobtrusively observe the changes in the client's behavior as a major means of evaluation. Anecdotal records, checklists, and rating scales may be used in conjunction with observation.[31] The evaluation should be recorded on the nurse's notes to facilitate continuity of teaching.

Methods of teaching

Informal and formal. The nurse may use both informal and formal methods of teaching. Much informal teaching can be done in conversations between nurse and client. Such teaching is frequently done in response to a client's questions or comments, is based on the client's interests and needs, and should be oriented to his future health needs as well as his present condition. Group teaching may also be done informally if the nurse watches for teaching opportunities. Such opportunities may arise while the nurse is caring for patients in a ward or making a home visit in the presence of the client's friends, neighbors, or relatives. Nutrition, pregnancy, child care, immunizations, or health problems of general interest might be discussed depending on the interests of group members. The nurse also teaches informally by setting an example.[32]

Lecture. Lectures, discussions, demonstrations, and role playing are methods of formal teaching. The lecture is an appropriate method to transmit large amounts of information to many people quickly; however, it has been defined as "a process by which facts are transmitted from the notebook of the instructor to the notebook of the student without passing through the mind of either."[33] Most people are not auditory learners and may be easily distracted from the lecture. Pictures, posters, flip charts, filmstrips, slides, and the chalkboard can be used to help hold the audience's attention. To guide lecture preparation Staton[34] recommends PEOPLE, an acronym for P, pinpoint the purpose and objectives; E, examine the audience—who are they and what is their purpose for attending the lecture? O, orient the lecture to the audience's knowledge and interest; P, partition the lecture into a few brief ideas—organization of information is important to make the lecture meaningful to the listener; L, limit the content. People are inclined to get bored with details and cannot remember facts that are presented too rapidly. A lecture that presents a lot of facts in rapid succession may be compared to holding a shallow pan under the water faucet and turning the water on full force. The water hits the pan and splashes out. Consequently, there is less water left in the pan than if the water had been turned on to a slow flow. E, examples. Verbal illustrations, examples, and stories help keep the audience's attention.

Discussion. If your subject demands reasoning and understanding, if you want to use the knowledge and skills the learners already possess, and if you can work with small groups, then you may find that group discussion will be advantageous as either a primary of supplemental method of instruction. Lecture, demonstration, or role playing may all be more meaningful when accompanied by a discussion, a method in which the teacher becomes an enabler, facilitator, guide, or advisor rather than a dispenser of knowledge. Quality rather than quantity is emphasized.

Group teaching has several advantages. It is a relatively economical method because it saves considerable time and energy to teach several people at once. It provides an opportunity to share ideas and experiences. When a person realizes others have similar problems, he may be more ready to discuss his. One person's question may be of interest to others and may help stimulate less vocal individuals to express their opinions. One disadvantage is that an individual's problem may get lost in the discussion, especially if the person is shy or the others are not interested.

In preparation for a group discussion the nurse should define and review the subject to be discussed and identify the desired learning outcomes. The group should know the subject topic so it does not spend most of the discussion time deciding what to talk about and can be prepared to discuss the subject. One to three days before the meeting the nurse should distribute appropriate information such as what will be discussed, by whom, when, and where. Less than a day usually allows too little time for preparation, and people tend to forget about the meeting if informed too far in advance. The nurse needs to prepare an agenda and then prepare a lesson plan from the agenda. The nurse is also responsible for preparing the place where the discussion will be held and should be in the room before the meeting begins to check the lighting, heat, and ventilation. It is appropriate to sit around a table or to arrange chairs in a circle because the personal touch provided by face-to-face communication is important. The nurse may greet people as they arrive and introduce them to each other. At first the nurse may be responsible for introducing the topic and initiating the discussion. The nurse then encourages others to participate, helps keep the discussion on the topic, and tactfully corrects errors and misunderstanding. At the end of the discussion a review of the major points covered is appropriate, and the time, place, and topic of the next meeting may be announced.[35]

Demonstration. The demonstration method is best suited to the teaching of motor skills. For better results, it may be accompanied with lecture and discussion. When preparing a demonstration, the nurse must determine the objectives, select and organize the content, select and assemble the equipment needed, and then rehearse the demonstration until it becomes automatic. Actually giving the talk out loud during rehearsal is important to identify the rough spots. The equipment should be tested and in good working order before the demonstration begins. The preparation of a handout outlining the procedure is useful, and the handout can be checked as a review of the procedure. It is appropriate to leave space on the handout for notes, since taking notes helps activate the student's mental processes and may help hold his concentration. When the demonstration is given, everyone should be able to see the equipment and hear the speaker. Learners should be able to handle the equipment and return the demonstration.[36]

Role playing. In role playing, a situation is described, characters are identified, and people are assigned roles and told to act the assigned parts. The learning is reinforced by a discussion and analysis of the drama. The nurse must first determine the objective of the drama and structure a situation to facilitate the desired learning behavior. The situation should be described in enough detail for everyone to imagine the same circumstances and should resemble conditions in the learners' daily lives. Roles must be established and participants selected. Players should have names different from their own, and their assigned characters should not be recognizable as their own. This practice should help reduce self-consciousness. A person should seldom play himself, since he will be more likely to hide rather than to express his feelings and may feel anxious about criticism and painful analysis of his behavior.

It is usually better for the nurse to assign people to roles rather than to ask for volunteers. The volunteer may identify better with the role but may use it to present his personal prejudices. The nurse should also avoid casting people in roles that will allow them to display conflicts of opinion that are known to exist between them and others. Preparing the audience and participants by reading the situation aloud, discussing the nature of the characters, and distributing a handout describing the situation and characters is appropriate. Then the situation should be acted out and analyzed. What happened? Why? What motives and feelings were involved? What results could be predicted from other variations in the situation? The situation may be repeated, but it would probably be better to use new situations to facilitate further learning.[37]

Tools for teaching

Chalkboard. The chalkboard is one of the most readily available teaching tools. When planning to use one, the nurse should make sure that it and chalk will be available. Unless there is a specific advantage to using colored chalk, as in illustrating the difference between arteries and veins, it is preferable to use hard white chalk, since it is easier to see and does not streak so much when erased. The nurse may put some material on the board before class or may wait until class is in session. When trying to illustrate a point in class, the crudity of the chalkboard illustration may help emphasize the points the teacher wants to receive the most attention. Disadvantages to the chalkboard are that it takes up valuable time to write on during class, and it takes the teacher's attention away from the students.

Bulletin boards. Bulletin boards are devices for displaying teaching materials. They can be used to supplement a nurse's teaching in class or, when placed in waiting rooms and hallways, can be used to reach people the nurse would not otherwise teach. The bulletin board should be placed in a well-lighted area where it can be seen by a large potential audience. It should be a comfortable height for the anticipated observers. The bulletin board will hopefully attract attention, stimulate thought, and perhaps raise further questions.

Felt or flannel boards. A felt or flannel board may be constructed by mounting a piece of felt or flannel on a board. By pasting sand paper, felt, or flannel cut to the size of the material to be displayed on that material, forms can be displayed by merely pressing them on the board. They can be easily removed by lifting them off the board. Because there are no tacks or magnets involved, the display material can be quickly put into place and removed while teaching. The display materials may be easily stored and used repeatedly.

Magnetic boards. A magnetic board is a small sheet of metal that may be attached to the wall or used with a stand. Display materials are held in place by the attraction between a small magnet and the sheet of metal. The display material can be placed on the board and the magnet on the display material. The material may be quickly changed. A disadvantage is that the small size of the boards usually limits the amount of material that can be displayed. An advantage of the smallness is that the board can be carried to the bedside or taken on a home visit.

Posters. Posters that are displayed on bulletin boards, felt boards, magnetic boards, or taped to doors and walls may be used to arouse interest in a health topic. They are often available at little or no cost and usually illustrate a single health principle.

Pictures. Pictures may be either photographs or taken from printed sources. They can visually present a realistic situation without background distractions. The printed material or photographs may be mounted on cardboard by rubber cement or dry mount methods to increase their durability. The nurse may want to permanently protect the picture by sealing a clear plastic laminating film over its surface.

Opaque projector. The opaque projector may be used to project a picture from a book or magazine directly on a screen. However, the page may need to be cut out and mounted to produce a good image. Visual aids can be improvised by projecting a picture on the chalkboard and drawing around it or by projecting it onto a piece of cardboard to make a poster. Use of the opaque projector requires little preparation; however, its disadvantages are that it is a large, bulky piece of equipment and requires considerable darkness in order to project a clear image. Since the development of the overhead projector, it is used less frequently.

Overhead projector. The overhead transparency projector is small, compact, lightweight, and easy to transport. It can be used without turning off the lights, and the staff member can face the audience while using it. It is easy to set up, focus, and use. A light shining from below the clear plastic transparency throws the lines on the screen. The teacher can sketch on the plastic during class much like using a chalkboard but without having to turn her back to the audience, or she may prepare transparencies before class. Instead of using an opaque projector, the teacher may cut a page from a book or magazine or photocopy the page and use a thermo process to make a permanent transparency.

Slides. Slides are still pictures that can be projected onto a screen. They can be shown to everyone in the class at once and can be discussed for varying lengths of time. They are easy to store and transport and can be used repeatedly; however, it takes considerable time to prepare them and expensive equipment to project them.

The 2 × 2 slide projector with a carrier that can hold up to 140 slides provides the teacher with a device that can impart a great deal of information and allows the teacher to set up a complete lesson with a written script to accompany it. The script may be put on tape and the voice and slides synchronized, or the projector can be operated by the tape. The slide carriers are numbered for each individual slide. Many of the slide projectors have remote control so the teacher can stand in front of the room and control the equipment while making the presentation.

Film strip. A film strip consists of a series of still pictures. Both commercial and teacher-made film strips are plentiful. Amateurs, using relatively inexpensive equipment, can make film strips that are tailored to a specific situation. The teacher can control the pace of the learning in a presentation without sound, whereas in a sound presentation in which the film is accompanied by a record or tape, she will have no control over speed of presentation.

Films. The 16 mm motion picture projector is one of the most utilized of the teaching aids. It is versatile, easy to operate, and can bring experiences into the classroom that cannot be brought in any other way. It can be used with large groups or smaller ones. There is a large selection of films to choose from on a rental basis or from the institution's film library. The nurse should preview the film to determine if it meets the teaching objectives and is appropriate for the audience. The classroom should be large so there is room for both the equipment and the audience. An electrical outlet is needed, of course, and an extension cord positioned out of the traffic pattern may be necessary. Seats should be a minimum 6 feet from the screen, and the room will need to be darkened. Films should be ordered well in advance with alternate dates specified and should be returned promptly.

The 8 mm projector may be used for small groups or in individual study carrels. Operation of this projector is simple, and it may be used for many more learning activities than the 16 mm projector. The films may be silent or have sound, and may be reel-to-reel type or cartridges. The small super 8, which is silent film with a cartridge load, enables students to study on their own.

Television. Television is a medium that incorporates motion and sound and in which color is feasible. It may be produced live or recorded. Television is an extremely expensive medium, however, requiring considerable skill and technical knowledge, and should be attempted only in consultation with experts.

Record player. The record player is being used less frequently with the increased use of tape recorders, although it is still a good way to introduce sound. The permanence of records prevents accidental erasures but may be a disadvantage, since records cannot be erased and reused. Record players are frequently used in conjunction with slides and film strips.

Tape recorder. The tape recorder is another way to introduce sound. Tapes may be prerecorded or recorded during class. The tapes can be erased and reused and are unfortunately sometimes erased inadvertently. Tape recorders come in reel or cassette types, and are operated by battery or electric current. The recorder is mobile, relatively inexpensive, and requires little storage space. Audiotapes are also inexpensive and easily stored. The tape recorder can help develop listening skills and is useful in preserving information for replay. If the instructor wishes to use a tape of a person's voice for teaching purposes, she should make certain she has the person's consent to do so. The mechanics of recording should not interfere with group interaction, and the group should be small enough for one stationary microphone to pick up all the voices.

Models and objects. Actual objects, rather than models, should be used when practical. It is often possible to use objects like bandages and syringes when teaching nursing procedures, to show a vaginal speculum when telling about pelvic examination, or various types of contraceptives when discussing birth control. Models are often used when the actual object would not be appropriate in the classroom. Models of human anatomy are commonly used. A doll may be used to demonstrate a baby bath. The nurse should make the necessary arrangements to use the objects and models and should have them ready before class.

Pamphlets. Pamphlets are often free or inexpensive and frequently can be obtained from voluntary health organizations. They generally discuss a single topic such as asthma, birth control pills, cancer, nutrition, or toilet training. Many pamphlets are written for the general public and are prepared for different reading levels and in different languages. The nurse must assess the client's reading level before determining which pamphlet is appropriate. Pamphlets may be used to stimulate interest in a subject or for later reference. They should not replace other teaching methods and tools, since the limited reading ability of many people restricts their use of pamphlets.

Flash cards. A flash card is a card of any size with a word, diagram, or picture on it that can be flashed to illustrate a point during class. Transparent plastic may be put over the flash card so the teacher can supplement the original by adding additional information with a grease pencil. The grease marks can be washed off and the flash card reused. Flash cards may also be used for drills such as vocabulary or arithmetic drills. The nurse can write symptoms on one side of the card and indicate what conditions these symptoms represent on the other. A student can then drill himself on whatever symptoms are presented.

Programmed instruction. Programmed instruction is self-instruction. It proceeds in a logical step-by-step progression through sometimes complex subject matter. Each segment of information is followed by a question concerning it; this unit constitutes a frame. The student is to study only one frame at a time. After he has answered the question, he is directed to uncover the correct answer, which is usually placed alongside the question. The programmed method makes the student an active part of the learning process. The immediate reinforcement for correct answers should help motivate him. The learner can progress through the program at his own rate.

Task analysis is the first step in the development of a programmed instruction. What does the student need to know or be able to do? After establishing the goals, the nurse can determine the specific behavioral objectives and conditions necessary to produce the desired behaviors. The objectives are divided into small units; examples and counterexamples for use in concept formation are determined. The response mode should be related to the behavior being taught and is consequently not always a paper and pencil response. There are a variety of programming methods and techniques being used. The development of programmed instruction should be done in conjunction with experts.

Games. Games can be a fun way to learn. Pin the tail on the donkey can help schoolchildren understand what it is like to be blind or have impaired vision. A bingo game in which food groups are listed across the top of the card with various foods listed under them can be developed to help students learn what foods belong in what food groups. Simulation games, which are imitations of real situations, can be used to promote learning. The simulation game should focus on the concepts and processes identified by task analysis and should deal with the critical elements of the processes.

The nurse should be familiar with various teaching tools, select the tool that will do the most good in a given situation, make the necessary arrangements for its use, make the presentation, give the students opportunities to apply their new learning, evaluate the teaching methods, and seek improvements in those methods.[38]

NOTES

1. Bower, F. L.: The process of planning nursing care, St. Louis, 1972. The C. V. Mosby Co., p. 110; Bratton, J. K.: A definition of comprehensive nursing care, Nurs. Outlook 9(8):481-482, 1961; Levine, M. E.: The pursuit of wholeness, Am. J. Nurs. 69(1):93-98, 1969.
2. Peabody, S. R.: Assessment and planning for continuity of care, Nurs. Clin. North Am. 4:309, June, 1969.
3. Dahlin, B.: Rehabilitation and the assessment of patient need, Nurs. Clin. North Am. 1:375-386, Sept., 1966.
4. Wolff, I. S.: Referral—a process and a skill, Nurs. Outlook 10(4):253-256, 1962; Brill, N. I.: Working with people, Philadelphia, 1973, J. B. Lippincott Co., pp. 191-195.
5. Mayers, M. G.: A systematic approach to the nursing care plan, New York, 1972, Appleton-Century-Crofts, p. 263; Fuerst, E. V., and Wolff, L. V.: Fundamentals of nursing, ed. 5, Philadelphia, 1974, J. B. Lippincott Co.
6. Bower, pp. 105-106; Little, D. E., and Carnevali, D. L.: Nursing care planning, Philadelphia, 1969, J. B. Lippincott Co., p. 187.
7. Phaneuf, M. C.: The nursing audit profile for excellence, New York, 1972, Appleton-Century-Crofts, p. 76.
8. Wahlstrom, E. D.: Initiating referrals: a hospital based system, Am. J. Nurs. 67(2):332-335, 1967.
9. Peabody, pp. 303-310.
10. Bernstein, L., and Dana, R. H.: Interviewing and the health professions, New York, 1970, Appleton-Century-Crofts, pp. 103-115. Discusses methods for implementing understanding; Hays, J. S., and Larson, K. A.: Interacting with patients, New York, 1963, Macmillan Publishing Co., Inc., pp. 7-23. Discusses and gives examples of twenty-five therapeutic techniques. Most of the book consists of process recordings of case studies that illustrate use of therapeutic and nontherapeutic techniques.
11. Bernstein and Dana, pp. 28-88. Discusses evaluative, hostile, reassuring, and probing responses; Hays and Larson, pp. 24-37. Identifies and discusses nineteen nontherapeutic techniques.
12. Skipper, J. K., Jr., Mauksch, H. O., and Tagliacozzo, D.: Some barriers to communication between patients and hospital functionaries, Nurs. Forum 2(1):14-23, 1963.
13. Champion, R. A.: Learning and activation, Sydney, Australia, 1969, John Wiley & Sons, Inc., pp. 1-2; Pohl, M. L.: Teaching function of the nursing practitioner, Dubuque, Iowa, 1968, William C. Brown Co., Publishers, p. 6; Redman, B. K.: The process of patient teaching in nursing, ed. 3, St. Louis, 1976, The C. V. Mosby Co., pp. 5-7.
14. Fylling, C. P.: Health education, Hospitals 49(7):95-97, 1975; Lazinski, H., and Oppeneer, J.: Hospitals offer employees health programs, Hospitals 48(22):66, 68, 1974; Williams, Z.: A hall of health, Hosp. Forum 17(14):4-5, 18, 1976; and Yeats, H. S.: Models for moppets, ONA J. 3(6):196, 1976.
15. Freeman, R. B.: Public health nursing practice, Philadelphia, 1963, W. B. Saunders Co., pp. 103-104; Pohl, pp. 48-53.
16. Pohl, p. 51; Schultz, E. D.: Television brings drama to clinic patients, Am. J. Nurs. 62(8):98-99, 1962; Robinson, G., and Filkins, M.: Group teaching with outpatients, Am. J. Nurs. 64(11):110-112, 1964.
17. Pohl, pp. 53-56; Marriner, A.: The role of the school nurse in health education, Am. J. Public Health 61:2155-2157, Nov., 1971.
18. Freeman, pp. 105-107.
19. Albert, S.: Storefront converted to health education center, Hospitals 49(4):57-59, 1975; Althafer, C., Butcher, R., and Fasburg, R. G.: Now it's health information by phone, tel-med, Am. Lung Assoc. Bull. 60:12-14, Jan.-Feb., 1974; Ward, B.: Carnival offers learning opportunities, Hospitals

49(12):72-73, 1975; Wilkinson, G. S., Mirand, E. A., and Graham, S.: Can dial: an experiment in health education and cancer control, Public Health Rep. **91**(3):218-222, 1976.

20. Pohl, pp. 1-10; Watson, D. L., and Tharp, R. G.: Self-directed behavior: self-modification for personal adjustment, Monterey, Calif., 1972, Brooks/Cole Publishing Co., pp. 26-46.
21. Pohl, pp. 8-9.
22. Frayer, D., et al.: Working paper 16: a schema for testing the level of concept mastery, Madison, Wis., 1969, University of Wisconsin, Wisconsin Research and Development Center for Cognitive Learning, pp. 1-31; Pohl, pp. 13-16.
23. Highet, G.: The art of teaching, New York, 1950, Vintage Books, p. 53; Pohl, pp. 16-23; Staton, T. F.: How to instruct successfully, New York, 1960, McGraw-Hill Book Co., p. 10; Redman, pp. 48-51.
24. Pohl, pp. 24-25.
25. Mohammed, M. F.: Patients' understanding of written health information, Nurs. Res. **13**:100-108, Spring, 1964.
26. Pohl, pp. 19-20, 24.
27. Mager, R. F.: Preparing instructional objectives, Belmont, Calif., 1962, Fearon Publishers, Inc., p. 12.
28. Bloom, B. S., et al.: Taxonomy of educational objectives: the classification of educational goals, Handbook I, Cognitive domain, New York, 1956, David McKay Co., Inc.; Krathwohl, D. R., Bloom, B. S., and Masia, B. B.: Taxonomy of educational objectives: the classification of educational goals, Handbook II, Affective domain, New York, 1956, David McKay Co., Inc.
29. Taba, H.: Curriculum development, New York, 1962, Harcourt Brace and World, Inc., pp. 267-289, 359.
30. Banathy, B. H.: Instructional systems, Belmont, Calif., 1968, Fearon Publishers, Inc., p. 60; Staton, p. 5.
31. Blood, D. F., and Budd, W. C.: Educational measurement and evaluation, New York, 1972, Harper & Row, Publishers, Inc., pp. 44-65; Redman, pp. 133-155.
32. Monteiro, L. A.: Notes on patient-teaching—a neglected area, Nurs. Forum **3**(1):26-33, 1964; Pohl, pp. 68-71.
33. Staton, p. 65.
34. Staton, pp. 65-82.
35. Hyman, R. T.: Ways of teaching, Philadelphia, 1970, J. B. Lippincott Co., p. 48; Pohl, pp. 72-74; Staton, pp. 97-113.
36. Pohl, pp. 75-78; Redman, pp. 117-119; Staton, pp. 83-96; Tobin, H. M., Yoder, P. S., Hull, P. K., and Scott, B. C.: The process of staff development, St. Louis, 1974, The C. V. Mosby Co., pp. 91-92.
37. Staton, pp. 124-156.
38. Hyman, pp. 186-199; Pohl, pp. 88-94; Popiel, E. S.: Nursing and the process of continuing education, St. Louis, 1977, The C. V. Mosby Co., pp. 101-109; Mechner, F.: Learning by doing through programmed instruction, Am. J. Nurs. **65**(5):98-104, 1965; Staton, pp. 173-177.

Selected readings

Ingeborg G. Mauksch and Miriam L. David predict that adoption of the nursing process as a way of professional life is the "Prescription for Survival." They discuss the rationale for the process and examine it through the use of a case study. Kathryn Buchanan Luciano further discusses the phases of the nursing process. Her case study illustrates the implementation of theory.

Donna Stulgis Zimmerman and Carol Gohrke Blainey demonstrate the use of the nursing process through a case presentation. Anita Havens discusses her use of problem solving in caring for an elderly depressed patient.

In "Talking with Patients," Hildegard E. Peplau expresses the need for the nurse to develop an awareness of her own communication patterns. The nurse is encouraged to replace social conversations with therapeutic communications. Phyllis Goldin and Barbara Russell further discuss the nature of social conversations and give examples of therapeutic communication techniques. Helon E. Hewitt and Betty L. Pesznecker discuss how commonly used nontherapeutic techniques are "Blocks to Communicating with Patients." They give examples of how changing the subject, stating one's own opinions, inappropriate reassurance, jumping to conclusions, and inappropriate use of nursing knowledge interfere with communications. Judith Petrello reports that patients do not understand many of the clinical terms nurses commonly use.

Dorothy T. Linehan interviewed 450 patients to learn "What Does the Patient Want to Know?" She informs her reader of numerous topics on which patients would like more information. James K. Skipper, Jr., Daisy L. Tagliacozzo, and Hans O. Mauksch found that communications between physicians, nurses, and patients help the patient secure information and help meet the patient's need for personal contact with hospital personnel.

PRESCRIPTION FOR SURVIVAL
Ingeborg G. Mauksch and Miriam L. David

The possibility that nursing as we know it today may not exist by the year 2000 is being voiced with increasing frequency.[1-3] The bases for these speculations range from a sense of superfluousness in the face of the emerging so-called "new" health professions to the fear that nursing's contribution to health and illness care may be eliminated by those more powerful within the decision-making group.

We believe that true nursing practice is a vital component of health and illness care and cannot be denied. It consists of a cure and a care component. The former serves to implement the physician's regimen, while the latter autonomously endeavors to meet the patient's (or client's) needs in health maintenance or to help him attain a higher level of health or achieve a dignified peaceful death.

Nursing's bad press certainly mirrors the truth. In objective self-examination we find, generally, that nursing really has not done its job. Not only has nursing not produced a visible autonomously effective practice, but the consumer, usually grateful, now does not seem to recognize nursing's worth. And certainly other health occupations seem to take little notice of nursing's contribution to health and illness care.

Nursing's most serious failure has taken place in hospitals where it reflects a bureaucratically oriented and organizationally constrained series of functions, largely generated by the orders of others. Nursing here lacks a design of cohesiveness and of continuity of care. It lacks a focal emphasis on primary care. Task orientation, adherence to outdated

Reprinted from American Journal of Nursing **72**(12):2189-2193, 1972. Copyright The American Journal of Nursing Company.

knowledge, a denial of accountability, and expedience born of lack of quantitative and qualitative controls characterize the delivery of nursing care in these settings.

Recent studies indicate that hospitals find it increasingly more difficult to maintain a stable nursing staff or, more significantly yet, to attract graduates of innovative, future-oriented nursing programs.

Young nurses from these programs are reluctant to function within such a system, and decline to be diverted into the management roles demanded of them. They prefer to work where they can function more autonomously and where they feel supported in their desire to practice in a patient-centered way. Some nurses are abandoning the old way of nursing and devising roles not necessarily new in content, but new in two other ways: care oriented to patients' needs, and the nursing process applied to this care.

RATIONALE FOR NURSING PROCESS

The nursing process focuses on the client (or patient) and his family. It is initiated through a comprehensive assessment which results in the identification of needs, their analysis, and their logical arrangement according to priorities. Subsequently, decisions are made regarding those needs which fall within the nurse's competence and which can be met within the context of the nurse-patient relationship. This is followed by goal setting, accomplished, when at all possible, jointly between nurse, client, and family.

Care is taken that goals are measurable, attainable, reasonable, and representative of the patient's aspirations. These goals are then implemented through a series of interventions, also called nursing orders or nursing actions. These, in aggregate, form the nursing care plan.

Concurrent evaluation of this process is imperative. At the time of the interruption of the nurse-client relationship, a major evaluative effort takes place. The final step is planning for "aftercare," a term covering a broad range of clients' needs and requiring from nurses knowledge and community contacts to maintain continuity of previously determined goals. Most significantly, however, these plans are designed to promote the client's own effort toward health-sustaining behavior.

We base our belief that the nursing process is a necessity on six major tenets which are the matrix of nursing's contribution to health care in the future:

1. The nursing process is a means of unifying the occupation, now sadly divided. It will bridge the distances between the greatly varying ideologies of nursing in hospitals and in other settings, and it will span the wide range between nurses with different kinds of education. One could liken this unifying effect to the use of a common language by heretofore multilingual people.

2. The nursing process demonstrates nursing's function through the use of science, art, humanity, and skills, a combination that is unique and unreplicated.

3. The nursing process restores nursing to its primary commitment, delivering care to people on a one-to-one basis, and thereby eliminates our present tendency to relinquish this overall function to those who are not prepared to fulfill it.

4. The nursing process promotes consumer satisfaction. By making the patient the undisputed focus of the endeavor, a nurse brings forth a one-to-one relationship in which the patient is an active partner and participates in crucial decision-making. The current much deplored anonymity and impersonality of health and illness care will finally be replaced by this personalized and individualized approach.

5. The nursing process provides a means of assessing nursing's economic contribution to the totality of patient care. Because evaluation is an integral component of the nursing process, both the effectiveness and the amount of nursing performance can be determined and economically valued.

6. The nursing process enables a nurse to realize her potential as an independent decision-maker who has command over competencies which heretofore were not used in carrying out predominantly assistance-type functions.

CHARACTERISTICS OF PRACTICE

Because the nursing process underlies nursing practice, it is important to understand the meaning of this concept. A practice is the delivery of a broad, knowledge-based service, designed to respond to a universal need of the society. Medical practice, legal practice, the practice of the clergy are a few examples. Many occupations which deliver a service through their practice are called professions.

The line between some service occupations and professions is a thin one, and it serves no purpose here to assert that nursing is or is not a profession.[4] We contend that the practice which nursing delivers must exhibit those characteristics which are usually ascribed to professional behavior. Let society decide, then, whether nursing deserves the label "professional." We suggest, therefore, that nursing practice must become noted for these characteristics:

accountability—a nurse considers herself the originator of her tasks and fully answerable for them.
primacy of client interest—the interest of the patient rather than the convenience of functionaries or the expediency of the institution is given first consideration.
scientific competence—use of the newest knowledge, made available through research.
peer review—validation of performance quality through approval by occupational peers rather than by institutional superordinates who may lack competence in practice or, worse yet, may not be nurses.
control over conditions of practice—a nurse decides or at least shares in the decision about the quantity and quality guidelines of her practice.

Hans Mauksch elaborates on this: . . . *the professional model is characterized by involving the assumption of responsibility for the conduct and the consequence of the task. In its inception it is guided by a determined and assessed need of the client as interpreted by the performer. . . . The client's needs represent the orientational base or the career of the professional task. The criteria which pattern the conduct of the professional task are principles of knowledge and selected appropriateness to the specific situation. The goal of the professional task is the reduction of the client's assessed problems. The rewards for the professionally performed tasks are consequence and effect, satisfaction, and peer approval.*[5]

In synthesis, these component parts of a practice become, operationally speaking, a process of care in the delivery of a service.

In studying the processes developed by other service occupations, one readily identifies their commonalities: a structure of need identification, process of data collection, and decision-making, and subsequently the implementation of a need-responding regimen.

The development of goals based on a comprehensive understanding of the client's needs and the striving to render individualized service further exemplify the very uniqueness of a practice responding to a societal mandate. Finally, there is the commonality of systematization. It provides for the universality of the process, which, by enabling the largest possible number of practitioners to share in it, invites them to strive for constant updating and improvement.

If, for example, we look at the process underlying legal practice, we recognize the above-described components. The practitioner (attorney) collects data by listening and questioning his client; he gathers the facts. He learns his client's needs and helps him formulate objectives to meet them within the feasibility of the circumstances. He prepares a brief, a carefully worded document, which describes the case. He then develops a plan of action, geared at resolution. The client must be able to agree with this course and to participate in the resolution, which may be a trial. This is a universal legal process, even though law itself may vary from country to country.

A PROCESS FOR PRACTICE EXAMINED

No occupation has found it easy to develop the process underlying its practice. If we look at nursing's past, we can understand why it has been particularly difficult for nursing. The circumstances of nursing's birth, which dictated that its practitioners undergo apprenticeship-type training, cast them as assistants to physicians. Furthermore, the very essence of a nurse's practice was obscured by the demand that she be the caretaker in a setting where she was virtually the only permanent functionary. Thus, she took care of everything and, by being all things to the patient as she assumed responsibility for him and for his environment, she embarked on a path of diffuse activity.

This role had no scientific basis; management, household arts, dietetic skills were but some of its components. The fledgling occupation was thus badly sidetracked from a direct approach to the development of a meaningful practice.

These conditions did not improve during nursing's infancy. Rather, they were reinforced, particularly through the depression years. It was then that nurses saw themselves as managers rather than primary care practitioners; the summit of professional aspiration was administration, not expert practice. Thus, nurses confused the purpose of their occupation, the delivery of nursing care to people, with managing the complex care in institutions.

Proverbially, adolescence is characterized by chaos; so it has been with nursing. As more and more nurses strove harder and harder to succeed in management, they passed on the essence of their practice to vocationally trained and on-the-job-schooled workers. Some nurses, however, began to search for the true meaning of nursing's practice. Reiter, Henderson, McCain, Johnson, and Smith are some of the many nurses who recognized the inappropriateness of nursing's management direction, and who conceptualized nursing as a "laying on of the hands" type practice.[6-11] They did so by describing and testing the nursing process.

We believe that application of the nursing process by some, even though few, practitioners marks the beginning of the occupation's maturity. Nursing has come of age. Like those arriving at a watershed, its practitioners must decide which stream to follow—that of management and subsequent oblivion, or that of primary practice and a burgeoning future.

What prevents nursing from developing a true practice? Manifestly, there are a number of obstacles to be overcome. Most important, perhaps, is our unwillingness to take risks and to plan.

Planning for the future is not a much-practiced behavior in this society. The inability to predict certain aspects of the future is often used to deny the desirability of planning in areas that can be effectively manipulated. Most of the time, it is easier to "cop out" by saying, "You can't tell what the future will bring so why bother to plan for it?"

The consequences of not planning despite meaningful indices to do so can be found in ecology, education, race relations, crime, and the conditions of the cities. On the other hand, where planning has taken place, its efficacy certainly is apparent: the legislation of social security, the creation of national libraries and galleries, the designation of wilderness areas and national forests, and the preservation of numerous historical sites, to mention a few. Each accomplishment was fraught with objections and required risk taking. So it will be with nursing.

Second, and again this is a barrier faced by the entire society in any endeavor, is resistance to change. "Human beings," states Etzioni, "are not very easily changed after all."[12] Nevertheless, change we must, in a range of areas.

Nurses will need to redefine themselves as human beings in order to become autonomous decision-making functionaries, for how else can their judgment become decisive, and their self-presentation worthy of note? Furthermore, nurses must see themselves as women, and acquire a stance of equality based on competence, taking advantage of the egalitarian climate which is sweeping our land. They will have to stop being submissive and quit playing the "nurse-doctor" game.[13] They must cease being self-sacrificial and self-effacing.

Today, women select and pursue careers as do men. If they are good at what they are doing, they will command the respect they deserve; it cannot be accorded them in any other way. Nurses must learn to behave as if they expect that this will be so. They must learn to rely on themselves, to build their identities upon their own achievements.

Lastly, nurses must place a value on their services by expecting and demanding appropriate remuneration. In a materialistic society such as ours, every service is translated into dollars and cents. Nurses have denied this, partly because they adhered to a fallacious interpretation of professionalism, partly because most are secondary wage earners who "do not need to earn so much"; and, lastly, because there have been no satisfactory means to assess the effectiveness of nursing in its proliferated diffuseness.[14]

The practice of nursing through implementation of the nursing process is really an altogether new style of functioning.[15] To make it nursing's new way of life will require a selling job. Each nurse must persuade her colleagues that implementing the nursing process is tantamount to nursing's survival!

The following excerpts from the written portion of one nursing process illustrate the various components discussed earlier. Appropriate charting of the process is essential. We encourage the methods recently described by Carlson and Schell and Campbell.[15,16]

Although similar care plans have been described, we do so again because we feel it is crucial that the nursing process be thoroughly understood and universally adopted. If this written, systematic approach to nursing care is adopted, the basic tenets of a practice—accountability, service to client, scientific competence, peer review, and control over conditions of practice—can be documented. If this process is not adopted, then we believe as does Bennett: "The reality for nursing will be that of the epitaph."[17] If nursing is to be viable and effective in the year 2000 implementation of the nursing process is mandatory. The time to begin is now.

EXCERPTS FROM THE CHART OF ONE NURSING PROCESS

ASSESSMENT—Ms. L., admitted for further evaluation of leukopenia and, secondarily, for evaluation of rheumatoid arthritis.

I. Personal data: Fourteenth hospital admission for this 58-year-old Caucasian woman who is married to a 69-year-old farmer who works in the field many hours daily. They have indoor plumbing and electricity. Their two sons (ages 20 and 19) live about 90 miles from here, in a town of 2,000.

II. Appearance on first sight: Ms. L. was lying supine in bed. . . . Extreme ulnar deviation of both wrists and obvious flexion contractures of all fingers, right more severe than left. Right leg remained flexed at the knee under the covers.

III. Understanding of illness: Ms. L.'s chief complaint is "pain and soreness in every joint." Apparently arthritis started 7 years ago. "I'm here now because I have only 3,500 white corpuscles." Says her gall bladder was removed 7 years ago. Takes 10-12 aspirin with 2 tablespoons Maalox every day for arthritic pain. Can do very little except feed herself and hold light magazines. Husband cooks, sons wash and iron. A woman comes in weekly to bathe her and do some cleaning.

IV. Expectations of stay: "My family didn't want me to come, said I shouldn't get all that radio-activity." (Small dose of radioactive lead used to determine white cell survival time.) "Yes, I'm a little afraid of it, but my doctor said it wouldn't do any damage. My arthritis is really what bothers me, but I don't expect them to do much for it."

V. Social and cultural history: "I used to keep house and work hard on the farm." Eighth grade education. Has no medical insurance. Is of Pentacostal faith and would like to see a minister. Significant others are her husband and her sons.

VI. Significant data:

A. Rest and sleep—"I'm in bed mostly because I can't get up by myself, and the men are gone all day. Sometimes they get me in a chair for a little while in the evening." No specific times for arising or going to sleep. No sleeping pills.

B. Elimination—Takes two Pericolace every other day and has bowel movement at least that often. Uses commode when husband helps her. Has recently had burning on urination and a sharp right flank pain. Urine has strong odor, dark brown color.

C. Respiration—Occasionally hyperventilates but can stop immediately when thinks of it. Sleeps on one pillow and a rubber ring under back of head. Does not smoke. No allergies.

D. Circulation—Pulse: 84, respiration: 18, blood pressure 130/90. About 7 years ago developed stasis ulcers on both ankles; recurrently has much pedal and ankle edema; told to wear elastic hose but neither she nor husband can put them on due to her arthritis. When legs are dependent, feet becomes extremely cyanotic; dorsalis pedis and posterior tibial pulses felt in right foot but not in left.

E. Nutrition—"I'm supposed to be on a 1,200 calorie diet but my husband doesn't fix it for me." Usually 3 meals per day with occasional snack at HS. Height: 5'8"; Weight: about 185. Wears upper dentures, which she takes out at night and soaks; does not wear lowers due to rubbing.

F. Skin integrity—Generally pale; ankles extremely discolored (brown, yellow) with several fresh scabs, fingernails and toenails long and brittle, unable to observe back at this time.

G. Senses—Wears glasses; has "clouds in front of my eyes"; taste, smell, hearing, touch intact; well oriented.

H. Activity—Unable to walk. States left hip is broken and prevents her turning on left side; needs help in most activities (sitting up, cutting food, getting to commode); extreme difficulty in flexing right arm; uses a rubber ring under head because "I have spurs on the back of my head." To pass time, Ms. L. watches TV. Has no radio at home. Occasionally reads light-weight magazines. "I'm content to be alone for the 7 or 8 hours while my family is in the field."

I. Interpersonal pattern—Ms. L. communicates easily and voluntarily maintains eye contact, can volunteer nothing which specifically upsets or makes her happy.

J. Dependency/independency pattern—Extremely dependent due to disability.

K. Emotional strengths/weaknesses—Ms. L. seems eager to be a "good patient," but has little hope that she can do much to improve her current level of functional ability. Although her family manages the household chores, she says they rarely assist her with any type of care and probably would not change their attitude even if encouraged by the health team. "They are all stubborn and have thick heads. They don't see much of a future for me."

Nursing goals and action

I. Promote optimal function (basic ADL)
1. Assist patient with activities: sitting up—turn to right side to eat—assist with food (cutting, positioning on plate, etc.)—assist to commode every afternoon for BM—daily sponge bath with good peri care in A.M.—assist getting onto bedpan (use fracture pan); wipe well following each voiding—draw sheet underneath patient to help pull up in bed—dentures out at HS to soak; help to put back in mouth in A.M. . . .
2. Encourage to do what she can: eat, drink (can hold cup if liquid is poured); can wash face, hands if given cloth, can rub cream on face, can use call light if it is in her hands—check for this every time in room.
3. Recommend consult to PT and OT to increase ability in ADL.

II. Relieve pain
1. Positioning: provide pillow on which to prop right knee, elevate head of bed (10°).
2. Back rub t.i.d. (8-4-HS)—turn to right side.
3. Obtain PRN order for analgesic.
4. Obtain PRN order for heating pad.

III. Treat bladder infection
1. Encourage fluids—at least 8 glasses water per 24 hours.
2. Record intake and output—observe frequency and character of voiding (urgency, dysuria).
3. Urine specimen for culture and sensitivity to lab.
4. Antibiotic as per physician's order.
5. Explain GI studies and prepare for.

IV. Promote bowel elimination
1. Give Pericolace as ordered.
2. Encourage fluids as above.
3. Assist to commode every day—about 2 P.M.

V. Promote circulation
1. Elastic hose to legs—take off and reapply every 8 hours.
2. Elevate foot of bed slightly.
3. Passive exercises with bath as patient tolerates.
4. Chair next to bed to rest feet on when in sitting position (e.g., when eating).

VI. Promote healthy skin
1. Lotion to ankles and legs when elastic hose removed.
2. Heel protectors and rubber donuts for elbows.
3. Sheepskin underneath buttocks.
4. Rubber donut under head.
5. Manicure and pedicure within next several days.
6. Observe for change in position and/or reposition at least every 4 hours (8-12-4-8).
7. Back rub—as above.

VII. Diversion
1. Sit and talk with patient as time allows—one-to-one.
2. Attempt to transfer patient into wheelchair every evening and wheel to TV lounge; encourage visiting with other patients.
3. Request radio from volunteers.
4. Provide light, easy-to-read magazines (*Woman's Day,* etc.).
5. Allow to call family once a day if desires.

VIII. Promote nutrition
1. Reduction diet (1,200 calorie)
2. Discuss advantages of losing weight with patient (increased mobility, less skin breakdown, etc.).
3. Dental consult to evaluate lower denture plate.
4. Diet instruction for husband and patient before discharge.
5. Weigh patient Mondays and Thursdays on bed scale.

Progress notes

Day 2—Goal VI. Promote healthy skin.

Except for lower legs, integument has good turgor and remains intact. Sheepskin was obtained for underneath buttocks, and heel and elbow protectors. Patient states, "They feel good." Powder applied to perineum and underneath breasts. Patient applied triamcinalone to face while sitting on side of bed.

Recommend: continue present nursing actions. Arrange for her to take elbow protectors home (has heel protectors at home).

Day 3—Goal I. Promote optimal function.

Patient is doing what she can: eating, pushing call bell, washing face, applying cream, reaching commode by pivoting on right foot. No response from physician regarding PT and OT consults. Continue to pursue matter.

Goal II. Relieve pain

On ASA regimen, standing. No complaint of pain to any extent since regimen begun. Heating pad is contraindicated. (Patient states, "I get red all over if I use one.")

Goal III. Treat bladder infection

Fluids exceeded 2,000 cc. per 24 hours yesterday. Voidings progressively lighter. Urine specimen sent. Antibiotic begun. Continue to offer water every 2 hours (patient prefers water over other liquids).

Goal IV. Promote bowel elimination

With Pericolace in A.M., patient had BM at 3 P.M. Assisted to commode by one person. Continue plan.

Goal V. Promote circulation

Elastic hose are very difficult to put on—tires patient greatly. Try removing and reapplying at bath time and HS only (not t.i.d.). Patient performing limited active exercises; encourage this. Continue passive exercises of other muscle groups.

Discharge summary

Prior to Ms. L.'s discharge, a team conference was held, attended by nurse who had followed patient through her hospital course, primary physician (an internist), dietitian, physical therapist who had worked with patient twice a day, and hospital chaplain who had visited her several times a week. After each member assessed Ms. L.'s current and potential abilities, a tentative plan of care at home was developed. The patient then joined the conference and helped make the final plan. The next time Mr. L. visited, the nurse discussed the plan with him. (Her sons had refused to participate in her care.)

Diet instruction and menu planning were provided by the dietitian. Finally, the county public health nurse was notified by telephone of Ms. L.'s impending discharge. A summary of the suggested care plan with certain orders from the physician were mailed to her. A visit in one month was scheduled in the outpatient department.

REFERENCES

1. Kramer, Marlene. Role conceptions of baccalaureate nurses and success in hospital nursing, *Nurs.Res.* **19**:428-439, Sept.-Oct. 1970.
2. ————. Current research. Special report. Nurse role deprivation—a symptom of needed change. *Soc.Sci.Med.* **2**:461-474, Dec. 1968.
3. Mauksch, I. G. *Science, Research, Politics and Nursing Care: Explorations in Strategy.* Paper presented at the fourth annual Nurse-Scientist Conference held April 2-3, 1971 at Denver, Colo.
4. Freidson, Eliot. *Profession of Medicine.* New York, Dodd, Mead and Co., 1970, pp. 77ff.
5. Mauksch, H. O. *Ideology, Interaction and Patient Care in Hospitals.* Paper presented at the Third International Conference on Social Science and Medicine, Elsinore, Denmark, Aug. 13-19, 1972.
6. Reiter, Frances. The nurse-clinician. *Am.J.Nurs.* **66**:274-280, Feb. 1966.
7. Johnson, D. E. Symposium on theory development in nursing; theory in nursing: borrowed and unique. *Nurs.Res.* **17**:206-209, May-June 1968.
8. Smith, D. M. Clinical nursing tool. *Am.J.Nurs.* **68**:2384-2388, Nov. 1968.
9. ————. Writing objectives as a nursing practice and skill. *Am.J.Nurs.* **71**:319-320, Feb. 1971.
10. McCain, R. F. Nursing by assessment—not intuition. *Am.J.Nurs.* **65**:82-84, Apr. 1965.

11. Henderson, Virginia. The nature of nursing. *Am.J.Nurs.* **64:**62-68, Aug. 1964.
12. Etzioni, Amitai. Human beings are not very easy to change after all. *Sat.Rev.* **55:**45-47, June 3, 1972.
13. Stein, L. I. The doctor-nurse game. *Am.J.Nurs.* **68:**101-105, Jan. 1968.
14. Jacox, Ada. Collective action and control of practice by professionals. *Nurs.Forum* **10**(3):239-257, 1971.
15. Carlson, Sylvia. A practical approach to the nursing process. *Am.J.Nurs.* **72:**1589-1591, Sept. 1972.
16. Schell, P. L., and Campbell, A. T. POMR—not just another way to chart. *Nurs.Outlook* **20:**510-514, Aug. 1972.
17. Bennett, L. R. This I believe . . . that nursing may become extinct. *Nurs.Outlook* **18:**28-32, Jan. 1970.

COMPONENTS OF PLANNED FAMILY-CENTERED CARE

Kathryn Buchanan Luciano

Planned family-centered care suggests a multidimensional, global concept of nursing care that embraces the family in their entirety during the total experience of illness and hospitalization. It suggests that nursing care is carried out through a many faceted approach and that care is goal-directed toward the family's well-being.

Components of family-centered care are reflected in the philosophies of the nurse, the nursing service department, and the hospital. We must consider the nature of the child and his family in their reaction to the stress of illness; we must look at the nature of the nurse and the values she sees as important in her role; and we must look at the nature of the interaction between the nurse and the family. A philosophy of family-centered care gives recognition to the worth of the individual child as a member of a family. This also means significant family members are included in establishing objectives to meet the health care needs of this child. It implies a systematic approach to the identification and resolution of family needs, and it demands an environment conducive to therapeutic relationships.

We're talking, also, of *planned* family-centered care. A serious look at this reveals the necessity of providing much more than unlimited visiting hours, a familiar teddy bear, or a bath given by Mommy. But, first of all, why do—or should—nurses plan care? We often assume that because activities of a nursing unit are coordinated, they are planned. Are we managing nursing care based on what must be *done* in an eight-hour shift or what the patient *needs* in an eight-hour shift? Observations of nurses in some hospital settings often show that nursing care is carried out by functions required for groups of patients rather than by care needed for individual patients and families. This is evidenced by all the baths being given at one time, by meals and feedings being completed at one time, and a host of other care requirements finished for the sake of the work activity itself rather than according to the child's usual daily activities of living. This functional nursing care is planned to enable nurses to meet schedules, whereas the primary focus for planning should be on the child and the nature of the therapeutic relationship between nurses and families.

In placing the emphasis on planning for family-centered care, how can nurses best

Reprinted from Nursing Clinics of North America 7(1):41-52, March, 1972. Published by W. B. Saunders Company, Philadelphia.

accomplish what may appear to be idealistic? Planning for care that is family-centered involves the same process that occurs for any patient of any age. However, it is broader in scope because of the fragile nature of the child's response and adaptation to the hospital environment. All nursing care, if it is to be effective in meeting the needs of the child and family, must proceed according to specific, sequential steps. Professional nursing care involves the nurse's engaging "in a knowledgeable, purposeful series of thoughts and actions which can be referred to as the nursing process."[3] The steps of this process are assessment, planning, intervention, and evaluation. Such an approach is essential if we are to be able to manage the multiplicity of problems and needs that patients present.

Much information from the behavioral and physical sciences has rapidly descended upon us, and we must utilize this knowledge to achieve family-centered care. No longer can we function solely through the traditional use of doctors' orders, intuition, and procedure manuals, although these will continue to be necessary for total care planning. We must become increasingly independent in our roles as practitioners and incorporate into our daily activities the scientific foundations upon which professional nursing exists.

ASSESSMENT

The first step toward providing family-centered care is assessment. By definition assessment is the appraisal of a child's condition and includes such factors as mental status, emotional status, sensory perception, and motor ability.[6] Because we are concerned about family-centered care, an assessment of family members is also needed. Assessment is a step involving the collection of data about the ill child and his family, the completion of a nursing interview or history, the identification of nursing problems, and the formulation of prime nursing care goals.

Four resources are available for making an assessment: the patient, his family, members of the health team, and the medical record. The tools of assessment include observation—perceptions from all senses, communication and interviewing, and the devices or equipment that give physiologic data about the patient, such as the thermometer, stethoscope, and laboratory tests.[3]

Case study

Eddie Anderson was a 9-year-old boy admitted to a medical ward with a diagnosis of suspected renal disease. He was accompanied to the nursing unit by his parents. The nurse's immediate objectives in seeing this family were directed toward relieving some of the initial fears and anxieties and learning as much as she could about Eddie and his parents.

Her first focus of attention was Eddie. The child should always be the center of the nurse's attention if this is where the parents' attention is. A "head to toe" assessment of Eddie's physical condition revealed a small, pale, weak-appearing child. His body lacked good muscle tone and he seemed to prefer lying flat in bed rather than sitting up. His abdomen was slightly distended and he admitted having minor flank pain. Vital signs were within normal limits. Mr. and Mrs. Anderson remained at Eddie's bedside. There was minimal conversation between Eddie and his parents; each seemed engrossed in his own thoughts.

When the nurse learned this was Eddie's first hospitalization and also detected that his parents seemed reluctant to discuss this in front of Eddie, she directed conversation to learning about Eddie's usual home routines, such as his food likes and dislikes, preferred diversional activities, and other essential points. It's a rare child or parent who doesn't respond to questions about the home situation, and this family was no exception. Eddie and his parents were quite involved in telling the nurse exactly what he did as a 9-year-old. There was even some kidding and joking. Tension in all family members appeared to be reduced. The nurse also learned Eddie's mother would spend the nights and mornings with him while daytime and evening visits would be shared by his grandmother and sister. The parents indicated they wanted to be involved with the direct care of Eddie.

Parent interviews and the completion of a nursing history as soon as possible after admission are invaluable in establishing a therapeutic nurse-family relationship. This first meeting sets the tone for the family's perception of the hospitalization and their ability to cope with the stress of illness. The very fact that a nurse is personally concerned about a child gives parents the encouragement and understanding they need.

Later in the day the nurse found Eddie asleep and thought this was a good opportunity to learn more about his parents and their feelings. She was interested in knowing how Eddie was prepared for hospitalization, what the family's knowledge of Eddie's diagnosis was, and what other persons made up this family unit. She learned from Mrs. Anderson that Eddie was told he needed to go to the hospital so the doctors could find out why his "side" hurt and he wasn't going to the bathroom as usual. His only responding comment was to ask if his Mom and Dad would be able to stay with him. Mrs. Anderson added that a friend of Eddie's had been in the hospital a month before for a tonsillectomy and had returned home full of "blood and guts" stories. She thought these stories might have made Eddie more fearful of coming to the hospital.

The nurse attempted to reassure Mrs. Anderson by telling her the staff tried to involve the children and their parents in all treatments and procedures by explaining what they were for and if there would be any discomfort. Mrs. Anderson continued by saying Eddie's older sister and grandmother were also quite worried about him. Eddie was very close to his grandmother, who lived with the family.

On the basis of two rather short but purposeful conversations with the Anderson family, the nurse was able to assess the family's status and identify the overt nursing care problems and needs. This assessment provided the beginning information required to initiate a nursing care plan. Communication is an essential aspect of assessment for it is the tool for determining the needs of the family as well as the methods for meeting those needs in a way acceptable to the family. Interactions between nurse and family must produce an empathetic relationship. This means the nurse begins to see the family's point of view and understands the meaning and response of this particular life experience. Since assessment is an ongoing process, this step necessitates ongoing communication with the family if changing health care needs are to be identified.

PLANNING AND INTERVENTION

The second and third steps of the nursing process are planning and intervention. Planning for nursing care and the determination of suitable approaches to identified or anticipated family needs are the basic reasons for a pediatric nurse's existence. But what exactly is the nurse, as a professional responsible for independent judgment and actions, expected to do?

First of all, we need to consider the importance of having a primary nurse assigned the responsibility for planning the care *and* the accountability for the kind of nursing care given to a patient. Just as the physician is answerable for the level of medical care he provides, so should the nurse be answerable for her care. This is not to say that only one nurse participates in the giving of care. Rather, it means one nurse has the ultimate responsibility of planning and seeing that others also participate in the planning and follow-through.

The first component of assessment identifies the factors that will dictate nursing care. Once nursing care problems have been stated and validated, attention must be directed toward formulating nursing objectives with the ultimate goal of mental and physical well-being of the family in mind. Nursing actions or intervention to assist the family in attaining these goals must be prescribed. Nursing interventions include both the dependent and independent functions of nursing, which are (1) the giving of strength and comfort to assist families in coping with problems, (2) safe and efficient performance of nursing techniques, (3) creation of an environment conducive to maintaining family integrity and unity, (4) protection of the patient from danger, injury, or risk, (5) teaching to provide knowledge, understanding, and skills, and (6) counseling and socializing to develop a trusting, goal-directed relationship with the family.[3]

Without planned nursing intervention care becomes detached from a goal of moving the family toward wellness. The most we could hope to achieve would be support of the medical program and some inconsistent T.L.C. (tender loving care). Another problem frequently seen is the limited time available for the professional nurse to carry out her own therapeutic plan of care. She finds herself depending on others, who may be less skilled than she is, to implement this plan. Systematically planned nursing care can be written and shared with others so that all staff support those objectives formulated for the individual family.

Meaningful objectives must be realistic and should take into account the needs and resources of the family. For example, a nursing objective and approach for teaching a mother the steps of injection technique are usually attainable. However, if the mother is a slow learner, works outside the home, or is otherwise not totally responsible for the 24-hour care of her child, objectives and approaches must consider what is reality for this family. Sometimes it is necessary for nursing plans to include grandmothers, uncles, or neighbors.

Objectives must take time limits into account. Some short-term objectives can be achieved in a few hours or a few days and may only require a few family contacts. Long-term objectives are difficult to achieve if the child and family are not going to be under a nurse's care for a significant period of time. Immediate or supporting goals should be set toward reaching a long-range objective. For example, an ultimate objective for a patient to effectively manage the outcome of diagnostic procedures will necessitate some short-range goals, such as his being able to understand the need and preparation for diagnostic procedures and to cope with the stress of the procedures. It is important to remember, also, that an ultimate goal of family well-being should not be lost sight of. Both the family and the nurse should recognize progress as short-term, contributing goals are reached.

Another consideration is the amount of family participation allowed. Maximum involvement of the child and his family is desirable to gain their cooperation with the plan of care and determine what is realistic. However, there are times when the child's or family's physical or mental condition or lack of knowledge for goal-setting restricts their involvement. For example, the parents of a child recently diagnosed as having cystic fibrosis will need to depend upon the nurse for setting short-term goals to prevent infection and to promote chest drainage. As the family's knowledge of the disease increases, their participation will be a prerequisite to effective care planning.

Objectives will determine the nursing approaches to be prescribed for the child and his family. Decisions for nursing intervention must be based on the unique or individual needs presented by them. Routine, ritualistic nursing care must be avoided in favor of the child's response and ability to cope with the hospital experience. Planned nursing approaches become hypotheses to test for reducing a problem. If they prove to be effective in meeting nursing objectives, then they are incorporated into a nursing care plan.[3]

The process of planning for family-centered care that is designed to meet health care needs must embody a multidiscipline approach. The talents and knowledge of health team members must be utilized so that planning and intervention coincide with demonstrated family needs and problems. It is a professional responsibility for the nurse to recognize the scope of problems that are best managed by allied health personnel, such as social workers, schoolteachers, physical therapists, occupational therapists, dietitians, and others. It is just as important that the nurse recognize her own limitations with family problems and seek advice and help from appropriate disciplines. Again in the case of a child with cystic fibrosis, the assessment and intervention of a physical therapist can be extremely meaningful to a nurse planning care that will include postural drainage. The assistance of the therapist will enable the nurse to meet the 24-hour needs of the patient for chest drainage.

A health team approach implies, also, that members talk together and plan together for goal-directed care. This should avoid fragmentation of care and prevent everyone from "doing their own thing." The nurse may often have to assume the coordinator role for the health team. Part of individualized care planning is the coordination and dovetailing of hospital services. Nursing is the only service constantly involved with direct patient care, and the effective utilization of health care services has to originate at the nursing unit level.

Case study

Like most children admitted to a hospital, Eddie Anderson was full of fear and anxiety, not knowing why he was so sick or what was going to happen to his body. His parents had an orientation to the hospital environment based on their own previous experiences, and this influenced their feelings and perceptions about this contact with health personnel. The ability of this family to withstand this stress of illness depended a great deal on the nurse. It is the nurse who stands between the family and the hospital environment. It is the nurse who is in the position to insure that physical care and emotional support make it possible for the family to cope with this experience of illness.

The reduction of anxiety and the maintenance of daily living routines were seen as immediate nursing goals for the Anderson family. Nursing intervention was planned on the basis of the initial assessment step and additional information obtained from other members of the health team. The nurse learned from the physician that Eddie was scheduled for an intravenous pyelogram the day after admission. A renal biopsy was to be performed two or three days later, and several laboratory tests

---

NURSING CARE PLAN

Nursing problem	Nursing approach
1. Eddie's first hospitalization (recently exposed to "horror" stories). Apprehensive.	1. Mother will stay at night and early morning. Grandmother & father will visit in evening. Encourage Eddie to verbalize fears; explain tests to him.
2. Admitted for diagnostic tests. Family apprehensive about scheduled tests. GOAL: To assist the family to cope with the stress of diagnostic procedures.	2. Allow family to express their feelings. Interpret tests after determining what M.D. told them.
3. Eddie: L flank area tender. Easily fatigued. Poor oral intake since onset of illness. *Food likes:* all juices, tacos, Rice Krispies, hot dogs. *Dislikes:* most vegetables, oatmeal, pork. GOAL: To maintain fluid and electrolyte balance with least expenditure of energy.	3. Allow Eddie to set his own pace. Mother will bring in books and games. Offer favorite juices q 2 °. Offer favorite foods but don't push. Family manages well in getting Eddie to eat. Monitor intake and output.
4. D.A.L.: bath, prayers at H.S., no violent TV shows.	4. Grandmother will manage his bath and prayers.

were ordered. A review of the history and physical examination form revealed that Mrs. Anderson's 16-year-old sister had died of glomerulonephritis four years ago. Eddie's sister and parents were in good health; his 66-year-old grandmother had some residual effects from a cerebral vascular accident occurring last year.

Eddie's physical examination revealed a loss of weight over the past month, easy fatigue, decreased urine output, and other findings suggestive of renal disease. Recording also included the fact that Eddie was usually an active, bright child who performed well in school.

Planning for family-centered care necessitates the setting of priorities for attention and care. All planning should consider the realities of staffing, the abilities of personnel giving patient care, and the most urgent needs of the child and his family. The nurse must decide what problems and needs the family can cope with themselves and which ones will require the assistance or intervention of the nurse.

Eddie's prime nursing care needs were concerned with preservation of physiologic systems and restoration of security and emotional well-being. His parents' prime needs were concerned with their understanding and feeling about the diagnosis of renal disease. Short-term goals for nursing intervention were determined, and these approaches were written into the care plan for use by all nursing personnel providing care to the family.

This particular care plan was prepared within a few hours after admission. It was expected that as other team members cared for Eddie and identified more needs, and as results of diagnostic tests were returned, his nursing care would change. Patients and families are never static, so their nursing care plans cannot be rigid and still remain effective.

Writing a care plan is no guarantee or final step in planning for continuity of care. Effective implementation of a family-centered approach to patient care demands not only that nurses familiarize themselves with family needs and problems but that they also follow through with written approaches. In Eddie's case, his usual activities of daily living included bedtime prayers, television restrictions, and evening baths. Nurses providing for these activities are working toward care planned to meet Eddie's needs; ignoring these activities as nonessential to Eddie's security results in mechanical care that is anything but individualized.

Effective nursing care planning involves the use of "tools" to assist the nurse in determining appropriate nursing interventions. The tools of assessment can be used on an ongoing basis for planning and intervention. The most important and dynamic tool is communication. Nurses find themselves constantly in conversation with other nurses, physicians, laboratory personnel, dietitians, social workers, and any number of other hospital personnel. The point here is the nature of all this communication and what the end result should be.

Planning for Eddie's care involved communications with radiology, laboratory, and dietary personnel and other nurses. Because a need to conserve energy had been identified for Eddie, his laboratory and radiology tests were scheduled for early morning when he would be well rested. The fact that his mother would be present in the morning was also a determining factor. A rest period was planned when Eddie returned to his room, and this subsequently provided him with necessary energy to sit up and eat lunch. How often do we see sleep periods, meal hours, and play activities interrupted for examinations, medications, tests and procedures? When are we going to review our planning and coordination of patient care so that it is more in keeping with the needs of the child and family and what they are able to tolerate?

Communication among nurses in both verbal and written form is of paramount importance if care is to see some continuity and be individualized. Nurses' notes and change-of-shift reports must reflect progress made toward achieving family goals. Nursing and health team conferences, both formal and informal, must be meaningful and directed toward creative patient care planning. Eddie's nursing care during his first 24 hours in the hospital was provided by a total of six nursing personnel. The need for communication is apparent in order that care be given on a continuous basis.

The results of Eddie's intravenous pyelogram were inconclusive and a renal biopsy was scheduled for his third hospital day. The family seemed to accept this since the need for a series of tests had already been discussed. Nurses made themselves available for preparation of the family and to allow for their expression of concerns and feelings. A short-term goal was established, namely that the Anderson family should know what to expect during Eddie's postoperative period. Nursing intervention included: (1) active listening to the family's verbalization about the renal biopsy and determining their perceptions of the physician's description of the operative procedure, (2) explaining the preoperative preparation to the family, and (3) explaining what could be expected postoperatively.

Preparing for surgery with the entire family (Eddie's sister was also present) enabled the nurse to focus on the family as a unit. The renal biopsy was a family event and a procedure affecting the mental and emotional status of each member. Exploring surgery with the family allows them the opportunity to react to it as a group and to utilize previously determined coping mechanisms. Eddie was also in a position to behave as he saw fit since he was within a supportive environment. His most intense fears of surgery included not being able to wake up and seeing a lot of blood, as his friend Tommy experienced after his tonsillectomy. Both the nurse and his parents were able to tell him that he would wake up and that he would be looked at frequently to make sure there wasn't any blood.

EVALUATION

Evaluation is the phase of the nursing process in which the nurse learns whether the nursing intervention hypothesized to meet the family's needs actually did meet those needs.[3] Nurses need to look critically at the care they plan and give in terms of its contribution to family well-being. If planned assessment and intervention are not practiced, the nurse has no basis on which to judge the effectiveness of her care.

The professional nurse has an obligation to the family, to the hospital, and to her profession to measure and document observable indications that nursing care was successful or unsuccessful in meeting preestablished goals. Nurses are continually being asked to define their role and its place within the other healing professions. Failure to evaluate care given by nurses is failure to seek both improved methods of family-centered care and increased autonomy in nursing.

Planning and intervention are not always successful in achieving goals related to the needs and problems of a family. Should nursing actions not meet the needs of the child or family, the nurse reassesses the situation and plans new approaches to the problems until the care does gratify the need.[3] This systematic approach to patient care and the recording of findings should contribute to the advancement of nursing practice and the achievement of family-centered care.

The only way to determine whether nursing actions taken have been effective is to observe the child's and family's responses. Using the tools of assessment, it is possible for nurses at least to notice obvious changes in the patient's condition or in family behavior. For example, observation of a child's physical condition will reveal whether nursing measures to insure an adequate fluid intake were successful. A plan to teach parents injection technique may be evaluated by observing the parents' return demonstration. Nursing interventions aimed at decreasing apprehension may be evaluated on the basis of the family's verbalization of feelings and their degree of orientation to reality.

When we think of the multiplicity of problems presented by the hospitalized child and his family, it seems very important that nursing begin to build a foundation on which to practice and plan care designed to meet the unique needs of a family. This can be done only by establishing criteria for nursing care. These criteria should be observed for the purpose of proving or disproving prescribed nursing actions. However, the uniqueness of families in their response to illness must determine the content of the nursing care plan. When care plans are found to be interchangeable among patients, then we are not adhering to the current concept of individualized care. Although commonalities are found to exist among patients, for example age, disease, and sex, the essence of nursing care is in knowing patients and families well enough to plan for care centered around them. An evaluation of the nursing care plan permits the nurse to judge herself as providing group-oriented or family-oriented nursing care.

Case study

The evaluation phase of Eddie's care was concerned with observing the response to the nursing intervention planned for him and his family. It was a step necessary to determine if the short-range goals had been achieved. The reality of most busy pediatric wards is that nurses are available to identify and meet most of the obvious problems while many covert needs go unnoted. Hopefully, the concept of a primary nurse ultimately responsible for care planning might increase the depth of a family assessment.

The initial steps of assessment, planning, and intervention dealt with the obvious needs of the Anderson family. Nursing approaches were aimed at reducing anxiety in the family members, providing care consistent with Eddie's usual home routines, and promoting physical comfort with a minimum expenditure of energy.

Specific responses observed and documented by nurses participating in his care included such things as these: (1) Eddie's oral intake improved. Rest periods prior to mealtimes gave him the needed strength to sit up and eat. On two occasions he was able to enjoy dinner with his family in the cafeteria. (2) There were no complaints of flank pain. The fact that this was identified as a problem on the care plan made personnel more aware of how they moved and touched Eddie. (3) The postoperative period was successful, with the family understanding and cooperating with the bed rest limitations and urine collections. (4) The family functioned as a unit. Eddie's parents, grandmother, and sister were frequent visitors with Mrs. Anderson staying all night. Care routines were planned with the family in mind and were mutually agreed upon by family and personnel. (5) Eddie seemed comfortable in his surroundings. This did not mean he really accepted and liked the hospital, but he began to develop some trust in the nursing staff. (6) Other family members looked to the nurses for support. They were able to verbalize their feelings and to ask questions, especially of the primary nurse.

These observations represent the evaluation of Eddie's first three or four days in the hospital. Although he remained a sick little boy, the beginnings of goal-directed care were established, and the goals established were planned and agreed upon between the family and the nurse.

SUMMARY

Family-centered nursing is a multi-dimensional approach to pediatric care. A systematic nursing process must be utilized to meet the dynamic needs of the hospitalized child and his family. Interventions must be planned on the basis of the family's perceptions about the child's illness and treatment and their ability to cope with this life experience. Nursing care activities need to be family-oriented, individualized, and coordinated. The implementation of family-centered care can offer the pediatric nurse a tremendous feeling of satisfaction by providing feedback and meaning to her goal-directed care.

REFERENCES

1. Komorita, Nori: Nursing diagnosis. Am. J. Nursing, 63:83-86, Dec., 1963.
2. Kron, Thora: Communication in Nursing. Philadelphia, W. B. Saunders Co., 1967.
3. Lewis, Lucile: This I believe . . . about the nursing process—key to care. Nursing Outlook, 16:26-29, May, 1968.
4. Linde, Shirley: When children need their parents most. Today's Health, 46:26-30, June, 1968.
5. Little, Dolores, and Carnevali, Doris: Nursing Care Planning. Philadelphia, J. B. Lippincott Co., 1969.
6. McCain, Faye: Nursing by assessment—not intuition. Am. J. Nursing, 65:82-84, April, 1965.
7. McPhetridge, L. Mae: Nursing history: One means to personalize care. Am. J. Nursing, 68:68-75, Jan,, 1968.
8. Petrillo, Madeline: Preventing hospital trauma in pediatric patients. Am. J. Nursing, 68:1469-1473, July, 1968.
9. Walker, Virginia: Nursing and Ritualistic Practice. New York, The Macmillan Co., 1967.
10. Zimmerman, Donna S., and Gohrke, Carol: The goal-directed nursing approach: It does work. Am. J. Nursing, 70:306-310, Feb., 1970.

THE GOAL-DIRECTED NURSING APPROACH: IT DOES WORK

Donna Stulgis Zimmerman and Carol Gohrke Blainey

The ever enlarging scope of nursing responsibilities has led us to a confrontation with routinized care.

We need to use a systematic approach to planning patient care, based on a scientific foundation, if we are to attack the multiplicity of problems which patients present. Such an approach is a process which encompasses four phases: assessment, goal setting and planning, implementation, and evaluation.

During the *first phase* all members of the nursing team, in cooperation with the professional nurse, gather information or data about the patient from all available resources. This information includes the patient's normal functioning, his present status, and tentative goals for his future level of function. The form of this assessment may involve one or more approaches. For example, the nurse may decide to assess the functioning of bodily systems; that is, she may ask herself, what is the patient's ability to exchange oxygen and carbon dioxide via the respiratory system? The nurse might also employ an assessment of the patient's activities of daily living, such as his sleep pattern.

Another approach might be a "head to toe" assessment. In this approach, general observations of the patient's condition are noted, as well as more specific ones. For example, the nurse would note the general signs and symptoms of fatigue as well as the specific sign of atrophy of the lower leg musculature.

The collected information is then organized and utilized in the identification of nursing problems. We define a nursing problem as a patient's need or potential need. Concomitant with the identification of the patient's needs is the setting of realistic goals for the resolution of the problem.

The *second phase* involves utilizing the collective knowledge and experience of all members of the nursing team and gathering current scientific information related to the identified problem. To illustrate, an assessment of a bedfast patient might include the aide's observation that the patient lies on his back without alteration of position for periods of up to four hours. This observation, coupled with additional data about the patient's age, nutritional status, and skin condition, would lead the nurse to define the problem as "maintenance of skin integrity and prevention of decubitus ulcers."

Scientific information which relates to decubitus ulcer formation has indicated that continuous pressure of one hour's duration causes beginning tissue breakdown.[1,2] Having determined this and gathered other information, this leads to the *third phase:* implementing nursing actions. For the problem described above, an action derived from the literature might be to turn the patient every hour, utilizing all four of his body surfaces in succession. In this third phase, careful communication and teaching are necessary to interpret the plan of care to all nursing team members involved in the patient's care.

The *final phase* of the process involves evaluating the effectiveness of the nursing action based on specific criteria. In the case of preventing decubitus ulcers, the criteria might include absence of redness and breaks in the skin. The appearance of these signs and

Reprinted from American Journal of Nursing **70**(2):306-310, 1970. Copyright The American Journal of Nursing Company.

symptoms would indicate a need for revision of therapy. This emphasizes the ongoing nature of this process.

This method of planning nursing therapy is applicable to patients wherever they are on the health continuum and in varying environments. The application of this process is illustrated by presentation of a patient with a diagnosis of systemic lupus erythematosus. This patient with a somewhat obscure diagnosis was chosen purposely to emphasize that it is not solely the patient's medical diagnosis that dictates nursing care. Rather, nursing care is determined by the needs manifested by the particular individual.

Prior to her illness, Mrs. W., a small, thin 28-year-old wife and mother, was an active participant in such activities as bowling, skiing, and sewing. On the first encounter with Mrs. W. one saw a pale, lethargic woman with a flat facial expression. With further inspection, we found diffuse symmetrical muscle wasting, sacral, foot, and ankle edema, and moderate abdominal distention.

While Mrs. W. presented a multiplicity of needs, only two—weakness and elimination—were selected to illustrate the use of the process, as well as the interrelationship of the patient's needs and the nurse's role in reinforcing the contributions made by other members of the health team. Other problems that Mrs. W. manifested which are not dealt with in this discussion included susceptibility to thrombus formation, alteration of body image and role, beginning formation of sacral decubitus ulcers, generalized edema and fluid and electrolyte disturbances secondary to impaired renal function. Problems of short-term duration that were resolved included diarrhea secondary to antacid therapy, with its associated fluid and electrolyte imbalance.

PROBLEM: WEAKNESS

Assessment. The first encounter with Mrs. W. suggested the likelihood of weakness as a possible problem. This led to the collection of additional information beyond the initial observation of lethargy and muscle wasting, with the purpose of validating or ruling out the presence of this problem.

On further investigation, it was learned that Mrs. W. had been on bed rest and steroid therapy for two months prior to this hospitalization. Yet, when she entered the hospital, Mrs. W. was encouraged to ambulate within her ability. Specific observations revealed interference with activities requiring minimal exertion. For example, she was unable to rise unaided from a sitting to a standing position and was unable to gradually lower herself back to a sitting position. Once erect, although she was able to walk, her walking was limited to a distance of 10 feet before she had to rest. When asked about her minimal activity even in bed, Mrs. W. stated, "Even turning to my side is exhausting." She also expressed frustration at not being able to do "the everyday things in life." The findings of an electromyelogram confirmed myopathy secondary to steroid therapy and the disease process.

In assessing Mrs. W.'s strengths, we noted that she was capable of some activities of daily living and had full range of motion in all her joints. The tentative goal formulated for her was the strengthening of muscles of the abdominal girdle and the extremities to minimize her frustration and to maximize her independence.

Planning. In an effort to find a scientific basis for intervention in this problem, we investigated literature on the causes and treatment of weakness and associated fatigue.

Muscle weakness in this patient was attributed to three factors: the disease process, prolonged bed rest, and steroid therapy. Data from 15 autopsies of persons who had lupus erythematosus revealed that 73 percent manifested muscle degeneration.[3] An earlier reference demonstrated a distinct relationship between immobilization and muscle strength, particularly in immobilized leg muscles.[4] Finally, we learned that muscle weakness from steroids is most prominent in the limbs and the abdominal musculature, to the point that activities requiring these muscles are hampered.[5]

In the area of nursing intervention for weakness, exercise has been cited as being most beneficial. Therefore, we investigated the uses of isometric exercises, since these exercises require less energy expenditure and equipment and can be supervised independently by nursing personnel.

A further basis for selecting isometric exercises was the fact that the patient was currently receiving isotonic exercises five times a week from a physical therapist. One study had demonstrated that isometric contraction of the forearm flexor muscle for six seconds twice daily resulted in increased muscle strength of from 17 to 20 percent.[6] Other findings from patients on bed rest for 60 days showed that a regimen of isometric exercises was sufficient to counteract the detrimental consequences of bed rest and inactivity.[7] Although exercise is recognized as therapy for weakness, it has been noted that prolonged and strong contraction of a muscle leads to muscle fatigue.[8]

Implementation. Nursing actions were directed toward (1) providing supplementary exercise, (2) facilitating movement in bed, and (3) preventing weakness and fatigue from overexertion. Mrs. W. was given written instructions and demonstrations, and then she redemonstrated, herself, the isometric exercises for the musculature of the arms, legs, and abdomen. She was helped to do these exercises twice a day on weekdays and three times a

ACTIVITY SCHEDULE FOR MRS. W.

Time	Activity
7:30	Awaken, void, wash face and hands T.P.R., weigh
7:45	*Rest*
8:15	Breakfast
9:15	Ambulate to B.R.; brush teeth
9:30	*Rest*
10:00	Physical therapy
11:00	*Rest*
12:00 noon	Lunch
12:30	*Rest*
1:00	Bath, linen change
2:00	*Rest*
2:30	Isometric exercises
2:45	*Rest*
3:30	Occupational therapy
4:15	*Rest*
5:00	Dinner
5:30	*Rest*
7:00	Visiting hours
8:30	Isometric exercises
9:00	Prepare for sleep, wash, brush teeth, massage
9:30	In bed for night

day on weekends when physical therapy was not available. Mrs. W. expressed satisfaction in doing these exercises, saying, "This is one thing I can do on my own to help myself."

As an additional means to encourage exercise and independence with less exertion, a trapeze and footboard were applied to her bed. In an effort to avoid overexertion, a schedule of daily activities was arranged with Mrs. W., including meals, exercises, physical therapy, and rest periods (see p. 168). Since physical therapy was available only in the mornings, it was agreed with Mrs. W. to schedule her bath after lunch to prevent overexertion.

Evaluation. Several measures were selected to evaluate the effectiveness of the nursing actions directed toward strengthening Mrs. W.'s musculature. These criteria included the following: (1) the distance Mrs. W. could walk, (2) the amount of assistance required by Mrs. W. to come to a standing or sitting position, (3) the consistency with which she performed the isometric exercises, (4) the frequency of use of the trapeze and footboard as a means to alter positions, and finally, (5) the incidence of frustration she expressed related to muscle weakness.

After six weeks with this plan in action, and despite further progression of her pathophysiology, Mrs. W. was able to walk unassisted for distances of up to 100 feet. Further, she was capable of standing and sitting without assistance, although this was not done with ease. She did the isometric exercises regularly, although at times she did require reminding and encouragement. She used the trapeze to assist herself in moving in bed and in coming to a sitting position. As Mrs. W.'s muscle strength increased, her comments related to frustration with the inability to perform daily tasks decreased.

While it is impossible to differentiate the contributions made by physical therapy and nursing, we believe that Mrs. W. would not have achieved this level of functioning without the supplementary nursing action.

PROBLEM: INADEQUATE ELIMINATION

Assessment. The problem of bowel elimination was manifested on admission by Mrs. W.'s complaints of constipation and inability to defecate. She reported that prior to her illness, she had had a daily bowel movement approximately 45 minutes after breakfast. She denied a history of constipation or diarrhea related to stress.

During her hospitalization, Mrs. W. was encouraged to use the toilet in the private bathroom adjoining her room. There, she was able to maintain an upright position but, because of her abdominal muscle weakness, she was unable to bear down with sufficient force to expel a stool of normal consistency.

Due to the problem of weakness, this patient spent the majority of her time in bed, and this in itself is known to decrease bowel motility. As a result of the additional problem of edema, Mrs. W.'s fluid intake was restricted to one liter a day.

Compounding the intake limitation was the fact that Mrs. W. was reluctant to take even this amount of fluid without encouragement. Her fluid intake was predominantly apple juice, ginger ale, and milk. She was receiving Colace (dioctyl sodium sulfosuccinate) 100 mg. daily which was given at 9 A.M., and milk of magnesia 30 cc. with cascara sagrada 5 cc. p.r.n. at bedtime to help alleviate her constipation.

In the assessment, Mrs. W.'s nutritional patterns were examined and a strength noted in that she consistently ate all of her general, low sodium diet. We assumed that Mrs. W. was receiving adequate bulk, since her stools were of normal size.

Planning. The long-term goal for Mrs. W.'s elimination was that she return to her normal defecation pattern of a daily bowel movement after breakfast. Collection of information related to bowel elimination again provided the guides to nursing action. It is well known that mass peristaltic movements from the upper intestines cause distention of the rectum and the urge to defecate. However, unless this urge is responded to in a few minutes it will disappear, leading to an accumulation of the wastes and constipation. Further, mass peristaltic movements usually occur after breakfast, and adequate fluid intake is essential to the prevention and treatment of constipation.[9] It is also suggested that the gastrocolic reflex may be augmented by hot coffee or warm water.[10]

The act of defecation requires the assistive contraction of several abdominal muscles as well as the contraction of the muscles of the pelvic floor.[11] Leaning forward from the hips while in a sitting position also assists in raising the intra-abdominal pressure. Others have concluded that regular abdominal exercises will enhance an individual's ability to "bear down," thus assisting with defecation.[10,12]

Yasuna, in studying stool softeners and laxatives, concluded that the primary action of stool softeners is that of decreasing the surface tension of the bowel. The peak action of stool softeners occurs six to eight hours after ingestion, whereas the peak action of milk of magnesia and cascara sagrada occurs approximately eight hours after ingestion. In conclusion, he suggests that if laxatives are given in combination with stool softeners, they should be administered at times that will allow their peak actions to coincide, so that the strong propulsive movements will occur in combination with the decreased surface tension.[13] The time-honored use of prunes and figs was also suggested as an adjunct.[10]

Implementation. Nursing actions focused on the following four areas: (1) taking advantage of mass peristaltic movements, (2) increasing intra-abdominal pressure, (3) increasing fluid intake within the ordered limitations, and (4) utilizing the complementary actions of the laxatives and the stool softener.

Mrs. W. was already including hot coffee with her breakfast, and prune juice was substituted for the morning apple juice. Forty minutes after breakfast she was assisted to the bathroom. We discussed with her the importance of heeding the stimulus to defecate and she was encouraged to call immediately for assistance whenever she felt the urge to evacuate.

Once positioned on the toilet, she was instructed to place her hands over her abdomen and lean forward from the hips in order to increase her intra-abdominal pressure. The nursing personnel remained with her when it was necessary to help her maintain this position. Mrs. W.'s isometric abdominal exercises also helped her with this problem and, in addition, she was encouraged to move in bed using the trapeze to increase the strength of her pelvic girdle musculature.

The desirability of having the peak actions of the stool softener and laxative coincide was discussed among the nursing personnel. As a result, it was agreed that the daily order of Colace would be given at 10 P.M. rather than the routine time of 9 A.M., since the milk of magnesia and cascara were given at bedtime. This enabled the peak actions of the medications to coincide at approximately the time of the morning meal when mass peristaltic movements are most likely to occur. This time was consistent with her normal bowel pattern.

Evaluation. We used two criteria to evaluate the success of nursing interventions: (1) that Mrs. W.'s bowel evacuation pattern returned to her prehospital evacuation pattern, and (2) that her stools should be of soft, formed consistency.

NURSING CARE PLAN

Problem/Goal	Nursing Actions
Weakness	1. Isometric exercises for arms, legs and abdomen b.i.d. 2:30 p.m. and 8:00 p.m.—remind and encourage patient.
Goal: decrease frustration, maximize independence	2. Physical therapy Monday through Friday 10 a.m. 3. Encourage use of footboard and trapeze. 4. Avoid rushing patient with *any* activity. 5. Observe planned rest periods—do not interrupt patient. 6. Follow planned schedule of activities—do not awaken until 7:30 a.m.
Inadequate bowel elimination	1. Encourage fluid consumption up to 1 liter limit 7-3 700 cc 3-11 250 cc 11-7 50 cc. 2. See that prune jce. and *hot* coffee included on breakfast tray.
Goal: return to normal defecation pattern	3. Assist patient to B.R. 40 minutes p̄ breakfast. 4. Positioning on toilet: assist patient to lean forward from hips while she applies external pressure over abdomen with hands. 5. Isometric exercise of abdomen as noted above. 6. Colace 100 mgm. 10 p.m., MoM 30 cc c̄ Cascara 5 cc @ 9 p.m. Evaluate need before giving.

For the first two weeks following the institution of these measures, little improvement of the problem was seen. However, after the third week, as Mrs. W.'s state of weakness began to show improvement with the concomitant increase in strength of the abdominal musculature, gradual improvement was observed. At this point, Mrs. W. was having daily, loose, semiformed stools, with the administration of Colace, milk of magnesia, and cascara each night. At the end of six weeks, Mrs. W. was able to have formed stools with the daily intake of prune juice but without the use of laxatives or stool softeners. The frequency of the stools varied from daily to every other day.

SUMMARY

It is our belief that the effectiveness of nursing care for this patient was enhanced by the utilization of a systematic process of assessment, goal setting, planning, implementation, and evaluation. Nursing care based solely on intuition or on routine carries no assurance that the individual needs of each patient will be met. This is not to imply that the nurse does not utilize her knowledge of specific disease entities and the associated nursing care. For example, in caring for a patient with external bile drainage following a cholecystectomy and common bile duct exploration, the nurse relies on her knowledge of the purpose, function, and location of the T-tube to guide observation and nursing care. Though the diagnosis is different, this patient might also manifest problems of weakness and inadequate bowel elimination similar to those of Mrs. W. Thus, if the nurse's focus is limited solely to nursing care as it relates to the cholecystectomy, it is probable that other needs will go undetected.

It is also our belief that the implementation of such a process promotes greater satisfaction for nursing personnel on all levels. A major strength is the goal-directedness of nursing care, and the fact that the nurse can use measurable criteria to demonstrate her contribution to the patient's well-being.

REFERENCES

1. Kosiak, Michael. Etiology of decubitus ulcers. Arch. Phys. Med. **42:**19, Jan. 1961.
2. Kottke, F. J., and Blanchard, R. S. Bedrest begets bedrest. Nurs. Forum **3**(3):59, 1964.
3. Lowman, E. W. Muscle, nerve and synovial changes in lupus erythematosus. Ann. Rheumat. Dis. **10:**19, Mar. 1951.
4. Deitrick, J. E., and others. Effects of immobilization upon various metabolic and physiologic functions of normal men. Amer. J. Med. **4:**18, Jan. 1948.
5. Harrison, T. R., and others, eds. Principles of Internal Medicine. 5th ed. New York, McGraw-Hill Book Co., 1966, p. 1315.
6. Hislop, Helen J. Quantitative changes in human muscular strength during isometric exercise. J. Amer. Phys. Ther. Ass. **43:**38, Jan. 1963.
7. Brannon, E. W., and others. Influence of specific exercises in the prevention of debilitating musculoskeletal disorders. Aerospace Med. **34:**905, Oct. 1963.
8. Guyton, A. C. Textbook of Medical Physiology. 3d ed. Philadelphia, Pa., W. B. Saunders Co., 1966, p. 99.
9. Bockus, H. L. Gastroenterology. 2d ed. Philadelphia, Pa., W. B. Saunders Co., 1964, Vol. 2, pp. 627-628.
10. Palmer, E. D. Clinical Gastroenterology. New York, Harper and Brothers, 1957, pp. 339-340.
11. Fuerst, Elinor, and Wolff, Luverne E. Fundamentals of Nursing. 3d ed. Philadelphia, Pa., J. B. Lippincott Co., 1964, p. 311.
12. Harmer, Bertha. Textbook of the Principles and Practices of Nursing. 5th ed. Revised by Virginia Henderson. New York, Macmillan Co., 1958, p. 436.
13. Yasuna, A. D., and Halpern, Alfred. Timed integration of stool hydration and peristaltic stimulation in constipation correction. Amer. J. Gastroenter. **28:**539, Nov. 1957.

CARE OF A DEPRESSED MEDICAL-SURGICAL PATIENT

Anita Havens

Mrs. R. was a 71-year-old patient from whom I learned the importance of a problem-solving approach to a problem that impedes many patients' return to health—depression.

I had cared for Mrs. R. at two different intervals. The first time, she was being treated for a myocardial infarction. She was then discharged to a recuperative home for further rehabilitation, but before she was able to leave the home she fell, fractured her hip, and was readmitted to the hospital for a hip nailing. At this time, I was again assigned to her care. Her discomfort and immobility were intensified by decubitus ulcers on the left buttock and both heels of her feet. She also had diabetes mellitus and glaucoma.

IDENTIFYING THE PROBLEM

It was not until Mrs. R.'s readmission that I detected any signs of depression. During her previous hospitalization, she had needed minimal support and encouragement; she had seemed very determined to recover. After her readmission, however, she seemed like quite a different person.

I readily observed signs which indicated the presence of depression: weariness, indecisiveness, a pessimistic outlook, feelings of sadness, hopelessness, emptiness, dissatisfaction, lack of belief that life can be worth living, frequent crying, inability to cope with small tasks, diminished appetite, complaints of fatigue, and increased desire for sleep with

Reprinted from American Journal of Nursing **70**(5):1070-1072, 1970. Copyright The American Journal of Nursing Company.

difficulty in staying asleep. Mrs. R.'s activities seemed flat, dull, and meaningless to her. She often verbalized a pessimistic attitude by saying she thought she would never get better, that she was not fit to go on living this way. She became frustrated during such small tasks as morning care and the use of the bedpan. At these times, she would become unable to cope with the situation and almost invariably began to cry. She lacked interest in her environment, became bored with the food, and awakened often during the night. Her diminished appetite and difficulty in sleeping had serious implications for her diabetes.

Mrs. R.'s depression was a problem for Mr. R. as well. Mrs. R. talked to me about one of his visits in which Mr. R. had become cross with her. It is not difficult for members of a family to become discouraged for lack of ways to support and encourage the patient.

Finally, Mrs. R.'s depression was also a problem for her nurses. I found it emotionally draining to constantly guard against becoming caught up in her depression. I also found difficult those moments when nothing I could do or say seemed to make a difference. It required much of my energy and imagination to answer her many calls for help in a truly empathetic and supportive manner.

In order to understand Mrs. R.'s depression and to formulate an approach to her care, it was necessary for me to consider the psychologic and sociologic factors which seemed to apply to her situation.

One authority says that depression is a response to a loss, actual, anticipated, or imagined, but always real and meaningful to the person.[1] I believe Mrs. R. was responding to the loss of physical health, one of the most real and meaningful things to anyone. This seemed evident each time she said, "I haven't been well in so long," and "I don't think I'll ever get my health back again." Mrs. R. grieved over the loss of her health and, I believe, became depressed in the process.

The same authority also says that depression comes when our expectations of the future become frustrated.[2] Mrs. R. had been recuperating from a myocardial infarction and was preparing to return home to her husband. She confided to me that she was anxious to return home for she missed him very much. When she fell and fractured her hip, and had to be readmitted to the hospital, her strongly felt expectations were shattered. This frustration of future expectations and the loss of health were, I believe, the major sources of her depression.

Sociologic factors also played a role, for Mrs. R. was Jewish. In a study entitled "Cultural Components in Response to Pain," Zborowski shows that a knowledge of group attitudes toward pain is extremely important to an understanding of individual reactions. He says that in his study the Jewish patient expressed his worries and anxieties to the extent that pain indicated a threat to his health.[3] Since Jewish persons are very health-centered, depression as a result of loss of health would be one of the symptoms to be expected in a Jewish patient.

Jewish patients are also very cure-oriented. Zborowski notes, ". . . the function of the pain reaction will be the mobilization of the efforts of the family and the doctor toward a complete cure. . . ."[4] This concern for a complete cure, so strong in Mrs. R., also played a part in producing her depression. She had diabetes and glaucoma, both of which are chronic conditions that can be controlled but not cured. Her myocardial infarction and fractured hip were conditions requiring long rehabilitation. Mrs. R. was very anxious to be able to walk again and she was impatient with the slow healing of her ulcers.

At times, when Mrs. R. became upset, and broke into tears or into moaning and sobbing, it was necessary for me to remember that members of the Jewish culture can be very emotional in their response to pain. Zborowski says that "both the Italians and Jews feel free to talk about their pain, complain about it and manifest their sufferings by groaning, moaning, crying, et cetera . . . they admit willingly that when they are in pain they do complain a great deal, call for help, and expect sympathy and assistance from other members of their immediate social environment. . . ."[5]

Gathering this related information was vital since it gave me the insight necessary to formulate a reasonable nursing care plan.

COURSE OF ACTION

In view of the information I had gathered, I began to formulate a plan of action to help Mrs. R. work through and handle her own depression. I realized that depression, like any other behavior, is an indication of a person's needs. I needed to recognize and give primary consideration to Mrs. R.'s needs and to keep from catching her feelings of helplessness in order to give her the support she needed.

My course of action contained three components: nursing intervention on my own behalf, nursing intervention on behalf of Mrs. R., and, at times, no intervention at all.

In order to help Mrs. R., I first had to identify and resolve some of my own feelings. From the beginning, I had no trouble in identifying with the patient's feelings. I felt that in her position, I, too, would have become very discouraged and pessimistic about the future. Perhaps one can overidentify, for I began to feel anxious and insecure about actually being able to help Mrs. R. How could I achieve the goals of my care plan when depression colored all of Mrs. R.'s words, actions, and reactions? I was frustrated. How could I use my time with her so that it would have maximum value for her?

From these feelings I knew I had two real needs: to achieve the goals set in my care plan, and to have faith: in my patient, that she could improve, and in myself, that I could help her. I knew that I had to set small immediate goals for my patient and to remember and believe in the determination she had demonstrated when I had cared for her previously. I also had to see my role as one of support and encouragement and to remember that it would take time for Mrs. R. to work through her depression.

After resolving some of my own feelings, I was in a better position to see the needs Mrs. R. expressed and to find the most effective ways to help her. Mrs. R. was partially immobile, so she needed to be somewhat dependent. However, she also needed small goals to fill her empty hopeless future. And, because of her Jewish background, she needed to be able to express her sufferings if and when she wished, and to feel that she was being treated and helped toward eventual recovery.

My intervention, therefore, was concerned with assistance that would help her help herself, with an attitude that was neither overly sympathetic or overly cheerful, and with reassurance that would direct her to the conclusion that success is possible, that her present state was being helped and would continue to be helped.

Finally, my course of action included no intervention at all. At times, I had to caution myself against trying to convince or persuade Mrs. R. of certain things. I had to remember to permit her to go at her own speed, to let her lead, to be cautious against forcing an issue and, at times, simply to permit her to drain off in tears or anger her depression and tension. I had to allow *her* to work through her own feelings, not to try to work them through for her.

NURSING ACTIVITY

In carrying out my plan of care, numerous nursing measures had to be tried.

Assistance. Comfort was of primary concern in caring for Mrs. R. Discomfort only heightened her suffering, thereby increasing her lack of desire to "go on living like this." When comfort measures were taken, such as pillow supports to keep pressure off the decubitus ulcers on her heels, her mood seemed to lift and she would remark, "Now, why didn't someone think of that all this time?"

Mrs. R. always complained about having to awaken so early for breakfast, for she was hardly awake enough to eat. Out of consideration for her feelings and because I knew she often had difficulty in getting to sleep and in staying asleep at night, I gave her time between breakfast and morning care for a short rest. This seemed to compensate a bit for the early breakfast.

I allowed her maximum independence in doing morning care, only washing her back and feet which she could not reach. Since the bedpan was so uncomfortable and irritating to her decubitus ulcer, she feared being left on it for very long. I always waited right outside the curtain for her to call me. Another time that assistance was very important was when Mrs. R. changed her position. Usually, she was able to do this on her own, but, at times, when she could not, she became frustrated to the point of tears. Helping her move about most efficiently, teaching her to use the trapeze and to use proper body mechanics in getting from bed to chair eliminated such frustrating occurrences.

The call bell close at hand and articles kept within Mrs. R.'s reach also prevented frustration. In addition, telling her the schedule for the day meant a great deal to Mrs. R. These measures of assistance helped her to keep trying. A little assistance when needed made her hopeless comment, "I can't go on any longer," less frequent.

Attitude. I tried to put Mrs. R.'s feelings first by letting her make some of the decisions. For example, I would say, "Would you like to rest now and do this later?" "Would you like to sit up for dinner or stay in bed?" "It's time to change your dressing now. Which side would be more comfortable for you to lie on while I change it?" Of course, when I gave her choices, I had to be prepared to accept her decision!

Listening was my main tool to convey an attitude of interest and understanding. I never ignored Mrs. R. or changed the subject when she verbalized her depression. I let her know that I understood her feelings and then I tried to suggest some other way of looking at things in order to try to pull her out of her depressed mood.

Now and then I made a point to sit with Mrs. R. just to chat and keep her company, since loneliness and boredom only add to an overall depression. In order to instill a feeling of self-esteem and of being needed, I questioned Mrs. R. about how her husband was getting along. When she said that he was tired of cooking and cleaning and that he had become cross with her, I commented that he missed her, that he was probably a little discouraged, and that he needed some support and encouragement from her.

Reassurance. I wanted to give Mrs. R. concrete reassurance and support so that she would have a more positive attitude toward her progress. When I took care of the decubitus ulcer on her buttock, I took advantage of this opportunity to explain how the treatment helped and to describe honestly the condition of the sore and its changes from day to day. I also instructed her about what she could do to hasten healing, namely, changing her position every two hours and eating meat and other high protein foods. I took an active interest in her rehabilitation at physical therapy, accompanying her when I could, praising her progress, and reminding her that this progress would be slow but steady. Since Mrs. R.'s roommate also had a fractured hip, I encouraged their relationship, not only as a source of company but also of support for one another. When the doctor approved, I asked the social worker to look for an opening for Mrs. R. in an extended care center. This measure helped Mrs. R. to look to the future and see the possibility of a change in her environment and a break in the monotony of her life.

Finally, there were times when I chose not to intervene at all, such as during some of Mrs. R.'s crying spells.

Sometimes her crying was "incongruous with the existing situation," sometimes very necessary, however, to drain off tension. At these times, I stayed with Mrs. R., but I said nothing to pacify her, for if such inner feelings are not allowed to be released, depression is only prolonged.[6,7]

EVALUATION OF PLAN

I had no pat list of techniques. Rather, I had to be constantly alert for opportunities to take measures toward my goals. I became more adept at this as I looked back on each day and evaluated how effectively I had handled each situation. My main guide was Mrs. R. herself. In considering her as an individual, I was able to judge what was and was not comforting and helpful to her. Since she had become better able to cope with her situation and to work through her depression, I believe my course of action was successful.

I learned that a problem-solving approach to patient care means considering the individual person in formulating and evaluating any plan of action and that when this is done, care will be effective.

REFERENCES

1. Neylan, Margaret P. Depressed patient. Amer. J. Nurs. **61**:77-78, July 1961.
2. *Ibid.,* p. 78.
3. Zborowski, Mark. Cultural components in response to pain. In Patients, Physicians and Illness, ed. by Gartly Jaco. Glencoe, Ill., Free Press, 1958, p. 257.
4. *Ibid.,* p. 263.
5. *Ibid.,* p. 262.
6. Ujhely, Gertrude B. When adult patients cry. Nurs. Clin. N. Amer. **2**:730, Dec. 1967.
7. Neylan, *op. cit.,* p. 78.

TALKING WITH PATIENTS

Hildegard E. Peplau

Talking with patients is easy when the nurse treats the patient as a chum and engages in a give-and-take of social chit-chat. But when the nurse sees her part in verbal interchanges with patients as a major component in direct nursing service, then she must recognize the

Reprinted from American Journal of Nursing **60**(7):964-966, 1960. Copyright The American Journal of Nursing Company.

complexity of the process. Social chit-chat is replaced by the responsible use of words which help to further the personal development of the patient.

It is this complexity which distinguishes the verbal part of the professional nurse's work from the verbal approach a layman might use toward a sick person. The layman most often is actually a friend or a member of the patient's family; the nurse is a stranger to the patient.

There are marked distinctions between a layman talking to a friend and a nurse talking to a stranger who is a patient. The role of friend has its own requirements. Friends trust each other, exchange confidences, advise each other, lend one another money. Since it takes time for friendship to develop, two friends learn enough about each other so that behavior becomes predictable to a degree; one friend will begin to take certain actions of the other for granted. Acceptance of such assumptions is often the basis of meaning on which conversation between two friends is built.

The nurse and patient are not friends; they are strangers to each other. If the nurse does not see the patient as a stranger, about whom she knows nothing but can learn much, then she is distorting the facts of the situation. She can distort in different ways. She might look upon the patient as a friend, seeking in him familiar elements that she has previously experienced with friends in other nonclinical situations. Or she can look upon the patient in light of her own need or wish to have friends, thus relating to him primarily to fulfill her own wishes. Such wishes for friends ought to be realized in the social life of the nurse outside the hospital. Another distortion is for the nurse to see the patient as a disease category. In this situation she searches only for familiar clinical signs which help her to feel able, and she misses the unfamiliar, the unique newness of the *person* who is a stranger.

When the nurse treats the patient as a friend, she puts herself in the role of friend to him. The actions of the friendship role come to be expected of the nurse by the patient. Often the nurse burdens the patient with her biography, even sharing her secrets or seeking advice about her personal affairs. The focus on the needs of the patient is lost. Many nurses rationalize their actions along these lines, saying "it is good for the patient to take his mind off himself." If this be the case there are innumerable nonpersonal subjects of common interest which might be a more useful focus for social conversations with patients than the personal life of the nurse.

When the nurse sees the patient as a stranger, her first verbal task is to help him get oriented to her, to the hospital, and to the tasks at hand. Here, the layman in the nurse often gets in the way. To get oriented to a stranger outside the hospital, most people use social chit-chat at first. The questions go something like this: "Where do you live, Mrs. Jones?" "Have you lived there long?" "Do you know Mrs. Smith down the street?" "She went to Jersey High School, did you?" "I did too; did you take cooking with Miss Main?" and so on. The process is largely one of locating common if elementary interests and experiences as a base from which friendship might later develop.

This approach works well among laymen. The professional nurse, however, is offering a direct and specialized experience from which, hopefully, the patient will learn something of lasting personal value with regard to health. The professional nursing focus is the needs of the patient. The relationship, if it is to be governed by sustained objectivity in the interest of the patient's learning, will be time-limited by the duration of the illness—it is a temporary, often brief relationship. The approach to the stranger must therefore be different in the nursing situation.

THE PATIENT IN FOCUS

When the focus is on the needs of the patient, then the time of the nurse must be used purposefully in the patient's interest. This is not to say that the nurse does not have needs. Of course she does, for she is human too. But her needs are met outside the sickroom. Inside the sickroom, the focus is on the patient.

In getting oriented to the nurse, the patient needs to know her name, he needs to know that she is a registered nurse, what she may be called upon to do, the time limits which govern the duration and frequency of his contacts with her, and what she will do with information which she gets from him.[1]

The patient may need validation of the self-evident. If he says "You have red hair" and the nurse has red hair, she can say "Yes, I do." But the patient does not need to know that all the women in the nurse's family for five generations back had red hair. If the patient notices a wedding ring on the nurse's finger and asks "Are you married," the nurse can reply "Yes, I am." But when she begins to describe the data and circumstances of the marriage this indicates pretty clearly that she is more interested in talking about herself than she is in the patient.

The nurse's biographical data is a burden to the patient who has no recourse but to translate the nursing situation into a social, chum-like one. Often the patient asks about the nurse's background primarily to test her capacity to focus on his needs and to find out whether she prefers instead to talk about herself. Since the patient must depend upon the nurse for many things, he will try to meet her needs so that he can feel safe with her. The nurse who can survive the patient's testing, and let him know clearly, simply, and directly that "this time is yours," will have offered the patient a unique experience with potential for learning.

Nurses should distinguish between a patient's demands and his needs. A demand is a request, a claim, or coercion to evoke some kind of response. In recognizing a need, on the other hand, the nurse draws her inference not only from such demands as the patient might make but also from her own observations and from other data.

A nurse does not meet the demands of a patient unless a valid need is represented in the demand. When a patient demands or asks persistently for biographical data from the nurse, she does not need to be pulled willy-nilly by these demands. She can say, quite simply, "Use this time to talk about you." Or she can ask gently, "What do you need this information for?" If the patient persists, the nurse might become more firm and ask, "Of what benefit to you would a review of my social life be?" or "I wonder what uses you would have for such personal information."

Of course, if the nurse is desperate for the patient's approval and uncertain about her professional role and its boundaries, then she will simply yield to the patient and answer any and all questions about her personal life. In a general hospital no great trauma will thereby accrue to the patient; only another opportunity for a patient to learn something of value about himself will have been missed. In psychiatric work, however, the nurse will have proved to the patient his belief that people are not interested in him—only in themselves.

If the nurse wishes to focus on the needs of the patient, then she must know how to

---

[1]Peplau, Hildegard E. Principles of psychiatric nursing. In American Handbook of Psychiatry, ed. by Silvano Arieti. New York, Basic Books, 1959, pp. 1840-1856.

listen and how to respond in ways that will further the patient's learning. There is a technique for creative listening. It is not just a matter of letting a patient ramble on as though the nurse had her hearing aid turned off. It is more like listening to music—for the themes and variations, for the nuances of meaning that are conveyed indirectly through sound or hint.

Teaching a nurse to listen can only be done in clinical seminars, where interfering factors in the individual can be revealed and looked at and, hopefully, deleted. But there are some general guidelines.

Patients frequently make such comments as "I'm not hungry," "I'm not sleeping," "I'm not feeling well," or "I'm not comfortable." In situations such as these the verbal response of the nurse should be used to help the patient describe what went on instead of opening further discussion of what did *not* occur. Comments such as "What did go on" (instead of sleep), "What do you feel," or "Are you saying you are uncomfortable" help the patient to think directly about what did happen or is occurring.

In these situations, the nurse often automatically asks "Why not?" More often than not a "why" question has an intimidating effect. It has a ring of familiarity and is frequently reminiscent of earlier experiences when mother or teacher reiterated "Why don't you do this" or "Why can't you tell me" or some similarly coercing "why" question. Moreover, if the patient knew why he wasn't hungry or sleeping or comfortable, he would most probably deal with the situation. A "why" question asks for reasons which the patient is not likely to know immediately. He can discover them with help. But, in order to discover them, the patient requires some raw data—he must recall, for example what actually went on, instead of sleep. The reasons can be generalized from these data; then the "why" question can be answered.

PERCEPTIVE DESCRIPTION

In order to understand the reasons for the patient's behavior, both the nurse and the patient must have descriptions of the patient's experience. Such descriptions are not as easy to secure as many nurses assume. A great many people are singularly lacking in skill, especially in describing personal perceptions of experience.

Many nurses themselves do not describe what they observe but record instead stereotyped clichés which condense and classify rather than describe their observations. Valuable data from which fresh insight about illness could be drawn are lost this way. Verbatim descriptions given by psychosomatic and psychiatric patients would provide nursing with a far more useful base for determining nursing practice than the current tendency to translate doctors' findings into nursing knowledge.

Such words as "what," "where," "when," and "who" will assist the nurse to elicit useful description. A few highly serviceable clichés like "Tell me about that," "Then what," "Go on," and "You will remember" will be convenient when a direct question seems inappropriate. Except in rare instances, the nurse will find patients eager to talk about themselves; when a patient is reluctant or definitely not eager, the nurse can show respect for privacy of thought and silently await initial comments from him.

Words such as "how" or "why" are quite challenging ones. Nurses who really consider their meaning use them sparingly. The nurse who asks a patient "How do you feel" really asks, in effect, "In what manner or by what process do you have a feeling?" It would be simpler and more direct to ask "What are your feelings this morning?" The phrase "how come" is a cliché that communicates even less about what the nurse is seeking. In general, "how" and "why" questions require the patient to analyze the data of his experience and to respond with a generalization about it.

QUESTIONS AND ANSWERS

A "how" question asks for the process, the operations, the steps by which something has occurred. A "why" question asks for reasons, causes, explanations, or conclusions. If a person has adequate information, and analytical abilities as well, then he can answer a "how" or a "why" question directly. If, on the other hand, a patient does not fulfill these two basic requirements, then a "how" or "why" question is a nonsense one which leaves him feeling inadequate, helpless, or powerless. The patient who is well educated and is quite aware of the cliché usage of "how" and "why" questions is more likely to consider as unknowing the nurse who uses these clichés.

One problem common to many patients in both general and psychiatric hospitals is the problem of self-identity; their answers to the question "who am I" have not yet been formulated. This problem is reflected in what the patient says. Through her responses, the nurse can further stalemate the patient in his struggle with this problem or she can assist in its solution. Self-identity is in part reflected in the use of personal pronouns. To speak for oneself requires use of such pronouns as "I," "me," "mine." When a patient speaks of himself as "you," or "one," the nurse ought to inquire about the referents. "You said 'one,' to whom does this refer?" In this way the nurse can help the patient to refer more directly to himself—to use the pronoun, "I."

TROUBLE WITH PRONOUNS

"We," "they," and "us" are similarly troublesome pronouns. Of course, there are group situations in which the group members know one another and, as "togetherness" evolves, they use "we," "us," or "they" to indicate they are speaking for others present or absent. When asked, "Whom do you mean by we" they can probably name the referent. That is, the speaker can tell you that he and Tom Jones were included in his use of "we."

But there are many patients who use these pronouns in a global way—they either have some difficulty or are completely unable to say whom they mean when they use "we" or "us." When a nurse is working with a patient who has this particular difficulty in self-identity, she has two tasks. First, she needs to raise the question, "Whom do you mean by we" (or us, or they). Secondly, she must be sure to speak only for herself and keep her identity clearly separate from that of the patient. In this instance, she would not use "we," "let's," or "our," as in the proverbial "We will now have our enema." Instead, she would say, "I have brought the enema you are to have."

Here is an example of a nurse reinforcing a patient's difficulty through the use of language:

A nurse said to a patient, "Let's go over what's been said and see if we have anything particular for us to discuss." The patient replied, "Oh, well, let's see what we'll see. Shall we watch for whether we are anxious between now and next week?" The merging of identity of nurse and patient—so that neither has the status of an independent person—is clear in this verbal interchange.

Magical or automatic knowing causes another communication problem. Magical knowing refers to knowing automatically—without asking, investigating, or finding out. Such phrases as "I know," "I see," "I understand" are included in this category when they precede rather than follow inquiry into a situation. Value terms such as "nice," "good," "bad" can also be used in such a way that consensus as to their meaning is assured rather than determined. For example, a patient said, "Well, last time my visitors were nice." The nurse responded, "Maybe today will go as well." This kind of verbal exchange shows the same limited communication inherent in such meaningless transactions as "Hello, how are you" to which the equally noncommunicative reply is "I'm fine, and you," and the final response is "I'm okay." Nothing has actually been said; these are merely words in juxtaposition.

The use of "they" as a pervasive global reference in which the identity of the referents is lost is typical of the patient diagnosed paranoiac. If you ask, "Who are they" the patient not only cannot tell you but may become quite anxious. If the nurse persists in asking, the "they" will become "other people," then a class of people as "my family" or "nurse" or "doctors," and finally names of particular people. Nurses should help more people become aware of the tendency toward loss of the referents by questioning "Who are they" whenever this pronoun is used.

SUMMARY

Talking with patients becomes productive when the nurse develops awareness of her own verbal patterns and then decides to take responsibility for her part in verbal interchanges with patients. When nursing is seen as an opportunity to further the patient's learning about himself, the focus in the nurse-patient relationship will be upon the patient—his needs, his difficulties, his lacks in interpersonal competence, his interest in living. What the nurse chooses to talk about during the relationship will be guided by her understanding of the scope and boundaries of nursing practice as a professional service.

THERAPEUTIC COMMUNICATION
Phyllis Goldin and Barbara Russell

An infant cries because he is hungry. Neighbors chat while having a cup of coffee. An executive dictates to his secretary. A country's emissary speaks at the United Nations. All are communicating, and the importance of this in today's sophisticated society cannot be overemphasized.

Rarely, in the life of an individual, does a day pass that he does not engage in social conversation: *Good morning.* (smile) *How are you?* (nod) *Just fine, thanks—and you? Couldn't be better.* (smile). Simple clichés with which we are all familiar.

The habit of social conversation is ingrained in our culture. As a rule, such conversation is a give-and-take process:
We went to Lake Tahoe for our vacation this year and. . . . Oh, you did! We flew to Hawaii for a week and had a wonderful time. . . . We took it easy for three weeks, fishing, hiking. . . .

The conversation shifts back and forth, focusing on no one particular contribution. But if we examine these statements the tendency toward "one upmanship" is obvious. The first person vacationed in Tahoe, the second flew to Hawaii for a week, but the first person had a three-week vacation.

One upmanship frequently occurs when two or three mothers talk about their children. Instead of actively listening, taking in, and understanding, the listener, instead, is contemplating the remarks he will make at the next pause!

The pleasant repartee of daily living has a definite and useful place in our culture. However, it also can be used to set the stage for truly therapeutic communication.

THERAPEUTIC COMMUNICATION

Therapeutic communication enables a nurse to know her patient as an individual and to discern his special needs. While she encourages him to express himself, she should bear in mind the ultimate purpose of such exploration: clearly and simply, to learn the patient's needs in order to give better nursing care. Any patient will sense if a nurse is merely trying to satisfy her curiosity. He probably will respond guardedly with a minimum of information.

Fear and anxiety use up a patient's energy. The nurse who helps a patient to verbalize such feelings and bring them into the open can help him redirect his energies to the cause of establishing good health.

If encouraged, a patient may voice his reaction to his illness or his feelings about his dependency upon others. By openly expressing himself and explaining to another how he feels, a patient's fleeting, nebulous thoughts must, of necessity, become precise words and structured sentences.

Words and sentences require organization of thought processes which help a patient center his attention around a particular idea for a period of time. The physical act of speaking requires a close examination of thought. It requires more time to speak than to think, and thoughts are heard by the speaker himself.

Through the use of therapeutic communication, a nurse is able to clear the way for her patient to make his own decisions and to come to his own conclusions. How much more meaningful such determinations are for him than if they had been made by another "for his own good!"

NONDIRECTIVE TECHNIQUES

The use of some pleasantries or social intercourse is necessary to establishing an initial rapport and create a climate for more meaningful conversation. When common ground has thus been reached, the patient may begin to move the conversation toward an area of concern to him. However, a patient may feel that the nurse's time is limited or that she is not genuinely interested in listening. Then he may not feel free to lead the conversation into more meaningful areas; instead, he may continue with social pleasantries. In this case, a broad opening statement by the nurse concerning a fact or facet of his behavior may be necessary to assure him that she is concerned. This in itself may move him to focus his conversation on himself. Such an opening statement should be nonthreatening to the patient:

I see from the doctor's orders you are going home today, or *You appear anxious,* or *Dr. Jones says you are interested in breast-feeding your baby,* or *You seem to be uncomfortable.*

Such questions as, "Isn't it wonderful that you are going home today?" or "Why are you so anxious?" demand an answer, whereas a simple statement allows the patient a choice of continuing or not.

Once the broad opening statement has been made by nurse or patient, the next step is to keep the communication flowing. Several techniques can be employed to accomplish this.

The patient is encouraged to go on when he feels his remarks are accepted and not judged or evaluated by the listener. This can be done by nonverbal and/or verbal means. For example, a nod of the head or such comments by the nurse as "Uh Huh!" "I see," "Yes."

Reflecting is another technique which keeps conversation flowing. The reflection may consist of a portion of the more significant points of a patient's cognitive dialogue as, for example,

Mrs. J.: I've had new pacemakers put in four times this year.
Nurse: Four times?
Mrs. J.: The wire keeps slipping out and I'm getting so disgusted.

The nurse also can encourage the patient to explore feeling tones through the use of reflection. For example, continuing the above conversation . . .

Nurse: You're disgusted?
Mrs. J.: Maybe that's not the word. I'm really afraid of where it is all going to end.

Her underlying fear becomes apparent.

Reflection gives feedback and essentially says, "Yes, I understand, you may continue if you wish." The questioning inflection in the nurse's voice asks, "Am I correct in what I understand you to say?"

The comment "Yes" by a patient only denotes that he believes the nurse has understood him correctly. However, a simple "yes" or "no" response to reflection may not necessarily be the end of a patient's reply to the statement.

Silence has advantages in therapeutic communication. A short pause after using reflection or other therapeutic techniques may encourage the patient to continue. He may need this time to consider what he has said and perhaps organize his thoughts for further communication. Silence also may be viewed as a kind of acceptance.

A nurse could well utilize this silent interval as an opportunity to formulate a response to her patient, instead of blurting out an immediate reaction. Open ended phrases, such as, "You were saying. . . ." "You want to go home because. . . ." "And then you. . . ." tend to encourage discussion by the patient in greater depth. Such phrases are particularly helpful when the conversation seems to be wandering away from the area of prime concern, or drifting into less meaningful communication. They also serve to emphasize to the patient that the nurse's interest in his concerns parallels his own.

The use of the word "feeling" when communicating often helps the patient to focus upon emotions rather than upon related factual information. For instance, "What are your feelings concerning your rehabilitation program?" or "How do you feel about going to a nursing home?" To be most effective, this technique requires a trusting relationship beyond just the initial rapport.

Summarizing a patient's dialogue is a method of mirroring his thoughts back to him.

Thus, he may see himself, his attitudes, his opinions, and his plans in a clearer light. By pinpointing his most salient remarks, the nurse clarifies their meaning both to the patient and to herself. If a patient is speaking of a problem and its related conditions, the nurse can crystallize this information for him, thereby enhancing his capability of making his own decisions.

As with reflecting, summarizing gives the patient feedback, apprising him of the listener's comprehension as well as his own thoughts. Where, however, reflection is brief, a reiteration of only a few words or an attitude, summarizing reviews an entire idea or thought.

A summarizing statement may begin with "Do I understand you to say . . . ?" "You seem to be saying that. . . ." "In other words you feel that. . . ."

In addition to the spoken word, much human communication is carried on in a nonverbal fashion. Therapeutic verbal communication should be accompanied by actions which enhance the desired atmosphere. Expression, stance, and gestures, all combine to relate information to the observer and reinforce or even negate the spoken word.

A nurse can learn a great deal about a patient by observing his behavior. Conversely, the patient can learn much about a nurse's understanding and interest level through her mannerisms. Seated with chair close to patient, leaning forward, interested facial expressions, and frequent eye contact, will denote a feeling of empathy with the patient. Hands should be still for finger tapping and other nervous gestures will be interpreted as impatience.

Nondirective techniques, in addition to allowing the patient freedom to talk, help to keep the nurse from inadvertently making value statements and judgmental comments, common in everyday conversation, which could easily be carried over to the patient-nurse interaction.

One student of nursing in analyzing her own communication said, "I needed to make a judgmental statement in order to protect myself." She was seeking protection from the reality of the situation when an attractive young teacher on a psychiatric unit told her he was taking LSD. Unable to reconcile the visual image with the verbal confrontation, she said, "No! You couldn't be taking drugs. You wouldn't do anything like that!"

Value judgments—positive or negative, such as "That's good" or "That's bad" are not conducive to a free atmosphere for communication. The nurse's value orientation may differ from that of the patient, and when expressed, may inhibit the patient from sharing his own views.

There is a tendency for nurses to respond with one of several clichés upon hearing of another's anxieties. "Don't worry. Everything is going to be all right." "Let's not talk about that just now." "You're lucky it wasn't worse." "Your doctor will take care of everything." "If you think you're bad off, look at the guy next to you."

Such remarks offer little solace to the patient and hinder further communication. Objectively considered, such clichés actually prove more soothing to the nurse than to the patient. Instead of conveying a message of comfort, they suggest, instead, an attitude of dismissal.

By relinquishing the automatic and stereotyped reactions of social communication, nurses can relate in more effective ways to patients. However, intellectual knowledge alone will not suffice. In order for communication techniques to be of value, they must be used, for it takes time and conscious effort to break old habits. But the self-discipline and energy required for this change become well worth the effort when a nurse receives the satisfaction of hearing a patient say, "Thanks for listening. Nobody else talks to me the way you do," or "I feel better, now."

Therapeutic communication becomes easier with use as it begins to replace old patterns of conversation. And when nondirective techniques are used in social settings, the user is often considered a "wonderful conversationalist!"

BLOCKS TO COMMUNICATING WITH PATIENTS

Helon E. Hewitt and Betty L. Pesznecker

Nurses who genuinely want to comfort patients or help them solve their problems often fail in their attempts. Ineffective communication may be the reason and it is often the nurse's own words inadvertent though they may be which block communication between herself and the patient.

To help nurses study their own interactions with patients, we have identified five major verbal blocks to effective communication. They are: changing the subject, stating one's own opinions and ideas about the patient and his situation, false or inappropriate reassurance, jumping to conclusions or offering solutions to the problem, and inappropriate use of medical facts or nursing knowledge. The classification is based on an original system developed by Joan Bachand.[1]

Once a nurse identifies one of these blocks in her interaction with a patient, exploration of possible reasons, which may have precipitated the verbal error, can provide her with the insight she needs to achieve effective communication. There are many reasons why she may have blocked her own good intentions. Her own anxiety, her attitudes about the patient, and her preconceived notions of how patients should behave are just a few. Before the nurse can deal with the underlying reason for poor communication she must be able to recognize when her own words cause the block.

CHANGING THE SUBJECT

In this category of verbal errors, the nurse shifts the focus of the conversation by directly changing the subject. Or she may shift the topic by responding to some insignificant aspect of the patient's conversation. The following example illustrates this.

Miss Brown: Good morning, Donald. How are you?
Donald: Hi (silence). Dr. Nash came in last night with Mrs. Robinson. He told me my mother died.
Miss Brown: I'm terribly sorry, Donald. Was she sick long?
Donald: Well, three months ago she told me her kidneys were all shot and the doctor said she had only three to six months to live. It was only three.
Miss Brown: It must have been quite a shock to you, Donald.

Reprinted from American Journal of Nursing **64**(7):101-103, 1964. Copyright The American Journal of Nursing Company.
[1]Bachand, Joan. Problematic Verbal Patterns of Student Nurses in Initial Interviews with Psychiatric Patients; A Tool and Its Application. Newark, N.J., Rutgers University, 1959. (Unpublished master's thesis.)

Donald: She was in the hospital when I had to come to the hospital, so I knew I might not see her again. (Donald began to cry.)

Miss Brown: I think maybe we'd better get started with your bath now, Donald. I'll get the linen to change your bed. (Donald continues to cry softly, and the nurse leaves the room.)

The nurse evidently could not respond to Donald's talk about his mother's death so she shifted to the safe topic of the bed bath. Perhaps her own anxiety concerning the subject of death was the cause.

Had Miss Brown been able to control her own anxiety, she might have been able to remain with Donald when he began to cry. Her physical presence could have conveyed to Donald that his feelings about his mother's death could be expressed freely. Verbal response from the nurse may not have been necessary at this point—just staying quietly with the boy.

In the next illustration, Miss Mills was not able to hear the patient's expression of concern because she was so preoccupied with a task she wanted to accomplish.

Miss Mills: Hello, Mrs. Long.

Mrs. Long: Yes?

Miss Mills: I'm Miss Mills. How are you feeling today?

Mrs. Long: Oh, pretty good. My back still gives me a lot of trouble.

Miss Mills: Oh. The doctor would like us to catheterize you for a urine specimen.

GIVING OWN OPINIONS

In this category, the nurse states her own opinions and ideas about the patient and his concerns in a way that hinders the exploration of the patient's problems. Such statements often have a moralizing tone.

In the following interaction, the nurse's ideas about how the patient should react to his hospital care blocked her from exploring how the patient thought and felt about his treatment.

Miss Lee: Good morning, Mr. Marsh. I will be taking care of you this morning. Would you like to wash before breakfast?

Mr. Marsh: Oh, I suppose (pause). I hope I don't get oatmeal again this morning. That is all they feed me for breakfast and I never get enough of anything.

Miss Lee: I know, Mr. Marsh, but you should be thankful that the doctors prescribed a special diet which will help you.

Mr. Marsh: I know! But it's no fun! I get hungry!

Miss Lee: Of course it's no fun but you'll be glad you kept on the diet when you begin getting well.

(After breakfast)

Miss Lee: Would you like your bath now?

Mr. Marsh: No, I want to rest. Besides, I don't want a bath. I don't need one every day. It takes too long to have a bath.

Miss Lee: It won't take long, Mr. Marsh. I'm sure you will feel much more comfortable and relaxed after you've had your bath.

Mr. Marsh: Oh yes, yes! Well, go ahead.

At first, Mr. Marsh was trying to express his feelings about his diet and some of the discomfort it caused. When the nurse replied that Mr. Marsh should appreciate the efforts of the doctors and nurses in his behalf, she stopped his expression of feeling. No doubt the nurse believed that all patients feel better after a bath. This attitude about patient care interfered with her ability to help Mr. Marsh talk about his need for rest and about the bath.

When Mr. Marsh said he never got enough of anything, Miss Lee might have explored this statement by saying, "Do you mean, Mr. Marsh, that you never get enough to eat?" This kind of question would have allowed the patient to further express his feelings about his diet or other concerns.

INAPPROPRIATE REASSURANCE

False or inappropriate comments made by the nurse can keep the patient from expressing his worry.

Mrs. Perry: Good morning, Mr. Cook, you look pretty fit. Feeling better today?
Mr. Cook: Yes, I just want to get out of this bed and go home. I can't take this lying around.
Mrs. Perry: Have you talked to your doctor about when you will be able to leave?
Mr. Cook: Oh, he doesn't say anything much. He keeps beating around the bush.
Mrs. Perry: Well, who knows, he may pleasantly surprise you soon. It probably won't be
  too much longer before you're on your way home. How about a bath, now?
Mr. Cook: O.K.

The conversation continued around the bath procedure and, interestingly, the patient did not again discuss his feelings about going home.

We can only speculate about the nurse's motivation. It is probable she sincerely wanted to relieve the patient of his anxiety. Perhaps this is often the reason for such inappropriate comments. Frequently, the nurse is unable to give an accurate answer to the patient's questions. Our data include many examples of nurses offering false reassurance and blocking communication with patients who question their prognosis, talk about death, or express fear of impending surgery. It is obvious the nurse cannot honestly answer a question about an uncertain outcome. These topics create a certain amount of anxiety within the nurse, and she sometimes feels more comfortable in cutting off the subject.

The nurse might have responded to Mr. Cook's concern about going home as follows:

Mr. Cook: I just want to get out of this bed and go home. I can't take this lying around.
Mrs. Perry: You're pretty anxious to get home, Mr. Cook?
Mr. Cook: I've got to get home! I've been off the job two weeks now and I don't know how
  much longer I'm going to have to be off. If I just knew how much longer it will be before
  I can go back to work . . .

By focusing on Mr. Cook's concern about going home, Mrs. Perry encouraged the patient to express concerns which he might otherwise have kept to himself.

JUMPING TO CONCLUSIONS

Jumping to conclusions or offering solutions prematurely to the problem is another error in communication. The nurse responds to a part of a situation or problem expressed by the patient as if the entire situation or problem had been stated. When a nurse reaches conclusions without exploring what the patient is trying to communicate, she tends to propose a quick—and perhaps not the best—solution to the problem.

The nurse entered the room of a patient who had suffered a fracture of the right forearm and left side of the pelvis and was complaining thus:

Mr. Cox: My back hurts.
Mrs. Ray: Your back will feel much better if you can turn on your side.
Mr. Cox: Which side?
Mrs. Ray: Well, the doctor said either side, so why not the side that hurts the least. Here, let me help you.
Mr. Cox: Oh! I can't! The pain!
Mrs. Ray: You must get off your back so something can be done to help it besides medicine. A rub would help a lot.
Mr. Cox: No. No. I can't do it. Stop! Impossible!

The nurse seemed to be preoccupied with completing a nursing task or finding a quick solution to the patient's problems as she perceived them. This preoccupation interfered with her exploring and clarifying the problem from the patient's point of view.

We can only speculate what the real problem or source of discomfort was for this patient. The location of his fractures could interfere with a comfortable position in bed. The patient appeared to be unable to tolerate the pain of changing positions and was experiencing pain in the recumbent position. This is not an uncommon nursing problem. There are times when such nursing measures as positioning and turning the patient must be enforced. When giving the physical care, however, emotional support must be considered too.

The foregoing illustration has a tone of aggressiveness on the part of the nurse. The patient was not allowed to verbalize his feelings about turning. Nor was he given the opportunity to express his feelings about being in such a miserable condition. Frequently, if the patient is allowed to reveal his feelings without the nurse interjecting her own ideas, directing, or attempting to control the patient, he will be able to clarify his thinking and feeling, for himself and as a result, modify his attitudes and behavior.

Mrs. Ray might have been less directive, allowing the patient to express more clearly his difficulty. The scene might have been as follows:

Mr. Cox: My back hurts.
Mrs. Ray: Where does it hurt?
Mr. Cox: All over, but mostly in the middle. Can't you do something?
Mrs. Ray: You're probably pretty uncomfortable from being flat so long. Perhaps if you can turn on your side, I could rub your back.

INAPPROPRIATE USE OF FACTS

The inappropriate use of medical facts or nursing knowledge is a common error. In order to teach or tell the patient before exploring how he thinks or feels about the topic being discussed, the nurse may state facts. The premature use of nursing or medical facts was used most frequently by nurses in an effort to change the behavior or attitude of a patient. The tone may be argumentative, since the nurse may be directly opposing or ignoring the views or feelings of the patient.

In the following example, a nurse used facts in an effort to persuade a patient with tuberculosis to change his behavior to be more in accord with his prescribed treatment.

Miss Hill: Good morning.
Mr. Leaf: Good morning. How are you?
Miss Hill: Oh, fine. How would you like your bed straightened?
Mr. Leaf: Fine. (He hopped out of bed into a chair.)
Miss Hill: (She began to straighten the bed.) Sit down and rest.

Mr. Leaf: I'm getting too fat. I need more exercise.

Miss Hill: You shouldn't worry about getting fat now. Get all the rest you can, so you will get well faster. Then you can gradually increase your exercise to decrease your weight.

Mr. Leaf: I don't need that much rest.

Miss Hill: Oh, but rest is probably the most important treatment for tuberculosis patients. You see, by resting, the lungs can be at rest, too and, therefore, healing takes place more rapidly.

Mr. Leaf: I don't care. I simply can't endure lying in bed when I don't feel badly.

Miss Hill: Well, you think about it.

The facts the nurse told the patient were logical, but they did not seem to help the patient become more comfortable or accept the prescribed rest. The patient apparently was having difficulty in assuming the role of patient. Perhaps he viewed resting in bed as becoming dependent, which he could not accept at that time. Although he indicated a greater concern about getting fat than resting, the nurse explained the logic of his rest treatment.

This mode of interaction tends to weaken the relationship between the nurse and patient. By allowing the patient to express his feelings, rather than opposing his ideas, the nurse would have created a more positive climate and a more therapeutic relationship.

The nurse might have conveyed more interest in the patient's feelings by responding directly to his comment, "I'm getting too fat and I need more exercise," by saying, "You seem concerned about the lack of exercise you have been allowed since your hospitalization." This would have allowed the patient to express more of his feelings about hospitalization and the restrictions on his activities imposed by illness.

We believe that nurses can use these categories to examine their own errors in response to patients. Speculation about the reasons can help the individual nurse to improve her ability to provide therapeutic nursing care for her patients.

YOUR PATIENTS HEAR YOU, BUT DO THEY UNDERSTAND?

Judith Petrello

Would you believe—when a nurse told a patient, "For a few days you will have to be checked for I and O," the patient thought she meant he could leave the hospital, but would have to be "in" and "out" for daily checkups? Would you believe—when a nurse tells patients, "Your pain results from a hematoma," 19 out of 20 of them don't understand? Well, you can believe it—a nurse's casual use of clinical words and abbreviations in conversing with patients usually confuses them and often causes them undue uncertainty and anxiety about their hospital stay.

Some clinical words are simply not part of laymen's vocabularies, for example, hematocrit, impaction, reflux, and hemorrhage. Others—such as elimination, culture, scrub, stool, traction, and sterile—mean one thing to a health-care professional and quite another to most patients. So the nurse who uses clinical language without consideration of the patient's possible misunderstanding or misinterpretation adds to the communication gap between staff and patients.

The extent of this communication gap was measured in a study conducted at a large medical center hospital. Nurses there cooperated by compiling a list of words and abbreviations frequently used in conversing with patients. From this list 40 words and 10 abbreviations were randomly selected. Each term in the list was read in a sentence to 200 hospitalized adult patients. Each patient was asked the meaning of the terms and whether nurses had used them in conversation with him or her.

The results: None of the 200 patients defined all the words and abbreviations correctly; however, they identified all the terms as ones used by nurses in conversation.

Fewer than 5% could define "hematoma"—one thought it meant "high blood pressure," another guessed "ulcer." Fewer than 10% defined "secretions," and answers ranged from "mysteries" to "scars." Relatively few were able to define "acute" (22%), "culture" (28%), and "traction" (19%). Only 11% understood the meaning of blood pressure—a number thought it referred to how hot the blood can get; one patient said when your blood is boiling you have high blood pressure; and another concluded it was a test to see how quickly you get mad. "Post-op" came in with a variety of interpretations including "postpone the operation," "propped up," and "Don't get near him, he's got some kind of disease." Only 21% grasped the meaning of "PO" while the other 79% bounced it all over the medical field and beyond: "prescription order," "personal only," "physical and oral," "passed over for a time," and "passed on."

Correct responses ranged from 41% for patients with 4 to 12 years of schooling to 68% for patients doing graduate work. Patients in private rooms had more correct responses (62%) than those in semi-private (58%) or on ward units (52%). Why? Perhaps because private-room patients have more one-to-one conversations with nurses. There's more opportunity for further clarification if the patient, at first, doesn't understand the nurse.

This study clearly demonstrates that hospitalized adults do not understand a great many of the terms being employed by nurses in "normal" conversations. Such communication blocks impede mutual understanding and can cause confusion, anxiety, and even antagonism between the patient and nurse. A patient-participant in the study commented, "One of the most frightening things about the hospital is not understanding what the doctors and nurses are saying." The nursing implications of that conclusion should be obvious.

With both patient and physician depending on the nurse for effective verbal communication, the clarity of the language she uses is imperative. The study suggests several ways to help nurses make their messages clear to patients. Just being aware that nonprofessionals may completely misunderstand the nurse's words and intentions is a good start. The nurse's selection of terms should be tailored to the patient's mental and emotional capabilities. These factors vary widely from patient to patient and even from time to time with the same patient.

But most important for the nurse in clinical practice is giving the patient time to react. The nurse can't do justice to her message simply by stating it and walking away. The feedback from the patient tells the nurse whether or not her message was received and understood. Negative feedback may be in the form of a puzzled look, or a question, statement, or inappropriate action that reveals some degree of confusion or misunderstanding. If she gets negative feedback, the nurse should repeat her message in simpler

WHICH COMMON CLINICAL WORDS PUZZLE PATIENTS?

Words	Correct	Partially correct	Incorrect	Do not know
Abscess	40%	21%	28%	9%
Acute	22	41	34	2
Allergic	96	—	4	—
Anesthesia	89	5	5	—
Bacteria	71	6	19	3
Benign	51	—	24	24
Biopsy	71	4	11	13
Bladder	59	—	39	1
Blood pressure	11	12	71	5
Blood sugar	59	6	23	11
Bowel	40	—	53	6
Buttock	94	—	4	1
Coma	77	—	22	—
Compress	38	31	26	3
Culture	28	48	14	9
Dehydrated	75	3	16	4
Dislocated	76	11	11	1
Elimination	47	2	28	22
Fasting	47	7	34	11
Gastric	42	—	35	23
Germs	57	21	21	—
Hallucination	64	2	29	4
Hematocrit	17	8	6	67
Hematoma	4	21	18	55
Hemorrhage	50	26	21	2
Immunization	76	1	14	8
Impaction	24	9	31	35
Inhalation	64	10	10	15
Intestines	73	5	18	3
Orally	87	—	12	1
Physical therapy	72	24	3	1
Secretions	9	12	51	27
Specimen	72	—	27	—
Spinal	83	—	15	1
Suction	41	11	13	34
Tendon	8	5	79	7
Therapy	70	22	6	—
Traction	19	38	41	1
Urine	79	5	15	—
Vitamin	22	28	48	1
Abbreviations				
CC	64	14	7	14
ECG	67	7	13	12
I&O	13	4	12	70
I.V.	93	1	2	4
OR	78	—	5	16
PO	21	—	17	61
Post-op	50	—	33	17
Prep	85	—	11	3
PT	79	3	7	10
TPR	21	44	12	22

Hospitalized patients' lack of understanding of clinical terms used by nurses is shown by the percentages in this table. The study included 200 adults, 50% of them high school graduates, 14% college graduates, 21% with some college training, and 15% with only 4 to 12 years of schooling. The terms were randomly selected from a list of 92 words and 26 abbreviations frequently used by staff nurses in talking to patients.

Fractional percentages are omitted, so the cumulative figures do not equal 100%.

terms, making every effort to avoid ambiguity and prevent anxiety in the patient. By immediately clarifying her statement, the nurse provides the information and support the patient needs—just what every nursing message is meant to do.

WHAT DOES THE PATIENT WANT TO KNOW?

Dorothy T. Linehan

What do patients want to know about their illnesses before they leave the hospital? This was the question to which we sought answers at the 250-bed Beverly Hospital, in Beverly, Massachusetts, and for which funds came from the Medical Foundation, Boston, and the Central North Shore United Fund of Beverly.

An advisory committee, whose enthusiasm and cooperation provided support and impetus throughout the project, included a trustee of the Beverly Hospital Research Foundation and the administrators of the various hospital departments: administration, medical services, nursing service, nursing schools, social service, and medical education.*

We started with the premise that at the time of discharge from the hospital, patients and their families have questions that often go unanswered; that many of these questions can be answered; and that if they are answered, a patient's recovery is speeded, his mind eased, and his opinion of the hospital and of health professionals enhanced.

Research on what the patient should know, how much he should be told, and by whom, as well as what he does know, has been explored from a professional point of view, but, as far as we could determine, "what the patient wants to know" has not.[1,2]

In order to design an interview schedule for the research project, I interviewed patients at random before they were discharged, asking open-end questions. During this time also I settled the question of what to wear, a nurse's uniform or a laboratory coat? I tried both. Since there seemed to be no noticeable difference in patients' reactions, I finally chose the laboratory coat and wore a name pin to show that I was a registered nurse. The coat became a conversation opener—both visitors and employees wanted to know what type of work I was doing and employees often would ask, "How is everything going?"

Every morning for five months I visited the wards to obtain a list of patients to be discharged from the head nurse. From this list, I selected patients for interview according to their availability and variation of diagnosis. It was not hard to talk with the patients. The magic word, "research," plus my obvious interest in them, was sufficient to elicit patients' questions and comments. From 88 open-end interviews the first formal questionnaire was developed and pretested. Three other schedules followed. These were tested on 108 additional patients, and then evaluated before the final interview schedule was prepared. A preliminary analysis of this exploratory phase led us to believe that patients liked to be interviewed. They did have questions and apparently they were willing to discuss them.

Our next step in the project was to determine the method of selecting patients to be

Reprinted from American Journal of Nursing 66(5):1066-1070, 1966. Copyright The American Journal of Nursing Company.
*Bernhard M. Kramer, Ph.D., associate professor of preventive medicine (social psychology), Tufts University School of Medicine, Boston, and the staff of the Medical Foundation, Inc. served as consultants. Richard E. Alt, the trustee on the advisory committee, also is president of the medical staff of the hospital.

interviewed, decide how to record the interviews, and to establish work procedures. A probability chart of daily admissions and discharges for one month was prepared to determine a numerical method of selection. We decided that it was possible to interview 3 to 7 patients each day. We excluded pediatric patients under 16 and, to avoid overloading the interviews with obstetrical patients, we selected every sixth obstetrical patient from the daily admission list and every third remaining patient, regardless of service. According to our probability chart, this would provide us with a backlog of approximately 35 patients to be interviewed and average 3 to 7 interviews a day. A card system of recording specific data was devised for my Kardex and used as a daily work sheet. A trial then was carried on for two weeks.

From the daily admission list, patients were selected, cards were started, rounds were made, and the data filled in from the patient's chart and placed in the working Kardex used on the wards. A notation in red written on the Kardex indicated that I wished to interview that particular patient during the 24 hours prior to his discharge.

Physicians did not use the ward Kardex and thus did not know that their patients had been selected for interview. Each morning, the head nurse was shown the cards of the patients marked for interview. She was able to tell me, at a glance, who was to be discharged. Rounds were made again in the afternoon. This cycle was repeated each day.

Check out time was 11:00 A.M., so interviews had to be obtained the day before or the morning of discharge. There were many reasons why some interviews were not obtained: evening, weekend, and holiday discharges; too many discharges at one time; meetings; a patient's death. All reasons were recorded.

DATA COLLECTION

Four hundred and fifty patients were interviewed from May 27, 1963 to January 31, 1964. An additional 537 patients had been listed for interview but were not questioned.

The interview schedule contained 44 questions plus a fact sheet for such specific data as age, religion, race, hospital accommodations, service, sex, and marital status. The first 20 questions explored the patient's ethnic, social, and educational background, and his knowledge of his illness. The next 5 questions were related to the time of admission to the hospital, leaving 19 questions for the time of discharge. For example: Do you have questions? What are the questions? Did you ask the questions? Whom do you ask or why didn't you ask? Was there anything you wish you had asked your doctor? I used the end page to note the observations and my evaluation of the reliability and medical sophistication of the interview.

Interviews averaged three per day with a time range of 10 minutes to one and one-half hours. Six patients refused to be interviewed: two were too ill, three would not answer "anything for anyone ever," and another thought I was from the credit office and could not be convinced otherwise. One interview form had to be torn up when the patient and his family changed their minds. Thus, there were 443 usable interviews from patients with a wide range of diagnoses, nationalities, ages, and occupations. Some were welfare patients, others were wealthy, some were unknown, and some V.I.P.'s.

Reactions to the interview schedule varied. Patients were interested, pleased to participate, and thought the purpose worthwhile, such as the young man whose friend had the same illness in another hospital. These men used to telephone each other every day to compare notes. One call came during the interview. Very importantly the patient announced to his friend, "I'm sorry, I can't talk to you now—I'm being *interviewed!*"

A few patients could see no sense to the interview, nor why it was being done. Some patients thought the interview was to elicit complaints, others were afraid to criticize their doctors; but most patients were glad of the opportunity to express their desires and opinions. Comments and questions came freely when patients were assured that interviews were confidential and that questions and remarks would never be individually identified even though they would be used in the final report.

It was hard to make the transition from nurse to researcher. However, as time went on, interviewing became easier and the frustration at not being allowed to answer patients' questions receded. Although my visits with patients were generally stimulating, there often were enervating moments.

One particular instance was the young man who had just been told that he had a fatal disease. He was full of questions: How long would he live? Would he have time to get his affairs in order? Could he continue to be a husband? Could he harm his wife or children? Would death be painful? Would he be helped when it was his time?

Of special interest, and to be considered in the final analysis, were 51 percent of the patients who had no questions, apparently because of fear, age, religion, trust in the physician, knowing their diagnosis or, not knowing *what* to ask, *how* to ask, or *whom* to ask. During the interviews some patients revealed why they did not ask questions:
I don't like to ask questions—I am timid. I was afraid of the answer. I assume he will before I leave. I know what is wrong with me—they know I know. I have faith in my doctor. How can you get hold of them to ask? I don't know what to ask him. If he doesn't tell me whom shall I ask? I was afraid they would think I was rushing them.

There were humorous incidents. I remember, especially, the pretty, dignified, sweet old lady, 70 years of age, who had no questions during the interview until I came to the very last question. "Getting back once again to the questions you might have had about your illness or your care, is there anything at all that you wished you had asked your doctor?" "Yes," she boomed, "What in hell am I in here for?"

Another was the sad, retiring, little old man who also had no questions, but just as I was leaving beckoned me to come close. Then he whispered, "You know I have trouble with my water works. Could I have a beer?"

It was not long before a pattern evolved from the recorded comments and questions. The questions fell into 17 categories related, in order of volume, to: activity, diagnosis, reasons why they did not ask, symptoms, suggestions, treatments, prognosis, medicines, operations, personal care, diet, problems, nursing care and nurses, miscellaneous, finances, marital relations, tests. There were 2,459 questions and comments, in addition to the 957 obtained in the exploratory phase of the study.

It would appear that most of the questions could be answered. The complaints seemed reasonable and most of them probably could be remedied. Patients wanted to know if they could lift, go upstairs, get into the bath tub, go outdoors, take a walk, have a highball. They asked:
What is wrong with me? Are they telling me the truth? Will it recur? What should I do about the dressing? How long will I need one? How long will I be on crutches or have the cast on? What did he do to me? What did he take out? Will there be any physical or psychological changes? What should I look for or expect? How long will I be out of work? Should I change jobs? What does "taking it easy" mean? How soon will I be normal? Will it harm me to have marital relations? Should I take the medicine I was taking before I came in?

How long should I continue on this medication? Why are the diets different from the ones my family doctor put me on? What should I eat to make milk? When can I take the baby outdoors? Why does it take so long to get an aspirin?

Patients wanted a chance to talk with their doctors other than at rounds, and apparently they disliked rounds. They wished privacy, especially when they had personal questions or when the doctors talked to them about their conditions. They wished for a greater display of interest in them as persons from doctors and nurses. They wanted to be talked to. They disliked the attitudes, casual responses, and evasive answers from doctors, interns, and nurses. They wanted simple answers, and fewer medical terms. They wanted more explanation of what was done to them and why; what to expect after an operation or treatment; more rapid reports of tests; better communication between doctors and families; more explanation of nursing procedures.

They also wanted more discharge information, especially the approximate date of discharge, in order to plan for transportation, husband's work, baby-sitters, help, and finances.

They wanted to talk alone with their doctors, if only for a moment, and wished the doctors did not "look out of the window, eat candy, or gaze in the mirror." They wanted to know who the head nurse was and they wanted to know why she didn't make rounds to ask if they had questions or worries and then relay these to the doctor. They would have liked the menu explained to them on admission—many did not know how to order. They would have liked more common names for foods; after all, "hamburger is still hamburger." They would have liked more privacy during the admission process, more explanation of costs, and how much their insurance would cover. They wished for better placement of patients in rooms in respect to age and condition. They disliked four-bed wards and said these were "not semiprivate."

Even though the questions were the main objective of the research project, the comments also were valuable. And when patients' reasons for not asking questions are examined, additional insight into attitudes and feelings may be gained. Replies to the question, "Can you suggest procedures for improving the ways in which patients can get answers to their questions?" focused mainly on the doctor and the difficulties in talking with him.

It was not until the question, "Did you talk to any of the following people about any question you might have about your condition?" (listing other patients, relatives, and hospital personnel) that nurses were mentioned. "The head nurse" seemed to release a spring.

Comments were numerous and unsolicited:

Nurses are not allowed to answer. Just ask the doctor; don't bother with the others, they don't know. I believe nurses are told not to answer you—but one nurse will tell you one thing and another something else. They don't seem to have much coordination—it is very upsetting to the patients. Ask, but you don't get any answer. Just regular nurses; I wouldn't know what they were. I figure they do just what they have to and that's all. Why can't one receive simple answers, especially from the head nurse? I feel she is qualified to communicate the answers and in a position to obtain them. I think nurses are not supposed to tell you; if they did they would lose their jobs. Be sure you go to the right person; some of the younger ones don't seem to care.

There were many favorable comments about the excellent nursing care given and the high caliber of nurses, all of which somewhat softened the critical comments. Nevertheless, the image patients had of hospital nurses in general became a major factor in the action phase of this study.

ACTION PHASE

The second objective of the study was to learn how difficult—or how easy—it was to get answers for patients and to determine who could give the answers. The patients' questions and their comments indicated that hospital personnel directly involved needed to be informed.

With the cooperation of department directors, 19 meetings were held with patients' doctors, residents, interns, nurses, dietitians, and other personnel from all administrative levels to present pertinent questions and comments and obtain reactions.

These were lively meetings. Many gripes were aired. Reactions ran the gamut of resentment, recrimination, and rationalization. Few comments and opinions of these groups would be new to members of the health professions, but the constant reiteration of the doctor-nurse-department relationship problems demonstrated that attitudes and concepts needed deeper introspection to improve communications, recognize and identify responsibilities, accept capabilities, and get back to the "team" which all seemed to desire. Personnel were disturbed by the patients' image of them. Their concern became a major factor in discussion and served to help them seek ways to improve their reflection.

After initial reactions subsided, all groups agreed that patients' questions should be answered. However, they disagreed about who was to answer the questions. Although there was agreement that answering many of the questions was primarily the responsibility of the patients' doctors, residents, interns, and nurses believed that they should be allowed to share this obligation. Residents, interns, and nurses wanted the attending physicians to serve as their teachers in determining what to discuss with patients in relation to activity, treatment, personal care, marital relations, and tests—areas in which they felt they could and would be able to counsel effectively.

Next, a liaison committee of physicians representing each service along with nurses from each department of nursing service and from nursing education was formed. This committee, in turn, worked with the paramedical groups through subcommittees. After five months of analysis and evaluation a *Check List for Patient's Discharge Instructions,* and a guide containing information about the discharge procedure, as well as a detailed report with recommendations were submitted to the advisory committee.

The advisory committee accepted the recommendations and with a few minor revisions recommended the following proposals. They also facilitated the implementation of a patient education program.

1. The responsibility for all patients' education emanates from the doctor. It is the consensus of the Advisory Committee that this responsibility could and should be shared and delegated in part to residents, nurses of head nurse stature, dietitians and to personnel on other allied services, utilizing their full capacities in patient education through planned patient-oriented education programs.

2. The *Check List for Patient's Discharge Instructions* be adopted and put into use as per instruction sheet.

3. The initial progress note should state the general plan for patient treatment or investigation as the case may be. At least the day before discharge, a progress note should be written containing the final diagnosis, the disposition of the patient, the medicines to be given, and the approximate date of office or house follow-up. These two notes, along with

the *Check List for Patient's Discharge Instructions,* would supply a large amount of valuable information.

4. We accept the expressed desire of all groups within the hospital for the need to improve communications and relationships. In order to do this, definite lines of communications must be established and adhered to. Only then can interdepartmental relationships be improved. In turn, informed department directors will then be held responsible for imparting communications to their personnel.

5. In order to implement the patient education program, the head nurse must be released from non-nursing duties so that she may assume her proper function and participate as a key person in the teaching programs.

6. There is a need for improved means of informing the patient of hospital operations and policies—preadmission, during hospitalization and pre- and post-discharge.

7. In order to further patient education as well as patient care, a position of education coordinator be established. The primary objectives shall be:

a. Provide, coordinate and channel patient education.

b. To keep personnel informed on new and changing patterns in patient education and care.

c. Fulfill agency's goal for improved patient care through an ongoing patient education program.

8. That the advisory committee and liaison committee on patient care and education be continued.

During the last month of the project, each group, including the board of directors, was informed of the results of the research project and the proposed implementation plan for a patient education program.

Beverly Hospital personnel have probed deeply for answers to needs and desires expressed by patients. They believe that patient education is an intrinsic part of the total care of the patient. They have devised a beginning tool, the *Check List for Patient's Discharge Instructions,* and have prepared the basic structure for implementing a patient education program. The Beverly Hospital and the Beverly Hospital Research Foundation have provided the means to implement and explore patient education within the hospital.

As a result of the survey there have been changes. Head nurses have been released from non-nursing duties and patient education is being incorporated into the inservice and ward teaching programs, and the *Check List for Patient's Discharge Instructions* is now a part of the chart and is being used and evaluated.

The dietary department has revitalized the nutrition clinic; a full-time dietitian has been employed to instruct inpatients at the bedside and at the nutrition clinic. Diet instructions are being adapted to individual patients with special attention to ethnic, financial, and dietary habits and a special diet card has been devised and placed on the tray of each patient on a special diet.

Administrative personnel are revising the patient handbook to provide the information requested by patients. Business office personnel are seeking new ways to answer patients' financial questions.

Interest and cooperation throughout the project was most gratifying, but the continued responsiveness of all groups is indeed rewarding.

CONCLUSION

It would be simple to conclude that only attending doctors are responsible for answering patients' questions and that patients themselves must assume responsibility for asking the questions. However, this survey demonstrated that such a simple conclusion is not satisfactory for doctors, other personnel, or even for the patients.

A major disclosure from patients' comments and study of the attitudes and opinions of personnel was that the capabilities of other members of the medical team were not being fully utilized in discharge instructions.

The survey does seem to suggest that there should be:

1. A place within the hospital where patients could call for information.

2. Exchange, among physicians, of their individual discharge instructions and patients' convalescent problems and anxieties; and some common basic discharge instructions for patients, particularly in the surgical area where the questions were more numerous.

3. A search for new methods of teaching patients, pictorially and verbally, through the use of charts, pamphlets, booklets, teaching machines, television, and, possibly, even the computer.

4. Patient education in the existing teaching programs of the hospitals, the medical and nursing schools, perhaps even extending into secondary schools.

5. Interchange of ideas and problems with community agencies for the advancement of patient education.

6. Comparison and evaluation of discharge information to patients in other institutions.

REFERENCES

1. Pratt, Lois, and others. Physicians' views on the level of medical information among patients. Amer. J. Public Health 47:1277-1283, Oct. 1957.
2. Dodge, Joan S. How much should the patient be told and by whom? Hospitals 37:66-79, 125, Dec. 16, 1963.

WHAT COMMUNICATION MEANS TO PATIENTS

James K. Skipper, Jr., Daisy L. Tagliacozzo, and Hans O. Mauksch

To hospitalized patients, communication with their nurses and physicians is extremely important. This fact is apparent in interviews conducted during the first phase of a research project designed to explore the patient's perception of the patient role.

The patients, a small sample of a patient population in a large, private, urban hospital, were interviewed using a semistructured technique, which allowed them freedom of expression. The 86 interviewees included men and women between the ages of 40 and 60. All were Caucasian, American born, married, and had had previous hospital experience. The two major disease categories were cardiovascular and gastrointestinal. A total of 132 interviews were conducted, and the fifth day of hospitalization was the mean date of interviewing. All interviews were recorded verbatim and had a mean length of one hour.

It is our thesis that communication had two primary meanings for the hospitalized patients: the securing of information, and interpersonal contact. The securing of information seemed to serve instrumental functions, while interpersonal contact had both instrumental and expressive functions. Expressive refers to action concerned with direct gratification, while instrumental refers to actions directed toward a future goal.

Probably in any culture illness brings a degree of fear and anxiety to the stricken individual. It also changes the expected behavior of the sick person. For instance, in our culture, one who is ill has the right to expect that others will allow him to deviate from his normal behavior but, at the same time, he must accept the obligation to get well.[1] This may be called the "illness" role. Because of the concerns that accompany illness and the pressure on him to recover, the sick person desires information about his illness.[2] For the hospitalized patient, the most reliable means of securing this information is communication with hospital personnel, especially the physician.

EXPLAINING THE ILLNESS

During the interviews, giving a "poor explanation" was the aspect of medical care patients criticized most. When questioned about what makes a good doctor, almost two out of three patients (65 percent) considered a good explanation of illness one of the most important qualities. Thirty-two percent emphasized that a good doctor should spend time answering patients' questions about their illness. The demand on physicians to give patients a full account of the nature and extent of their illness and progress seemed to have several functions for the patient.

First, for some, a good explanation seemed to put the patient more at ease. One said, "I have to have an explanation. I just could not live with it any other way. I can live with anything I can understand." Another said, "My physician has upset me. It drives me nuts. What's up? I don't know what's up. It's driving me crazy."

Second, for some patients, communication with the physician allowed them to know that he understood their illness and was using his skills to facilitate their recovery. This bolstered the patients' trust and helped them to cooperate.

When asked, "What can be done to increase the patient's confidence in the doctor?" one patient said, "I think doctors should tell patients the truth, because I think that builds a lot of confidence." A second said, "I like them to tell me what's wrong with me and no beating around the bush. I feel I would cooperate much more with the doctor then."

Finally, a good explanation of his illness helped the patient assess his rights. Patients characteristically had difficulties defining their rights in the hospital. Almost one quarter (23 percent) admitted that they didn't know what their rights were, and over 10 percent stated categorically that they did not have any rights. Most patients determined rights by how ill they deemed themselves to be. "The sicker I am the more I should get." Therefore, it was very important for patients to receive some information about their illness.

A patient paused a long time when asked, "What are your rights as a patient?" Then he said, "Well this is hard to answer. It depends on how sick you are." Another illustration of this is, "It depends on how sick you are. As I say, I'm sure that when you are very sick, most of the care goes to you. If you are not sick you simply have to exercise some patience."

FEARS ABOUT MISTAKES

Not only were patients concerned with receiving information about their illness, but also about the technical and medical procedures, their medicines, and generally what was going to happen to them, and when. In these matters patients desired communications with both physicians and nurses.

Information about these matters served several functions for the patient. Even though every patient in the sample had had previous hospital experience, they lacked knowledge about technical medical procedures and found it difficult to foresee forthcoming events. Many times patients were taken by surprise. At times anxiety and fear was the result of patients' lack of psychological preparation.

"If they would tell you ahead of time the house doctor or the intern will be in to give you a complete examination, you expect it. But I didn't expect it and that embarrassed me."

"Certainly I would prefer being told beforehand. That way you can prepare for it. That does make a lot of difference in a person's attitude."

Patients were often preoccupied with safety in the hospital and many feared being neglected or being the subject of gross mistakes. Patients often related stories of previous hospital experiences of themselves or acquaintances who had been wheeled to the operating room instead of the x-ray department, received the wrong medicine, or not gotten their medicine on time.

"You feel that something may happen to you if you do not get the things the doctor ordered on time and if they forget the medicine or give you the wrong medicine as it happened two weeks ago. You lose confidence and you feel you can't trust them."

Patients wanted information about what was supposed to be happening to them so that they would have more control over the situation and would be better able to protect themselves from errors. "I always ask questions because maybe they are doing the wrong thing." "If you don't watch them they will bring you the wrong medicine. You have to watch and take care of yourself to get well."

In addition to the expectations surrounding the illness role, a person is faced with another new set of rights and obligations when he becomes a patient in a hospital. These stem from the nature of the social organization of the hospital. Like any other organization, the hospital has certain regulations and customs. These standard operating procedures allow hospital personnel to carry on their jobs in a relatively predictable manner. Patients, of course, are expected to comply with established procedures and to behave appropriately. This may be called the "hospitalized patient" role. Although the patient entering the hospital may have some idea of what he may expect of others and what they may expect of him, the interviews indicated that many did not.

Patients manifested a desire to understand the rules of the game. For instance, what do various nurses and doctors really expect of me, which of the hospital regulations may be stretched a bit, who can I turn to for help with personal problems, how promptly will nurses answer my call, how do I identify the head nurse?

This appears to be more of a problem for patients in private rooms. In a ward, the patient, through informal communication with other patients, learns the reality of the hospital situation. As Barnes has described the typical ward:

Patients have an almost uncanny knack of finding out exactly what is going on. . . . Information is passed along a sort of secret "bush" telegraph and very little escapes their eyes. This seems to be true regardless of the type of ward or the type of illness of the patient.[2]

In the hospital studied, patients were isolated from most other patients and informal communication was severely limited. Therefore, the hospitalized patient was very dependent on the more formal channels of communication with hospital employees and doctors. "Well I think maybe a lot of patients coming to the hospital know very little about the hospital. As I mentioned before—if the nurses can just explain things to you."

Can a doctor help the patient in his adjustment to hospitalization? the interviewer asked. "Oh yes, by explaining to the patient the trouble there is in not having enough people around to help you. I think it is important to explain to the patient about his hospitalization."

INTERPERSONAL CONTACT

To secure information, patients wanted communication with hospital employees and physicians through direct personal contact. However, patients desired such communication for other reasons also. Many patients reported that the days passed slowly for them, that there was little to occupy their time. Others felt extremely lonely and wished they "just had somebody to talk to." For this type of communication, patients looked especially to nurses.

"What is a really nice nurse?" the interviewer asked. "One that is willing to say a few words to you. After all when you are in the hospital it helps some people to have nurses that make occasional remarks whether it's about the weather or anything else."

"What should a patient expect from his nurse?" was another question. "She should be ready to talk to the patient when she is around and ready to take a joke and joke back."

Communications of this kind with the nurse seemed to be, from the point of view of some patients, strictly expressive. It was concerned with direct gratification as an end in itself as contrasted to the more instrumental desire for information. This is illustrated nicely by the meaning patients ascribed to nurses' smiles. "It just makes them a little more cheerful. It takes them out of the gloom." "The patient feels that his day is a much better one when a nurse comes in with a smile. You feel things don't look so bad." "If a grouchy nurse comes in the morning your day is ruined—I mean if she snaps at you."

At the same time, this typically expressive type of communication may be a means toward an instrumental end for the patient. For example, patients manifested a strong sense of obligation toward both the doctor and the nurse to be cooperative, to be considerate, especially of the doctor, and not to be demanding, and not to be dependent, especially with the nurse.

REJECTION

Although patients tried at all times to adhere to this hospitalized patient role, they often said that the sick patient is sometimes not himself. They expressed some anxiety over being rejected by hospital personnel (especially the nurse) for not being a "good patient." The nice, kind, patient, and tolerant nurse was able to indicate to the patient that his occasional deviations from being a good patient were understood.

It is interesting and important to note that in this case the nurse's smile may be more instrumental to the patient than it is expressive, for here it takes on an added symbolic meaning. For example, "So when the nurse comes in here and she has a smile on her face, I know that she's willing to do anything."

Another says, "But a patient who really feels bad and needs assistance from a nurse, well that really makes a difference. If the nurse is cooperative in that way and gives him a smile or runs into the room once in a while it makes him feel good. She doesn't tire of that. She's not dissatisfied with the patient."

FEELINGS ABOUT SAFETY

The possibility of rejection is closely related to a patient's preoccupation with safety and it must be elaborated here. First, it must be understood that the most common belief

The nursing process

expressed by almost every patient interviewed was that both doctors and nurses were very busy, rushed, and overworked, and really did not have enough time to take care of all their patients. Furthermore, patients recognized the bureaucratic nature of the hospital with its complexity.

Some patients believed that some doctors and nurses had little interest in their patients and were not as dedicated as they might be. A few patients insisted that some doctors were only interested in making money. Therefore, these patients believed that they must be on guard against being neglected or being the subject of gross mistakes which would hamper chances of getting well.

Even though many times patients were afraid for their safety in the hospital, relatively few comments showed concern about the knowledge, skill, and training of nurses and doctors. It seemed that patients, being laymen, found themselves unable to judge either the hospital or nurses and physicians on strictly technical grounds. Freidson came to essentially the same conclusion in his study of subscribers to a prepaid medical plan.[3] For instance, in our study, in defining criteria for evaluating nurses and doctors, "personalized care" was mentioned by 89 percent of the patients for doctors and 81 percent for nurses.

These percentages must be evaluated very carefully. We do not think that they mean that the patients felt personalized care was a more important facet of total patient care than knowledge and skill. On the contrary, we postulated that being unable to judge the knowledge and skill of hospital personnel, patients used personalized care as an indication that their doctors and nurses were technically competent, dedicated, and interested in their patients. In other words, in this case, communications were not sought for direct gratification but for the much more instrumental function of a sign of safety. Thus, it was symbolic meaning which these patients attached to the communication of personalized care which made it so important for them.

SUMMARY

The 132 interviews revealed that communication with physicians and nurses was of great importance to the patients. It meant, first, the securing of information and, second, interpersonal contact. Patients desired information about their illness, technical procedures, and the general social organization of the hospital. When received, this type of information seemed to help stem patients' anxieties over their illnesses. It also aided patients to learn what nurses and physicians expected of them.

Patients desired personal contact with hospital personnel because they needed attention. They wanted someone to talk to, to help pass the time, and keep them from feeling lonely, and to be kind to them and give them emotional support. Patients used this type of communication as a sign that not only were their nurses and physicians dedicated and interested in their care and cure and would not reject them, but also that these persons were technically qualified, possessing the knowledge and skill to get them well.

REFERENCES

1. Parsons, Talcott, and Fox, Renee. Illness, therapy and the modern urban American family. In Patients, Physicians and Illness, ed. by E. G. Jaco, Glencoe, Ill., Free Press, 1958, pp. 234-245.
2. Barnes, Elizabeth. People in Hospital. London, Macmillan and Co., Ltd., 1961, pp. 15, 88.
3. Freidson, Eliot. Patients' Views of Medical Practice. New York, Russell Sage Foundation, 1961, p. 175.

SUGGESTED READINGS for Chapter 4

BOOKS

Auld, M. E., and Birum, L. H., editors: The challenge of nursing, St. Louis, 1973, The C. V. Mosby Co. Unit III is a collection of articles related to nursing process.

Banathy, B. H.: Instructional systems, Belmont, Calif., 1968, Fearon Publishers, Inc. Discusses systems for education and learning, formulation of objectives, analysis of learning tasks, design of the system, implementation, and quality control.

Beland, I.: Clinical nursing: pathophysiological and psychological approaches, New York, 1970, Macmillan Publishing Co., Inc. A medical-surgical textbook.

Benjamin, A.: The helping interview, Boston, 1969, Houghton Mifflin Co. Discusses the conditions, stages, and philosophies of interviewing, recording, types of questions and communication, responses and leads.

Bermosk, L. S., and Mordan, M. J.: Interviewing in nursing, New York, 1964, Macmillan Publishing Co., Inc. Discusses interviewing, climate for interviewing, and the role of the nurse.

Bernstein, L., and Dana, R. H.: Interviewing and the health professions, New York, 1970, Appleton-Century-Crofts. Discusses interviewing techniques, evaluative, hostile, reassuring, probing, and understanding responses, emotional reactions to illness, death, and dying.

Bird, B.: Talking with patients, Philadelphia, 1955, J. B. Lippincott Co. Discusses communication with adults and children.

Blood, D. F., and Budd, W. C.: Educational measurement and evaluation, New York, 1972, Harper & Row, Publishers. Discusses the nature of educational measurement, validity, educational objectives, observational tests, paper-and-pencil tests, objective examinations, item analysis, standardized tests, statistical treatment of test scores, grading, and reporting.

Bloom, B. S.: Taxonomy of educational objectives: the classification of educational goals, Handbook I, Cognitive domain, New York, 1956, David McKay Co., Inc. Discusses cognitive domain—knowledge, comprehension, application, analysis, synthesis, and evaluation.

Bower, F. L.: The process of planning nursing care: a model for practice, ed. 2, St. Louis, 1972, The C. V. Mosby Co. Discusses planning individualized nursing care, identifying nursing problems, selecting nursing actions, formulat-

ing evaluative criteria, and implementing the nursing care plan.

Brill, N. I.: Working with people: the helping process, Philadelphia, 1973, J. B. Lippincott Co. Discusses understanding ourselves, the human condition, institutions, communications, dealing with dependency, an eclectic approach, and integrating the personal and professional self.

Byers, V. B.: Nursing observation, Dubuque, Iowa, 1968, William C. Brown Co., Publishers. Discusses the role of observation in nursing practice; observation of patients in their environment—voice, eyes, gait, appetite, elimination, sleep; observation of signs and symptoms—pain, hemorrhage, edema, dizziness; observations related to nursing activities—admitting and bathing the patient; applications of observation to patient situations.

Byrne, M. L., and Thompson, L. F.: Key concepts for the study and practice of nursing, ed. 2, St. Louis, 1978, The C. V. Mosby Co. Discusses following concepts: organismic behavior, basic human needs, level of wellness, adaptation, behavioral patterning, steady state, stress, behavioral stability continuum, structural variable, and the consequences of an act. Presents a working model for assessing patient's needs and predicting the effects of nursing care.

Champion, R. A.: Learning and activation, New York, 1969, John Wiley & Sons, Inc. Discusses the nature and measurement of learning, types of learning situations, basic features of learning, activation, complex learning phenomena, retention and forgetting.

Collins, M.: Communications in health care: understanding and implementing effective human relations, St. Louis, 1977, The C. V. Mosby Co. Explains a therapeutic relationship and presents exercises for analysis.

Dale, E.: Audiovisual methods in teaching, New York, 1969, Holt, Rinehart, & Winston, Inc. Discusses the theory and practice, media and materials of audiovisual teaching, systems, and technology in teaching.

De Vito, J. A., editor: Communication: concepts and processes, Englewood Cliffs, N.J., 1976, Prentice-Hall, Inc. A collection of articles about communications.

Eckelberry, G. K.: Administration of comprehensive nursing care, New York, 1971, Appleton-Century-Crofts. Discusses comprehension of nursing care, personal frame of reference, identifying nursing needs, nursing diagnosis, planning of nursing care, care plan, implementing and evaluating care, groups who work together, and coordination.

Ellis, H. C.: Fundamentals of human learning and cognition, Dubuque, Iowa, 1972, William C. Brown Co., Publishers. Discusses the elements of conditioning, characteristics of verbal learning, processes in verbal learning, transfer of training, memory, concept and perceptual learning, problem solving, and motor skills.

Freeman, R. B.: Community health nursing practice, Philadelphia, 1970, W. B. Saunders Co. A basic community health nursing textbook that includes a discussion on working with groups.

French, R. M.: The nurse's guide to diagnostic procedures, New York, 1971, McGraw-Hill Book Co. Discusses numerous diagnostic tests.

Fuerst, E. V., and Wolff, L. V.: Fundamentals of nursing, ed. 5, Philadelphia, 1974, J. B. Lippincott Co. Discusses the practice of nursing, nursing implementation, nursing responsibilities in relation to therapeutic agents and measures, and to assisting the physician.

Giffin, K., and Patton, B. R.: Fundamentals of interpersonal communication, New York, 1971, Harper & Row, Publishers. Discusses interpersonal communication.

Hays, J. S., and Larson, K. H.: Interacting with patients, New York, 1963, Macmillan Publishing Co., Inc. Identifies, illustrates, and discusses twenty-five therapeutic techniques and nineteen nontherapeutic techniques. Most of the book consists of process recordings of case studies that illustrate therapeutic and nontherapeutic communication.

Hein, E. C.: Communication in nursing practice, Boston, 1973, Little, Brown & Co. Discusses therapeutic communication, channels of communication, feedback.

Highet, G.: The art of teaching, New York, 1950, Vintage Books. Discusses the qualities and abilities of a good teacher, methods of teaching, great teachers and their pupils, and teaching in everyday life.

Hyman, R. T.: Ways of teaching, Philadelphia, 1970, J. B. Lippincott Co. Discusses discussion, recitation and lecture, role playing, questioning, and observing.

Johnson, M. M., Davis, M. L. C., and Bilitch, M. J.: Problem solving in nursing practice, Dubuque, Iowa, 1970, William C. Brown Co., Publishers. Discusses an overview of problem solving, patient problems vs. nursing problems,

problem assessment, problem statement, and solving problem.

Johnson, S. R., and Johnson, R. B.: Developing individualized instructional material: a self-instructional material in itself, Palo Alto, Calif., 1970, Westinghouse Learning Press. Discusses the taxonomy of educational objectives, criterion measures, format checklist, methods of instruction, and cost comparisons.

Kemp, J. E.: Planning and producing audiovisual materials, Scranton, Pa., 1963, Chandler Publishing Co. Describes how to plan and produce audiovisual materials.

Krathwohl, D. R., et al.: Taxonomy of educational objectives: the classification of educational goals, Handbook II, Affective domain, New York, 1956, David McKay Co., Inc. Discusses affective domain—receiving, responding, valuing, organization, and characterization by a value.

Kron, T.: Communication in nursing, Philadelphia, 1972, W. B. Saunders Co. Discusses the elements of communication, thinking, perceiving, doing, listening, speaking, reading, writing, and keys to effective communication.

Lewis, G.: Nurse-patient communication, Dubuque, Iowa, 1969, William C. Brown Co., Publishers. An introduction to the study of communication. Emphasizes nonverbal communication within the framework of senses.

Little, D. E., and Carnevali, D.: Nursing care planning, Philadelphia, 1969, J. B. Lippincott Co. Discusses current concepts and rationale for planning patient care, relationship of the philosophy of patient care to nursing care plans, processes used in care planning, nursing history, nursing care plans, revisions of nursing care plans, nursing care plan forms, activating a nursing care plan system, and teaching planning of nursing care.

Lockerby, F.: Communication for nurses, St. Louis, 1968, The C. V. Mosby Co. Discusses communication, observation, listening, speaking, and writing.

Mager, R. F.: Preparing instructional objectives, Belmont, Calif., 1962, Fearon Publishers, Inc. Discusses the development of objectives, stating terminal behavior, conditions, and the criteria of acceptable behavior.

Mager, R. F.: Developing attitude toward learning, Belmont, Calif., 1968, Fearon Publishers, Inc. Discusses developing objectives, approaches, and evaluation.

Maloney, E., editor: Interpersonal relations, Dubuque, Iowa, 1966, William C. Brown Co.,

Publishers. A collection of articles on interpersonal relations.

Mayers, M. G.: A systematic approach to the nursing care plan, New York, 1972, Appleton-Century-Crofts. Discusses systematic problem solving, the problem as a basis for care planning, the expected outcome as a standard for evaluation, nursing action as a strategy for solving problems, the patient's response as a test of good planning, nursing history, communicating patient care information, implementing nursing care planning, and current trends for improved patient care. Care planning in hospitals, institutions, community agencies, and nursing education are considered.

McCroskey, J. C., Larson, C. E., and Knapp, M. L.: An introduction to interpersonal communication, Englewood Cliffs, N.J., 1971, Prentice-Hall, Inc. Discusses interpersonal communication.

McKeachie, W. J.: Teaching tips: a guidebook for the beginning college teacher, Lexington, Mass., 1969, D. C. Heath & Co. Discusses preparing a course, meeting the class for the first time, numerous teaching methods and tools, counseling, research, and evaluation.

O'Brien, M.: Communications and relationships in nursing, St. Louis, 1978, The C. V. Mosby Co. Discusses verbal and nonverbal communication, effective communication, perception, writing, and communication as it relates to patient care and administration.

Orlando, I. J.: The dynamic nurse-patient relationship, New York, 1961, G. P. Putnam's Sons. Discusses function, process, and principles of nurse-patient relationship; rich with illustrations.

Peplau, H. E.: Interpersonal relations in nursing, New York, 1952, G. P. Putnam's Sons. Studies nursing as an interpersonal process. Discusses phases of the nurse-patient relationship and roles in nursing; influences of human needs, interferences to achievement of goals, opposing goals, unexplained discomfort in nursing situations. Identifies the psychological tasks of the sick role.

Peplau, H. E.: Basic principles of patient counselling, Philadelphia, 1964, Smith Kline & French Laboratories. Presents extracts from two clinical nursing workshops in psychiatric hospitals. Discusses a form of counseling interviews and principles for nurse-counselor. Principles discussed in detail include: setting an example for the patient, maintaining a professional attitude, respecting the patient, assessing the patient's

intellectual competence, guiding the patient to reinterpret his experiences rationally, asking sensible questions to aid description, and studying and applying theory in counseling.

Phaneuf, M. C.: The nursing audit profile for excellence, New York, 1972, Appleton-Century-Crofts. Describes some problems of evaluating quality of nursing care, what an audit is and is not, the audit instrument, planning for auditing, orientation of the audit committee, the auditing process, influences of auditing. Appendices contain a table of random numbers, suggested readings, and explanations of audit schedule components and audit forms.

Pluckhan, M. L.: Human communication: the matrix of nursing, New York, 1978, McGraw-Hill Book Co. Integrates general and technical aspects of human communication.

Pohl, M. L.: Teaching function of the nursing practitioner, Dubuque, Iowa, 1968, William C. Brown Co., Publishers. Discusses teaching as a function of nursing, principles of teaching and learning, problems of teaching and learning in nursing settings, subject matter, teaching methods and materials, and planning for teaching.

Popiel, E. S., editor: Nursing and the process of continuing education, ed. 2, St. Louis, 1977, The C. V. Mosby Co. A collection of papers related to continuing education.

Redman, B. K.: The process of patient teaching in nursing, ed. 3, St. Louis, 1976, The C. V. Mosby Co. Discusses teaching in nursing, the teaching-learning process, readiness, objectives, principles of learning, teaching methods, and evaluation.

Reilly, D. E.: Behavioral objectives in nursing: evaluation of learner attainment, New York, 1975, Appleton-Century-Crofts. Details the development of behavioral objectives, the taxonomy of educational objectives, and evaluation.

Saxton, D. F., and Hyland, P. A.: Planning and implementing nursing intervention, St. Louis, 1975, The C. V. Mosby Co. Uses stress-adaptation and patient needs as the theoretical framework for nursing intervention.

Seedor, M. M.: Aids to diagnosis: a programed unit in fundamentals of nursing, New York, 1964, Teachers College Press, Columbia University. Presents a programmed unit in fundamentals of nursing; discusses vital signs, observation, physical examination, and laboratory tests.

Sierra-Franco, M. H.: Therapeutic communication in nursing, New York, 1978, McGraw-Hill

Book Co. Provides a programmed self-instruction about communicating with patients.

Skipper, J. K., Jr., and Leonard, R. C., editors: Social interaction and patient care, Philadelphia, 1965, J. B. Lippincott Co. A collection of articles about social and psychological aspects of the nurse's role, the importance of communication, the patient's view of his situation, structural and cultural content of patient care, the role and status relationships between doctor, nurse, and patient.

Staton, T. F.: How to instruct successfully, New York, 1960, McGraw-Hill Book Co., Inc. Discusses the nature of learning, psychological factors underlying learning, planning for instruction, numerous teaching methods and tools, evaluation, and counseling.

Sullivan, H. S.: The psychiatric interview, New York, 1954, W. W. Norton & Co., Inc. Discusses basic concepts, technical considerations, structuring, early stages, detailed inquiry, and termination of the interview process.

Sundeen, S. J., Stuart, G. W., Rankin, E. D., and Cohen, S. P.: Nurse-client interaction: implementing the nursing process, St. Louis, 1976, The C. V. Mosby Co. Discusses communication, the nurse-client relationship, and the helping relationship.

Taba, H.: Curriculum development: theory and practice, New York, 1962, Harcourt, Brace and World, Inc. Discusses the foundations for and process of curriculum planning, the design of curriculum, and strategies of changing the curriculum.

Tobin, H. M., et al.: The process of staff development: components for change, St. Louis, 1974, The C. V. Mosby Co. Discusses continuing education and staff development, the history of staff development, adult learning, motivation, organization, philosophy, purpose, and goals, identifying learning needs, designing and implementing learning offerings, selecting teaching methods and aids, and evaluation.

Travelbee, J.: Interpersonal aspects of nursing, Philadelphia, 1966, F. A. Davis Co. Discusses the nature of nursing, nurse-patient relationships, and nursing intervention. Explores the concepts human being, patient, nurse, illness, suffering, communication.

Vitale, B. A., Latterner, N. S., and Nugent, P. M.: A problem solving approach to nursing care plans: a program, ed. 2, St. Louis, 1978, The C. V. Mosby Co. Stresses data collection and classification, making deductions, the nursing diagnosis and hypothesis, hypothesis imple-

mentation, and evaluation in a program text form. Presents numerous case studies.

Watson, D. L., and Tharp, R. G.: Self-directed behavior: self-modification for personal adjustment, Monterey, Calif., 1972, Brooks/Cole Publishing Co. Discusses behavior modification.

Yura, H., and Walsh, M. B., editors: The nursing process, Washington, D.C., 1967, The Catholic University of America Press. Discusses assessing patient needs, planning to meet those needs, implementing, and evaluating plan of care.

Yura, H., and Walsh, M. B.: The nursing process: assessing, planning, implementing, evaluating, New York, 1973, Appleton-Century-Crofts. Discusses components of the nursing process.

PERIODICALS
Continuity of care

Bielski, M. T.: Continuity of care for the patient with coronary heart disease, Nurs. Clin. North Am. 7:413-421, Sept., 1972. Stresses continuity of care in a system of coronary care.

Cucuzzo, R. A.: Method discharge planning, Superv. Nurse 7(1):43-45, 1976. Illustrates the use of problem-oriented medical records system for discharge planning.

Dahlin, B.: Rehabilitation and the assessment of patient need, Nurs. Clin. North Am. 1:375-386, Sept., 1966. Discusses assessment related to rehabilitation and the continuity of care.

Deakers, L. P.: Continuity of family-centered nursing care between the hospital and the home, Nurs. Clin. North Am. 7:83-93, March, 1972. Stresses that discharge planning begins on the day of admission and the degree of continuity provided depends on the ability of health team to work together.

Discharge planning, Utah Nurse 23:16, Spring, 1972. Discusses how to approach discharge planning.

Jennings, C. P.: Discharge planning and the government, Superv. Nurse 8(3):48-52, 1977. Outlines the regulatory process of discharge planning.

La Montagne, M. E., and McKeehan, K. M.: Profile of a continuing care program emphasizing discharge planning, J. Nurs. Adm. 5(8): 22-33, 1975. Defines continuity as a circular process, itemizes guidelines for implementing a continuing care program, and presents a patient care referral form.

Mehaffy, N. L.: Assessment and communication for continuity of care for the surgical patient,

Nurs. Clin. North Am. **10**(4):625-633, 1974. Describes preoperative assessment, nursing care plan, documentation of care in OR, evaluation, and results of changes in the assessment and communication patterns.

Peabody, S. R.: Assessment and planning for continuity of care, Nurs. Clin. North Am. **4**:303-310, June, 1969. Describes planning of the continuing care program and assessment of patient care needs.

Stillar, E. M.: Continuity of care, Nurs. Outlook **10**(9):584-585, 1962. Identifies contributions of the rehabilitation nurse to continuity of care in the hospital setting.

Health teaching

Agrafitis, P. C.: Teaching parents about Pierre Robin syndrome, Am. J. Nurs. **72**(11):2040-2041, 1972. Discusses information about Pierre Robin syndrome and describes the teaching aid used to teach parents.

Albert, S.: Storefront converted to health education center, Hospitals **49**(4):57-59, 1975. Gives details of a storefront health education center that provides information, screening, and referrals to New York City residents.

Allison, S. E.: A framework for nursing action in a nurse-conducted diabetic management clinic, J. Nurs. Adm. **3**(4):53-60, 1973. Uses Orem's self-care concept as a framework for diabetic control in adult patients.

Althafer, C., Butcher, R., and Fosburg, R. G.: Now it's health information by phone, tel-med, Am. Lung Assoc. Bull. **60**:12-14, Jan.-Feb., 1974. Discusses the use of the San Diego County Medical Society's medical tape library to answer questions about health by phone.

Amend, E. L.: A parent education program in a children's hospital, Nurs. Outlook **14**(4):53-56, 1966. Discusses orientation sessions, the open visiting schedule, and planned instruction for parents.

Ardell, D. B.: A case for hospital action, Hosp. Forum **28**(14):9-10, 1976. Identifies ways hospitals can promote wellness.

Bille, D.: A study of patients' knowledge in relation to teaching format and compliance, Superv. Nurse **8**(3):55-62, 1977. Stresses individualizing in hospital-patient teaching.

Borgman, M. F.: Exercise + health maintenance, J. Nurs. Educ. **16**(1):6-10, 1977. Presents a teaching plan with competency-based objectives.

Boyle, M. T., and Kaufman, A.: Strep screening to prevent rheumatic fever, Am. J. Nurs. **75**(9): 1487-1488, 1975. Nursing students did a clinical community experience by culturing throats of a large Puerto Rican population to prevent rheumatic heart disease.

Bruess, C. E.: Professional preparation of the health educator, J. Sch. Health **46**(7):418-421, 1976. Defines health educator, identifies skills and knowledge needed, and lists functions of the health educator.

Bruess, C. E., and Gay, J. E.: Professional preparation of the health educator: a report of a forum sponsored by the ASHA committee on college health education and professional preparation, J. Sch. Health **46**(4):222-225, 1976. Discusses the preparation of health educators.

Bryan, N. E.: Every nurse a teacher, Aust. Nurses' J. **4**(1):31-33, 1974. Stresses the importance of the nurse helping people recognize their health needs and ways to meet them.

Buford, L. M.: Group education to reduce overweight: classes for mentally handicapped children, Am. J. Nurs. **75**(11):1994-1995, 1975. School nurse educated and motivated fifteen students and their parents toward weight reduction. Discusses student activities.

Burnside, I. M.: Things my nursing instructor never taught me, Nurs. Outlook **11**(2):124-125, 1963. Discusses improvisation in extended nursing care program for the chronically ill.

Claxton, I.: Nurses explain hospitals to children, Hospitals **49**(13):41-42, 1975. Describes an orientation program taught by Children's Hospital nurses to second graders in the St. Paul area. Children are told about what happens in hospitals from admission through discharge to dispel their fears.

Coalville—an experiment in family planning, Nurs. Times **70**(37):1428, 1974. Describes an experiment in family planning.

Communications: nursing instructions to patients, The Regan Report on Nursing Law **16**(3):2, 1975. Presents a legal case that emphasizes the need for nurses to give explanations to patients when something is required of the patient for his treatment.

Crate, M. A.: Nursing functions in adaptation to chronic illness, Am. J. Nurs. **65**(10):72-76, 1965. Discusses four phases of adaptation and the nurse's role during each phase.

Crow, M., Bradshaw, B. R., and Guest, F.: True to life: a relevant approach to patient education, Am. J. Public Health **62**:1328-1330, 1972. Discusses the development of a magazine resembling confession magazines in order to reach women in family planning program.

Daniel, M. C.: Special programs on health and safety, Occup. Health Nurs. **22**(3):14-15, 1974. Outlines safety and health education for employees and the community.

Deeley, T. J.: Carcinoma of the bronchus—the future, Nurs. Times **72**(8):314-315, 1976. Describes education, prevention, diagnosis, and treatment of bronchial carcinoma.

De Grave, G., Riordan, B., and Mathias, R.: Sex education for delinquent boys—unveiling the taboo, Nursing '76 **6**(6):22-25, 1976. Discusses and evaluates a sex education program.

Dickinson, F. S.: National agency to be health education troubleshooter, Hospitals **50**(9):69-71, 1976. The National Center for Health Education in New York City will study consumer motivation and third-party payment for patient education. Describes the center.

Dixon, G., and Rickard, K.: Nutrition education for young patients, Children Today **4**(1):7-11, 1975. Describes nutrition educational projects.

Downs, F. S., and Fernbach, V.: Experimental evaluation of a prenatal leaflet series, Nurs. Res. **22**(6):498-506, 1973. Research report indicates no significant difference in information level among groups who read pamphlets and those who did not. Level of education made a difference in correct responses to questions.

Einstein, S., Lavenhar, M., and Garitano, W. W.: Drug abuse education and the multiplier effect: an experience in training 109 teachers, J. Sch. Health **42**:609-613, Dec., 1972. Discusses training teachers to teach about drug abuse.

Epstein, J. B., Magrowski, W. D., and McPhail, C. W. B.: The role of radio and TV spot announcements in public health education, Can. J. Public Health **66**(5):396-398, 1975. Encourages the use of mass media for health education.

Evans, M. W.: An introduction to health education in hospital, Nurs. Mirror **139**(15):49-50, 1974. Mentions primary, secondary, and tertiary health education and teaching individuals and groups. Describes hospital involvement in health education of hospitalized patients, hospital staff, and the community served by the hospital.

Farquhar, J. W.: Perspectives on coronary risk. Part I. You can cut the odds on coronary risk, RN **40**(2):23-26, 1977. Identifies roles for the nurse in coronary care education.

Feldstein, M., and Swabb, L.: The use of the "micro-unit" in health education, J. Sch. Health **42**:105-108, Feb., 1972. Discusses how micro-unit can be used to integrate health education material into what students are already studying.

Fitzpatrick, D.: I need a friend, J. Pract. Nurs. **25**(5):35, 1975. Two student nurses taught 374 elementary students how to give mouth-to-mouth resuscitation in two hours. Outlines class activities.

Flowers, L. K.: The development of a program for treating obesity, Hosp. Community Psychiatry **27**(5):342-345, 1976. Evaluates a weight control class and discusses the changes made to make the class more successful.

Fuhrman, R. R., and McWilliams, M.: Consumer management program aims for total health education, Hospitals **50**(16):86-89, 1976. Describes a program that uses community resources to provide educational services to the medical center. Senior dietetic students use a mobile nutrition cart to teach nutrition to patients in waiting rooms.

Fusillo, A. E., and Beloian, A. M.: Consumer nutrition knowledge and self-reported food shopping behavior, Am. J. Public Health **67**(9):846-850, 1977. Report of a research study that found nutrition knowledge, food beliefs, and reported shopping behavior to have a positive, linear association.

Fylling, C. P.: Health education, Hospitals **49**(7):95-97, 1975. Indicates that the trend is for the American Hospital Association to stress promotion, organization, implementation, and evaluation of health education by health care institutions.

Galli, N.: Foundations of health education, J. Sch. Health **46**(3):158-165, 1976. Presents sociocultural, psychobehavioral, educational, legal, and scientific foundations of health education.

Galton, L.: Questions patients want to ask about their health and how you can answer them, Nursing '77 **7**(4):54-59, 1977. Lists questions and answers.

Green, L. W.: The potential of health education includes cost effectiveness, Hospitals **50**(9):57-61, 1976. Indicates that health education can promote cost effectiveness by reducing broken appointments, unpaid bills, and malpractice suits, and by gaining community support, speeding diagnosis, and increasing patient compliance.

Green, L. W.: Evaluation and measurement: some dilemmas for health education, Am. J. Public Health **67**(2):155-161, 1977. Identifies and discusses problems of evaluating health education.

Gross, D., and O'Rourke, T. W.: Research and the future of health education, J. Sch. Health **45**(1):30-32, 1975. Discusses benefits of research to health education.

Grover, P. L., and Miller, J.: Guidelines for making

health education work, Public Health Rep. **91**(3):249-253, 1976. Lists media guidelines and interpersonal and environmental factors associated with health education.

Hammond, E.: Home care and improvisations, Nurs. Outlook **12**(4):49-51, 1964. Describes improvisations in home care for cancer patients.

Haskin, J., Hawley, N. R., and Weinberger, J. B.: Project teen concern: an educational approach to the prevention of venereal disease and premature parenthood, J. Sch. Health **46**(4):231-234, 1976. Describes the educational approach used by the San Francisco Unified School District to help prevent venereal disease and early pregnancy.

Hassett, M.: Teaching hemodialysis to the family unit, Nurs. Clin. North Am. **7**:349-362, June, 1972. Discusses how dialysis center became home teaching center.

Hellman, S.: The health educator—a resource for nurses, Superv. Nurse **7**(9):18-22, 1976. Advocates the use of health educators for patient teaching and patient education program planning.

Hoeper, B. E.: A lesson in positive health, Nurs. Outlook **8**(11):614-615, 1960. Describes how some industrial nurses implemented new philosophy that increased emphasis on health maintenance, health counseling, cooperation with family physician and community agencies, health and safety education.

Hollister, W. G., and Edgerton, J. W.: Teaching relationship-building skills, Am. J. Public Health **64**:41-46, Jan., 1974. Reveals approach to teaching skills in building interpersonal relations.

Hopp, J. W.: Values clarification and the school nurse, J. Sch. Health **45**(7):410-413, 1975. School nurses used values clarification techniques. Gives examples.

Horner, A. L., and Jennings, M.: Before patients go home, Am. J. Nurs. **61**(6):62-63, 1961. Describes how family member is instructed about home nursing before disabled patients are released from hospital.

Horridge, D.: The louse war, Nurs. Mirror **144**(3): 58-59, 1977. Discusses health education, treatment, follow up, and the role of the community nurse in the war against lice.

Hurd, G. G.: Teaching the hemiplegic self-care, Am. J. Nurs. **62**(9):64-68, 1962. Uses case study to illustrate four-step method of teaching—preparation, demonstration, practice, and evaluation.

Hutchison, D. J.: An editorial exploration: health education an institutional responsibility, J. Con-tin. Educ. Nurs. **6**(2):3-5, 1975. Lists national developments in health education.

Iverson, D. C., and Hosokawa, M. C.: Health education research: accomplishment or exercise, J. Sch. Health **45**(3):154-156, 1975. Identifies areas needing research.

Jacobson, L. D.: Ethanol education today, J. Sch. Health **43**:36-39, Jan., 1973. Presents concepts, useful teaching points, and techniques for ethanol education.

Jamplis, R. W.: The practicing physician and patient education, Hosp. Practice **10**(10):93-99, 1975. Describes the Patient Education Center in Palo Alto, California, where physicians prescribe health education and health educators provide it.

Jones, P., and Oertel, W.: Developing patient teaching objectives + techniques: a self-instructional program, Nurse Educator **2**(5):3-18, 1977. Provides a self-instructional program for the development of clear, measurable patient-teaching objectives and determination of teaching techniques.

Kahn, A. N.: Group education for the overweight, Am. J. Nurs. **78**(2):254, 1978. Describes a seven-week session to increase understanding of self-image and to identify nonphysiological blocks to weight loss.

Kanaaneh, H. A., and Rabi, S. A.: The eradication of a large scabies outbreak using community-side health education, Am. J. Public Health **66**(6):564-567, 1976. Describes the eradication of a scabies epidemic in an Arabic village.

Kinsella, C.: Educational television for a hospital system, Am. J. Nurs. **64**(1):72-76, 1964. Discusses use of open circuit television for in-service education.

Koons, S. B.: The future of cancer nursing, RN **39**(8):23-34, 1976. Identifies future objectives for oncology nurses, one of which is preventive teaching.

Kopelke, C. E.: Group education to reduce overweight . . . in a blue-collar community, Am. J. Nurs. **75**(11):1993-1995, 1975. Presents a weight reduction program based on basic health education and resocialization.

Kratzer, J. B.: What does your patient need to know? Nursing '77 **7**(12):82, 84, 1977. Advises consideration of what your patient needs to know in making a teaching plan.

Kratzer, J. B., and Rauschenberger, D. S.: What to teach your patient about his duodenal ulcer, Nursing '78 **8**(1):54-56, 1978. Presents a case and identifies teaching content.

Krysan, G. S.: How do we teach four million diabetics? Am. J. Nurs. **65**(11):105-107, 1965.

Discusses nurse's role in four categories of teaching services—assessment and counseling, teaching self-care, coordinating community services, and follow-up. Stresses use of group teaching.

Kucha, D.: The health education of patients: assessing their needs, Superv. Nurse **5**:26-35, April, 1974. Discusses how to assess patients' learning needs.

Kucha, D.: The health education of patients: development of a system, part 1, Superv. Nurse **5**:8-21, May, 1974. Discusses planning as a subsystem in health education.

Kucha, D.: The health education of patients: development of a system, part 2, Superv. Nurse **5**:8-15, June, 1974. Outlines planning, programming, and budgeting for an outpatient health information and management system. Presents a planning process flow chart.

Kyle, J. R., and Savino, A. B.: Teaching parents behavior modification, Nurs. Outlook **21**(11): 717-720, 1973. Describes group instruction used to teach behavior modification.

Laugharne, E.: The tri-hospital/diabetes education centre, Dimens. Health Care **52**(3):43-44, 1975. Describes a diabetes education center that stresses good basic nutrition. Three of Toronto's teaching hospitals sponsor the center.

Lazinski, H., and Oppeneer, J.: Hospitals offer employees health programs, Hospitals **48**(22): 66, 68, 1974. Hospital offers courses to teach employees about risk factors in heart disease. Recommends that nurses initiate preventive programs for employees.

Lee, E. A.: Health education, Hospitals **48**(7): 133-139, 1974. Identifies needs for health education.

Lexow, G. A., and Aronson, S. S.: Health advocacy: a need, a concept, a model, Children Today **4**(1):2-6, 36, 1975. Describes a health-advocacy training program.

Lynch, L. R.: The conceptual approach to teaching health education, J. Sch. Health **43**:130-132, Feb., 1973. Conceptual approach was used to help students arrive at self-understanding.

Major, D. M.: Nursing school courses for non-nurses, Nurs. Outlook **22**(12):769-772, 1974. School of nursing offers courses in sex education, drugs, nutrition, and legal dimensions of human service programs to students from various disciplines.

Marriner, A.: Sex education for parents, Am. J. Public Health **61**:2031-2037, Oct., 1971. Discusses the need for sex education, theoretical preparation of parents and teachers, teaching techniques, gives suggestions, and answers questions commonly asked by intermediate students.

Marriner, A.: The role of the school nurse in health education, Am. J. Public Health **61**: 2155-2157, Nov., 1971. Discusses numerous aspects of the role of school nurse in health education.

Mechner, F.: Learning by doing through programmed instruction, Am. J. Nurs. **65**(5):98-104, 1965. Describes programmed instruction, gives several examples, and suggests some of its uses.

Melody, M. M., and Carrington, L. G.: Poster explosion, Am. J. Nurs. **62**(8):92-93, 1962. Describes posters that illustrate the team approach to improved patient care.

Milio, N.: A broad perspective on health: a teaching-learning tool, Nurs. Outlook **24**(3): 160-163, 1976. Presents a frame of reference for planning health education.

Milio, N.: A framework for prevention: changing health-damaging to health-generating life patterns, Am. J. Public Health **66**(5):435-439, 1976. Indicates that the impact of health education depends on the ease of availability of alternative health-promoting options.

Moarefi, A.: The corner-stone, World Health, pp. 30-33, Aug.-Sept., 1975. Discusses health education in the Navajo culture.

Mohammed, M. F.: Patients' understanding of written health information, Nurs. Res. **13**:100-108, Spring, 1964. Study indicates that 43% of patients tested were unable to profit from written health materials; many others are unable to profit from materials as they are currently used.

Monteiro, L.: Notes on patient teaching—a neglected area, Nurs. Forum **3**(1):26-33, 1964. Stresses formal and informal types of teaching.

Morris, A. G.: The use of the well-baby clinic to promote early intellectual development via parent education, Am. J. Public Health **66**(1):73-74, 1976. Suggests that parent-education programs as part of well-baby clinics can promote intellectual growth.

Murray, R., and Zenter, J.: Guidelines for more effective health teaching, Nursing '76 **6**(2):44-53, 1976. Lists guidelines for effective teaching. Discusses teaching in general.

Neeman, R. L., and Neeman, M.: Complexities of smoking education, J. Sch. Health **45**(1):17-23, 1975. Recommends a movement by nonsmokers against smoking.

Norman, M.: Health education in schools, Nurs. Times **71**(16):620-621, 1975. Recommends that health education be integrated in school classes and be taught by a health educator.

Nuttelman, D.: Instructional objectives, Superv. Nurse **8**(11):35-44, 1977. Discusses how, when, and why to write behavioral objectives.

Ogden, H. G.: Health education: a federal overview, Public Health Rep. **91**(3):109-205, 1976. Historical review of federal input in health education.

Pallan, P.: Community planned health care, Dimens. Health Serv. **52**(4):15-16, 1975. Emphasizes the importance of community involvement in health project or program planning.

Pasternack, S. B.: Annual well-child visits, Am. J. Nurs. **74**(8):1472-1475, 1974. Stresses counseling and health promotion.

Pidgeon, V. A.: Characteristics of children's thinking and implications for health teaching, Matern. Child Nurs. J. **6**(1):1-8, 1977. Discusses characteristics of the preschool, school, and adolescent child's thinking in relation to health education.

Pierre, R. S., and Lawrence, P. S.: Reducing smoking using positive self-management, J. Sch. Health **45**(1):7-9, 1975. Recommends using positive self-management such as positive peer reinforcement, reading a list of the positive outcomes of stopping smoking, and aversion techniques.

Piper, G. W., Jones, J. A., and Matthews, V. L.: The Saskatoon smoking study: results of the second year, Can. J. Public Health **65**(2):127-129, 1974. Research report of a smoking education program for eighth grade students that utilized peer pressure.

Porter, C. S.: Grade school children's perceptions of their internal body parts, Nurs. Res. **23**(5):384-391, 1974. Research using a projective technique found elementary school children most often draw the cardiovascular, gastrointestinal, and musculoskeletal systems. They know more about their internal body parts than previous studies indicated, and boys named more parts than girls.

Prave, M., et al.: Lumbar pain linked to hypokinesia, Can. Nurse **70**(11):27-31, 1974. Inactivity can cause chronic lumbar pain. Reports research findings. Illustrates and describes exercises.

Price, B. N.: Dermatitis in industry, Occup. Health Nurs. **22**(3):16-18, 1974. Discusses causes, control, and incidence of occupational dermatitis.

Rabinowitz, H. S., and Zimmerli, W. H.: Teaching-learning mechanisms in consumer health education, Public Health Rep. **91**(3):211-217, 1976. Study reports that students influenced teacher and parents' behaviors more than teachers and parents influenced the students.

Redman, B. K.: Client education therapy in treatment and prevention of cardiovascular diseases, Cardiovasc. Nurs. **10**(1):1-6, 1974; Colo. Nurse **74**(7):6-9, 1974. Discusses teaching for behavioral change, major issues in patient education, and future directions of patient education.

Richie, N. D.: Some guidelines for conducting a health fair, Public Health Rep. **91**(3):261-264, 1976. Outlines purposes, timing, site selection, financing, inviting agencies to participate, publicity, attracting children, physical layout, giveaways, thanking participants, and evaluating a health fair.

Robinson, A. M.: The RN's goal: under 90 mm. Hg diastolic, RN **37**(5):43-49, 1974. Discusses the role of the nurse in hypertension screening and treatment programs.

Robinson, G., and Filkins, M.: Group teaching with outpatients, Am. J. Nurs. **64**(11):110-112, 1964. Describes how to use waiting time for clinic appointments for health education.

Robinson, H. L.: Learning to count the calories, Nurs. Times **71**(27):1062-1064, 1975. Presents a diary of a discussion group for ten pupils with weight problems.

Robinson, W.: A health farm, Nurs. Mirror **141**(24):52-53, 1975. Describes a medically supervised and disciplined environment to help clients learn healthful habits.

Rosenberg, S., and Judkins, B. A.: Federal programs make education an integral part of patient care, Hospitals **50**(9):62-65, 1976. Discusses family teaching activities, physical assessment and patient teaching, and coordinated patient-family education as an outgrowth of Medicare/Medicaid promotion of patient and family education in long-term care facilities. Includes discussion on extension services.

Rosenstock, I. M.: What research in motivation suggests for public health, Am. J. Public Health **50**:295-302, March, 1960. Discusses motivation for participation in public health programs.

Schroeder, J.: This rehab program turns cardiac patients into athletes, RN **39**(9):68-73, 1976. Gives an exercise program for cardiac patients.

Schweer, S. F., and Dayani, E. C.: The extended role of professional nursing-patient education, Int. Nurs. Rev. **20**(6):174-175, 1973. Stresses the importance of patient education and preparation of professionals for that task.

Schulz, E. D.: Television brings drama to clinic patients, Am. J. Nurs. 62(8):98-99, 1962. Uses closed circuit television to teach health to young mothers in health center waiting room. It conserves the nurse's time and enables large numbers of patients to learn more about health.

Sessoms, D.: A safety project in elementary school, Am. J. Nurs. 60(9):1288-1289, 1960. Describes safety education offered by the school nurse.

Sexton, D.: A nurse shows how to help the patient stop smoking, Am. Lung Assoc. Bull. 61:10-11, May, 1975. Suggests helping the smoker find his own motive to stop smoking and support his efforts. The sense of how well he feels when he is not smoking can be motivating.

Shapiro, I. S.: HMOs and health education, Am. J. Public Health 65(5):469-473, 1975. Describes health education in the structure and functioning of health maintenance organizations.

Shea, K. M., et al.: Teaching a patient to live with adrenal insufficiency, Am. J. Nurs. 65(12):80-85, 1965. Presents detailed teaching guide, patient's questions and nurse's answers.

Simmons, J.: Making health education work, Am. J. Public Health 65:1-49, Oct., 1975. Report of health education in health program development with primary attention on programming for low-income and minority groups. Discusses initiating, developing, implementing, and assessing a health education program, participation, and gaining and maintaining support.

Simon, R. K., and Moyer, D. H.: A preliminary assessment of a cooperative drug education pilot project in the middle school, J. Sch. Health 46(6):325-328, 1976. Reports assessment of a pilot drug education project and recommends that trained people give factual information about drugs.

Snegroff, S.: Venereal disease education: facts are not enough, J. Sch. Health 45(1):37-39, 1975. Stresses the importance of dealing with motives as well as giving information.

Somers, A. R.: Consumer health education—to know or to die, Hospitals 50(9):52-56, 1976. Advocates consumer health education as a responsibility of hospitals.

Southall, C.: Innovative school nursing in Harlem: family life and sex education, Am. J. Nurs. 77(9):1473-1474, 1977. Describes a sex education program for black fifth and sixth graders that strives to improve intrafamily and positive self-directed behaviors.

Stewart, R. F.: Education for health maintenance, Occup. Health Nurs. 22(6):14-17, 1974. Discusses the nurse's role in teaching, objectives as a teaching base, and motivation for learning.

Stillman, M. J.: Women's health beliefs about breast cancer and breast self-examination, Nurs. Res. 26(2):121-127, 1977. Presents a research report about breast self-examination with implications for health education.

Sturdevant, B., and Patterson, R.: Helping patients do their "homework," Superv. Nurse 8(4):72-73, 1977. Advocates using the nursing process for patient teaching and gives sample teaching plans.

Swisher, J. D.: Mental health—the core of preventive health education, J. Sch. Health 46(7):386-391, 1976. Outlines mental health education strategies for personal, interpersonal, extrapersonal, and health problem skills.

Terry, D. E., and Woodward, L. H.: A five-year plan for designing and implementing a statewide health education curriculum in Maryland, J. Sch. Health 46(5):282-285, 1976. Gives the six phases of planning and implementing the health education curriculum.

Thygerson, A. L.: Safety in health education: some precautions, J. Sch. Health 74(9):508-510, 1974. Discusses use of statistics, scare techniques, and rules to teach safety and gives examples of changing rules to conceptual statements.

Tinch, J.: For sickness or for health? Nurs. Mirror 140(17):71-72, 1975. Stresses the importance of nursing education making health teaching a priority for promotion of health, prevention of disease, and rehabilitation, as well as during illness.

Tipping, J. R.: Fighting the stigma—the role of mass education, Nurs. Mirror 142(10):60-61, 1976. Discusses mass education about leprosy.

Van Mondfrans, A. P., Sorenson, C., and Reed, C. L.: Mediated approaches to learning: live or taped? Nurs. Outlook 20(10):652-653, 1972. Indicates that videotapes are superior to live presentations for demonstration of various nursing procedures.

Varvaro, F. F.: Teaching the patient about open heart surgery, Am. J. Nurs. 65(10):111-115, 1965. Outlines in detail a teaching program for patients about to have open-heart surgery.

Wang, V. L.: Application of social science theories to family planning health education in the People's Republic of China, Am. J. Public Health 66(5):440-445, 1976. Presents a health education model and discusses Lewin's theory of group decision and social change.

Ward, B.: Carnival offers learning opportunities,

Hospitals **49**(12):72-73, 1975. Describes a children's health carnival coordinated by the Department of Community Health Education at Morristown Memorial Hospital, New Jersey.

Weaver, B., and Williams, E. L.: Teaching the tuberculosis patient, Am. J. Nurs. **63**(12):80-82, 1963. Describes how patient's guide booklet and the patient teaching notebook are used for patient, staff, and student teaching.

Werden, P.: Health education for Indian students, J. Sch. Health **74**(6):319-323, 1974. Discusses health education for Indians.

Wilkinson, G. S., Mirand, E. A., and Graham, S.: Can-dial: an experiment in health education and cancer control, Public Health Rep. **91**(3):218-222, 1976. Library tapes are played over the telephone to give information about cancer. Reviews promotion costs and evaluation of the program.

Williams, Z.: A hall of health, Hosp. Forum **18**(14):4-5, 18, 1976. Describes a Hall of Health, a community health education project at Alta Balts Hospital in Berkeley, California, and lists the purposes of the project.

Woods, H.: Preventing blindness: a lot more than meets the eye, J. Pract. Nurs. **24**(11):28-29, 34, 1974. Discusses cataracts, glaucoma, and symptoms of eye problems in children. Stresses observation and teaching.

Wu, R.: Explaining treatments to young children, Am. J. Nurs. **65**(7):71-73, 1965. Offers suggestions for preparation of young child at level of his understanding.

Yankauer, A., et al.: What mothers say about childbearing and parents classes, Nurs. Outlook **8**(10):563-565, 1960. Discusses childbearing classes and offers suggestions for improvement.

Yeats, H. S.: Models for moppets, ONA J. **3**(6):196, 1976. Describes a community resource day held at Shriners' Hospital for Crippled Children in San Francisco.

Implementation

Bratton, J. K.: A definition of comprehensive nursing care, Nurs. Outlook **9**(8):481-482, 1961. Discusses the faculty's development of definition and gives five-paragraph definition of comprehensive nursing care.

Chamings, P. A.: Need a little help . . ., Am. J. Nurs. **69**(9):1918-1920, 1969. Tells how nursing team planned time schedule for difficult patient, and modified it in light of his needs; found that meeting them helped remove his difficult label.

Howitz, I. A.: Unrecognized cues on the case of Mr. X, Am. J. Nurs. **68**(10):2133-2134, 1968.

Case study illustrates how nurse met goals she set for patient but not patient's goals.

Levine, M. E.: The pursuit of wholeness, Am. J. Nurs. **69**(1):93-98, 1969. Discusses dynamic physiological exchange, levels of organismic response, use of perceptual systems, holistic approach.

Marquand, C. J.: Planned nursing care applied, N.Z. Nurs. J. **63**:11-14, May, 1970. Discusses development and implementation of nursing care plans through team nursing.

Theis, C., and Harrington, H.: Three factors that affect practice: communications, assignments, attitudes, Am. J. Nurs. **68**(7):1478-1482, 1968. Compares the effect of hospital environments on job satisfaction.

Referrals

Furbank, M. E.: A nursing referral system: admissions, transfers, and discharge to and from hospital, Nurs. Times **72**(11):41-44, 1976. Presents findings of a survey about the need for a referral form, a nursing referral form for admission, discharge, and transfer of patients, and guidelines for the use of the referral form.

Park, W. E.: Patient transfer form, Am. J. Nurs. **67**(8):1665-1668, 1967. Describes transfer communications form that contains information required under Medicare.

Wahlstrom, E. D.: Initiating referrals: a hospital based system, Am. J. Nurs. **67**(2):332-335, 1967. Describes the referral system for home nursing care at veterans administration hospital.

Weston, J. L.: Initiating referrals: a health department approach, Am. J. Nurs. **67**(2):332-335, 1967. Describes informal sessions that provide initial contacts for counseling and referrals for mothers in hospital obstetric ward.

Will, M. B.: Referral: a process, not a form, Nursing '77 **7**(12):44-45, 1977. Stresses the importance of follow-through.

Wolff, I. S.: Referral—a process and a skill, Nurs. Outlook **10**(4):253-256, 1962. Discusses the importance of referral being merited, practical, and fitted to the client's individuality.

Therapeutic communication

Aguilera, D. C.: Sociocultural factors: barriers to therapeutic intervention, J. Psychiatr. Nurs. **8**:14-18, Sept.-Oct., 1970. Discusses sociocultural factors and crisis intervention.

Alexander, M. M., and Brown, M. S.: Physical examination. II. History-taking, Nursing '73 **3**(8):35-39, 1973. Discusses history taking as part of the diagnostic workup, ways of conducting interview, kinds of interviews. Gives two examples of histories.

Behringer, S. M.: You and your aphasic patients: speech pathologist's view: how the nurse can help, RN **37**(3):43-53, 1974. Itemizes what to observe for a language evaluation and gives general pointers for working with aphasic patients.

Bender, R. E.: Communicating with the deaf, Am. J. Nurs. **66**(4):757-760, 1966. Gives pointers about how to talk with deaf persons.

Brunner, N. A.: Communications in nursing service administration, J. Nurs. Adm. **7**(8):29-32, 1977. Outlines accurate transfer, correct interpretation, and desired behavioral change aspects of communication.

Chapanis, A.: Interactive human communication, Sci. Am. **232**(3):36-42, 1975. Discusses studies about how people communicate and the development of a conversational computer.

Cohen, M. S.: Easy to listen to, Am. J. Nurs. **66**(9):1999-2001, 1966. Discusses how loudness, rate, pitch, and timbre affect speaking voice; suggests using a tape recorder to improve voice quality.

Cosper, B.: How well do patients understand hospital jargon? Am. J. Nurs. **77**(12):1932-1934, 1977. Research reports about patient understanding of the following terms: abdomen, void, NPO, emesis basin, injection, OR, temp, preop, force fluids, sutures, catheterize, ambulate, and constipated. Makes four recommendations.

Craytor, J. K.: Talking with persons who have cancer, Am. J. Nurs. **69**(4):744-748, 1969. Discusses techniques for communicating with cancer patients.

Creighton, H.: Law and the nurse supervisor: nurses' failure to communicate, Superv. Nurse **8**(12):10-11, 1977. Stresses the importance of nurses reporting to doctors.

Cuthbert, B. L.: Switch off, tune in, turn on, Am. J. Nurs. **69**(6):1206-1211, 1969. Author suggests we interrupt old reflex reactions that allow us to avoid an uncomfortable situation, tune in to what patient is asking, and help the nurse and patient turn negative personal feelings into positive, useful responses.

Davis, A. J.: The skills of communication, Am. J. Nurs. **63**(1):66-70, 1963. Discusses skills of communication.

Donn, M.: Communication—the key to preparation for surgery, Nurs. Mirror **143**(7):46-47, 1976. Discusses the importance of communication in preoperative and postoperative care.

Drummond, E. E.: Communication and comfort for the dying patient, Nurs. Clin. North Am. **5**:55-63, March, 1970. Communication aids physical, emotional, and spiritual comfort.

Elder, R. G.: What is the patient saying? Nurs. Forum **2**(1):24-37, 1963. Study indicates that most patients did not adequately communicate their needs during initial communication with nurses.

Eldred, S. H.: Improving nurse-patient communication, Am. J. Nurs. **60**(11):1600-1602, 1960. Discusses the language, kinesics, and vocalizations of interpersonal communication.

Ellis, G. L.: Communications and interdepartmental relationships, Nurs. Forum **5**(4):82-89, 1966. Discusses the aspects of interdepartmental communications; lists seven steps to improve organized communications.

Epstein, C.: Breaking the barriers to communications on the health team, Nursing '74 **4**(9):65-68, 1974. Indicates that communications must be improved by breaking through hierarchies and traditions for a health team to function well.

Gilmore, S. E.: Your aphasic patient: comprehending . . . communicating, J. Pract. Nurs. **25**(10):18-19, 1975. Stresses the importance of maintaining the aphasic patient's independence and self-esteem by encouraging his participation with others.

Goda, S.: Communicating with the aphasic or dysarthric patient, Am. J. Nurs. **63**(7):80-84, 1963. Illustrates assessment tool and stresses the importance of assessing both ability to express and receive language.

Greenhill, M.: Interviewing with a purpose, Am. J. Nurs. **56**(10):1259-1262, 1956. Discusses interviewing techniques, rationale, setting, and goals for interview.

Hemion, R. P.: Family nurse therapist: a model of communication, J. Psychiatr. Nurs. **12**(6):10-13, 1974. Stresses the importance of communication in family therapy.

Hull, R. H., and Traynor, R. H.: Restoring communication in the hearing impaired elderly, Nurs. Care **10**(6):14-15, 32, 1977. Discusses how to work with the hard of hearing elderly.

Hutton, G. A.: It all began with talk, Am. J. Nurs. **63**(12):107-108, 1963. Talk therapy with individuals was used to remotivate long-term patients on a minimal care unit.

Jourard, S. M.: The bedside manner, Am. J. Nurs. **60**(1):63-66, 1970. Discusses reasons nurses develop modes of behavior that interfere with giving successful nursing care; mentions ways to improve nurse-patient relationships.

Klagsbrun, S. C.: Communications in the treatment of cancer, Am. J. Nurs. **71**(5):944-948, 1971. Stresses the importance of discussing the patient's questions and concerns.

Kohut, S. A.: Guidelines for using interpreters, Hosp. Prog. **56**(4):39-40, 1975. Lists guidelines for using interpreters.

Kroah, J.: Strategies for interviewing in language and thought disorders, J. Psychiatr. Nurs. **12**(2): 3-9, 1974. Discusses the language and thought process of the schizophrenic; identifies and illustrates forms of the schizophrenic's speech and offers strategies for intervention.

Leonard, C. V.: Treating the suicidal patient: a communication approach, J. Psychiatr. Nurs. **13**(2):19-22, 1975. Discusses the process of problem-solving for helping the patient connect his depression with specific incidents.

Lewis, G. K.: Communication: a factor in meeting emotional crises, Nurs. Outlook **13**(8):36-39, 1965. Discusses the use of communication with patients experiencing a crisis.

Licker, L., et al.: It's the staff that keeps the patients talking, J. Psychiatr. Nurs. **14**(5):11-14, 1976. Research report indicates that patient verbalization correlates with the amount of conversation from the staff.

Madore, C. E., and Deutsch, Y. B.: Talking with parents, Am. J. Nurs. **62**(11):108-111, 1962. Discusses how the nurse can evoke responses from parents that will help them find and investigate problems.

Miltz, R. J.: Nurses improve their personal communication, Superv. Nurse **8**(12):13-15, 1977. Discusses how to use the communication, teach-reteach, and immediate feedback techniques during micro-teaching to improve communications.

Mitchell, A. C.: Barriers to therapeutic communication with black clients, Nurs. Outlook **26**(2): 109-112, 1978. Identifies language, culture, and perception of therapy differences as barriers to communication with black clients.

Mulrooney, J.: Deaf-patient care: a special concern to me, RN **39**(6):69-70, 1976. A deaf nurse discusses patient communication with the nurse. Illustrates some sign language.

Munn, H. E.: Communication between patients, nurses, physicians and surgeons, Hosp. Topics **55**(2):6-7, 1977. Briefly discusses communication.

Murray, J. B.: Self-knowledge and the nursing interview, Nurs. Forum **2**(1):68-79, 1963. Discusses communication skills and stresses the importance of self-awareness. See pp. 45-49.

Nelson, J.: You and your aphasic patients: pa-

tient's view: "they talk more," RN **37**(3):42, 72-77, 1974. An RN discusses her experience as a stroke patient with aphasia.

Newman, M. A.: Identifying and meeting patient's needs in short-span nurse-patient relationships, Nurs. Forum **5**(1):76-86, 1966. Stresses the importance of effective communication.

Padberg, J.: "Bargaining" to improve communications in conjoint family therapy, Perspect. Psychiatr. Care **13**(2):68-72, 1975. Outlines the steps in the bargaining process and presents a case.

Paynick, M. L.: Cultural barriers to nurse communication, Am. J. Nurs. **64**(2):87-90, 1964. Studies how unfamiliar beliefs and language of tuberculous patients in New Mexico influence the patient's response to the nurse.

Robinson, A. M.: Communicating with schizophrenic patients, Am. J. Nurs. **60**(8):1120-1123, 1960. Suggests love as an important element for interpersonal communication with schizophrenic patients.

Rudolph: The art of patient interviews, Physician's World **1**:56+, April, 1973. Discusses interviewing techniques.

Sabatino, L.: Do's and dont's of deaf-patient care, RN **39**(6):64-68, 1976. Lists ways to make communication with a deaf person easier.

Scarlett, M. R.: Her only disease was a language barrier, RN **39**(2):69-72, 1976. Presents a case study in which a student nurse believed that a specific patient's weepiness and loss of appetite were due to communication problems instead of mental illness.

Sharp, C.: First or last name? Am. J. Nurs. **71**(5):958-959, 1971. A student interviewed forty patients and found that even if they expressed a preference for first or last name, they indicated that name usage was relatively unimportant to them.

Sheahan, J.: Communication skills and assessment learning, Nurs. Times **72**(40):1570-1572, 1976. Discusses communication as it relates to teaching and the assessment of learning.

Skipper, J. K., Jr., Mauksch, H. O., and Tagliacozzo, D.: Some barriers to communication between patients and hospital functionaries, Nurs. Forum **2**(1):14-23, 1963. Discusses the factors that inhibit patients from initiating communication with nurses and physicians.

Smith, C. M.: Identifying blocks to communication in health care settings and a workshop plan, J. Contin. Educ. Nurs. **8**(2):26-32, 1977. Identifies (1) lack of understanding of the language, (2) differences in relating to the sensory world,

(3) high anxiety, (4) preconceptions and stereotypes, and (5) a tendency to evaluate others as stumbling blocks to communications. Describes a communication workshop.

Smith, E. C.: Are you really communicating? Am. J. Nurs. **77**(12):1966-1968, 1977. Stresses that although children may seem to understand, they may have inaccurate meanings for words. The nurse needs to be aware of the child's concepts.

Stollak, G. E.: Learning to communicate with children, Children Today **4**(2):12-14, 40, 1975. Describes a course that facilitates the development of communication skills with children.

Swanson, A. R.: Communicating with depressed persons, Perspect. Psychiatr. Care **13**(2):63-67, 1975. Discusses problematic verbal and non-verbal messages, dynamics of verbal messages and depression, and communication in treatment.

Thomas, B. J.: Clues to patients' behavior, Am. J. Nurs. **63**(7):100-102, 1963. Applies psychiatric nursing principles to medical-surgical nursing.

Thomas, M. D., Baker, J. M., and Estes, N. J.:
Anger: a tool for developing self-awareness, Am. J. Nurs. **70**(12):2586-2590, 1970. Offers guidelines for intervention with angry patients.

Underwood, P. R.: Communication through role playing, Am. J. Nurs. **71**(6):1184-1186, 1971. Suggests role playing as an interpersonal technique for some situations.

Velazquez, J. M.: Alienation, Am. J. Nurs. **69**(2):301-304, 1969. Discusses how nurses can reduce patient alienation by monitoring their own behavior and eradicating those behaviors that estrange patients.

What if your patient is also deaf? RN **39**(6):59-63, 1976. Suggests measures to improve care of deaf patients and illustrates some sign language.

Wilson, J. M.: Communicating with the dying, J. Med. Ethics **1**:18-21, 1975. Discusses communicating with dying patients.

Young, J. J., and Golding, A. M. B.: The need to communicate, Nurs. Times **70**(15):566-567, 1974. Identifies some communication problems in psychiatric hospitals and suggests solutions.

CHAPTER 5

EVALUATION

Evaluation is the process of assessing (1) the patient's progress toward health goals, (2) the quality of patient care in an institution, (3) the quality of individual nursing care through self-evaluation, as well as (4) overall personnel performance. Its value cannot be overemphasized.

EVALUATION OF PATIENT PROGRESS

The consequences of nursing intervention can be positive or negative, anticipated or unexpected. The effects of intervention must be evaluated periodically and the nursing implementation changed accordingly. The frequency of reevaluation depends on the situation. A patient in an intensive care unit needs more frequent reevaluation than one in a long-term rehabilitation ward.[1] In general, the nurse is constantly reevaluating her assigned patient's progress toward the patient's and nurse's mutually defined goals. The patient's behavior is compared with the terminal behavior described in the objectives of the nursing care plan and with the baseline data on the nursing history to determine the patient's progress.

NURSING AUDIT

Phaneuf has done extensive work with the nursing audit method. She defines the nursing audit as the nurse's formal, systematic, written appraisal of the quality of nursing service indicated in care records of discharged patients. (See pp. 240-245.) Her audit plan uses the functions of nursing as stated by Lesnik and Anderson in *Nursing Practice and the Law*.[2] These functions include (1) application and execution of physician's legal orders, (2) observations of symptoms and reactions, (3) supervision of the patient, (4) supervision of those participating in care, (5) reporting and recording, (6) application of nursing procedures and techniques, and (7) promotion of health by direction and teaching.[3] The seven roles are the dependent and independent nursing functions that are reflected in most nurse practice acts. Phaneuf has developed fifty components and descriptive statements of these seven functions. Her detailed description of these functions helps auditors evaluate the quality of nursing care by focusing their attention on the patient rather than on the nursing specialties or the nurses who administer the care.

The first step in the nursing audit is the selection and orientation of an audit committee that represents administrative, supervisory, and staff personnel. The size of the committee varies with the amount of work to be done, but it should have at least three members. On occasion all records of patients with a specific diagnosis or those who are assigned to a particular ward may be evaluated. It is preferable, however, to direct the audit toward an inclusive view of nursing service by randomly selecting a certain percent of charts from the year's closed cases. The chairman of the committee assigns records of discharged patients to each committee member who should require about 15 minutes to audit a record.

There should be no indication on the patient's care record that it has been audited. The audit is a tool for administrative, supervisory, and staff personnel only and should be placed under administrative care. It improves patient care by revealing serious problems and will reveal significant weaknesses in performance even in prestigious agencies. Audits have revealed weaknesses in an understanding of the pathophysiological process, failure to use patient's health history when planning care, the ignoring of secondary diagnoses, and fragmentary observation of symptoms and reactions. The single dependent nursing function, which is carrying out the physician's orders, is shown to be the best-executed function.[4]

The nursing service of the Veterans Administrative Hospital, Batavia, New York, expanded its auditing beyond the evaluation of patient care records by taking this method to the bedside. Initially a group of supervisors and head nurses identified nursing care of acutely ill patients, nursing care plans, and nurses' notes as areas that would provide an index to the quality of patient care. Then statements of standards of performance were developed to provide a pattern for the format of the audit. The committee decided that a clean body, clean hair and scalp, clean area between toes, clean and trimmed fingernails and toenails, and other specific criteria are indicators that the patient is receiving an acceptable standard of care. On the audit form, these indicators were translated into questions. The auditing nurse marked yes, no, or not applicable in columns beside the question. The staff felt that auditing three random patients per unit per month was adequate to determine the quality of care given. Committee members, including all levels of professional nurses, do monthly audits on wards other than those to which they are assigned. The three scores per month are averaged to give the ward a rating. These ratings are compiled for all units and distributed to each ward. Scores are posted to stimulate competition, increase motivation, and improve performance.[5]

In 1972 Congress amended the Social Security Act, mandating the formation of Professional Standards Review Organizations to review the quality and expense of care given to clients of Medicare, Medicaid, and Maternal Child Health programs. Consequently, health facilities developed quality control programs. Many books and articles have subsequently been published that address the structure, process, and outcome frameworks for studying quality assurance, standard of care, criteria, tools, collection and analysis of data, and corrective actions.

SYSTEMS ANALYSIS

A system is a set of interrelated, interdependent, or interacting elements organized into a complex whole. Purpose, process, and content have been identified by Banathy[6] as the three main aspects of systems. The purpose gives direction to the system, identifies what is to be done, and determines the operations and functions that comprise the processes necessary to accomplish the purpose. The parts that comprise the system are the content. The content is chosen for its ability to perform the processes required to accomplish the purpose of the system.

There are systems within systems. For instance, respiration and digestion are subsystems within the total body system. Each subsystem has its own distinct objectives that should contribute to the overall goals of the system. Society is a suprasystem of the health care system. It is also a suprasystem for education, religion, business, and politics. Each subsystem receives its purpose from the suprasystem but also has its own purpose, process, and content that help achieve the purpose of the suprasystem. Each subsystem can be further divided into more subsystems. Subsystems of the health care system include nursing, medicine, dentistry, pharmacy, dietetics, physical therapy, occupational therapy, and social welfare. Each of the interdependent subsystems is fairly distinguishable but contributes to the integration and unity of the suprasystem. Assessment, planning, implementation, and evaluation comprise the nursing process, which is utilized to accomplish the purposes of the nursing subsystem.

Systems may be closed or open. A closed system is self-contained and isolated from its environment. Most systems are open, or influenced by the environment, resulting in a dynamic equilibrium. The human organism is an example of an open system that tries to maintain a steady state. The energy taken in or absorbed by the system is called input; the energy that passes from the system is called output. The continuous inflow and outflow of an open system assist in the maintenance of equilibrium. The temperature-regulating system of the body is an example of the system's attempt to maintain equilibrium. The body increases its heat production by shivering when in a cool environment and cools itself by sweating in a hot environment.[7]

Systems may be deterministic or probabilistic. In a deterministic system the parts interact in a predictable way. When given the state of the system and knowledge of its dynamic network, one can predict the next state without risk of error. In a probabilistic system, however, no precise prediction can be made. Because machines operate on deterministic systems, they may be adjusted with predictable outcome, but predicting how a human being will react under certain circumstances is probabilistic.[8]

Systems analysis involves dividing a whole into its component parts to evaluate and manipulate the relationships. The system is evaluated by measuring critical variables, exposing problems, and predicting the consequences of various alternatives.[9] The nurse applies systems analysis to her daily assignment, ward activities, and the functioning of the entire institution or community health care system. Systems analysis requires accurate information systems, is closely related to flow charting, can use computer processing, and may involve other sophisticated management techniques that are beyond the scope of this book.

EVALUATION OF PERSONNEL

Personnel are evaluated in an effort to maintain and improve their performance. Evaluation makes the employer and employee aware of important factors in the job description and also provides administrative information for promotions, terminations, and references requested by other employers.[10]

If a discrepancy exists between actual and desired performance, the supervisor must identify and determine the importance of the discrepancy. Is it a training problem due to a skill deficiency? Did the person once have that skill? Does the skill need to be used frequently or infrequently? If the skill is used infrequently, the employee may need a regular schedule or practice. If the skill has deteriorated despite frequent use, periodic feedback should help maintain an adequate level of performance. The supervisor considers the need for on-the-job training, formal training, or the need to change job requirements or the worker's title. The supervisor should consider the following: What are the obstacles to desired behavior? Does it matter if the performance meets the desired standard? Do working conditions make it painful for an employee to carry out the desired performance and more rewarding to perform in a less desirable manner?[11]

Job descriptions inform employees of the responsibilities for each title. Standards of performance and criteria for measuring that performance increase the validity and objectivity of evaluation. Involvement of personnel in the evaluation process increases commitment to it and facilitates utilization of the results. Frequent feedback about performance reinforces desired behaviors and increases the individual's awareness of her need for improvement. Constructive criticism coupled with suggestions for improvement help the employee change her behavior to a more acceptable level of performance.[12]

Evaluative data should contain only factual information on both strong and weak attributes of the employee. Data should be collected in sufficient quantity from a variety of situations to determine the characteristic behavior of the person being evaluated.[13]

Evaluation may be carried out through a variety of methods. An anecdotal record, in which the evaluator objectively describes behavior she has observed, is one of the least structured techniques. If interpretation is to be included in the anecdotal record, it should be separated from the objective description. Anecdotal notes are kept in the employee's folder. Although they provide a systematic procedure for recording observations, anecdotal notes do not ensure that the observations will be systematic or directed toward relevant behaviors. Time sampling makes the observations more systematic. When using this method, the supervisor sets aside time specifically for observation, divides the time among personnel, and concentrates on a specific individual for a short time.

In another evaluation method, the critical incident rating, job requirements, and objectives must first be defined. With this evaluative method the supervisor looks for examples of how the employee is meeting or failing to meet the objectives. If using a checklist, she records the presence or absence of a specific behavior. When a rating scale is used, the behavior is registered at a point along a continuum to indicate qualitative differences in performance.[14]

Wandelt and Stewart[15] have developed the Slater nursing competencies rating scale. It is designed to rate the nursing process as care is being delivered. It lists numerous behaviors of the nurse under six categories: psychosocial, individual; psychosocial, group; physical; general; communication; and professional implications.

SELF-EVALUATION

From formal evaluations the employee receives an indication of how others perceive her. Self-evaluation is equally important. Nurses should constantly evaluate their own performances, determine their own strengths and weaknesses, consider how they might have done a task better, use the analysis for future reference, and seek help to improve their performances. This is critically important because the quality of patient care depends on the quality of those giving the care and their effective use of the nursing process.

NOTES

1. Byrne, M. L., and Thompson, L. F.: Key concepts for the study and practice of nursing, St. Louis, 1972, The C. V. Mosby Co., pp. 74-75.
2. Lesnik, M. J., and Anderson, B. E.: Nursing practice and the law, ed. 2, Philadelphia, 1955, J. B. Lippincott Co.
3. Phaneuf, M. C.: Quality of care: problems of measurement. I. How one public health nursing agency is using the nursing audit, Am. J. Public Health 59:1828, Oct., 1969. This list can be found in several books and articles, but this particular list is from the Phaneuf article.
4. Donabedian, A.: Quality of care: problems of measurement. II. Some issues in evaluating the quality of nursing care, Am. J. Public Health 59:1833-1836, Oct., 1969; Phaneuf, M. C.: Analysis of a nursing audit, Nurs. Outlook 16(1):57-60, 1968; Phaneuf, M. C.: Quality of care: Problems of measurement. I. How one public health nursing agency is using the nursing audit, Am. J. Public Health 59:1827-1832, Oct., 1969; Phaneuf, M. C.: The nursing audit for evaluation of patient care, Nurs. Outlook 14(6):51-54, 1966; Phaneuf, M. C.: A nursing audit method, Nurs. Outlook 12(5): 42-45, 1964; Phaneuf, M. C.: The nursing audit, New York, 1972, Appleton-Century-Crofts.
5. McGuire, R. L.: Bedside nursing audit, Am. J. Nurs. 68(10):2146-2148, 1968.
6. Banathy, B. H.: Instructional systems, Belmont, Calif., 1968, Fearon Publishers, Inc., p. 4.
7. Yura, H., and Walsh, M. B.: The nursing process: assessing, planning, implementing, evaluating, New York, 1973, Appleton-Century-Crofts, pp. 36-43.
8. Hicks, H. G.: The management of organizations: a systems and human resources approach, New York, 1972, McGraw-Hill Book Co., pp. 461-470; McFarland, D. E.: Management: principles and practices, New York, 1974, Macmillan Publishing Co., Inc., pp. 80-82.
9. Finch, J.: Systems analysis: a logical approach to professional nursing care, Nurs. Forum 8(2):176-188, 1969; Pierce, L. M.: A patient-care model, Am. J. Nurs. 69(8):1700-1704, 1969.

10. Cochran, T. C., and Hansen, P. J.: Developing an evaluation tool by group action, Am. J. Nurs. 62(3):94-97, 1962.
11. Mager, R. F., and Pipe, P.: Analyzing performance problems, Belmont, Calif., 1970, Fearon Publishers, Inc.
12. Douglass, L. M., and Bevis, E. O.: Nursing leadership in action: principles and application to staff situations, St. Louis, 1974, The C. V. Mosby Co., pp. 123-132.
13. Kron, T.: The management of patient care, Philadelphia, 1971, W. B. Saunders Co., pp. 155-157.
14. Beyers, M., and Phillips, C.: Nursing management for patient care, Boston, 1971, Little, Brown & Co., pp. 157-158; Blood, D. F., and Budd, W. C.: Educational measurement and evaluation, New York, 1972, Harper & Row, Publishers, pp. 44-65.
15. Wandelt, M. A., and Stewart, D. S.: Slater nursing competencies rating scale, New York, 1975, Appleton-Century-Crofts.

Selected readings

Barbara J. Stevens analyzes the trends in nursing care management and discusses quality control in detail. Carol A. Lindeman lists and discusses the steps in tool development for measuring quality of nursing care. Maria C. Phaneuf lists seven functions with their fifty components and descriptive statements to be used by audit committees on closed records. Mary Jane Munley describes "An Evaluation of Nursing Care by Direct Observation" that benefits current patients and emphasizes the nurse's accountability. Betty Jane Ryan discusses the fundamentals of general systems theory and their application, with control measures, to a nursing care plan system.

ANALYSIS OF TRENDS IN NURSING CARE MANAGEMENT

Barbara J. Stevens

Within the last ten years there has been great growth in the measuring, i.e., quantifying of nursing care. Ideally, if quantification can be done accurately, it should give a scientific base from which to solve many present nursing problems. For example, quantification should give a basis by which to *evaluate* whether care requirements have in fact been met, *relate* staffing patterns to care requirements, and *compare* the staffing patterns and quality of nursing care among institutions.

In actual practice, most quantification on nursing care has not yet reached a level at which it serves as a basis for decision-making by administrators of nursing care. Indeed, many a director finds herself in the role of apologist when her institution fails to remain within the normal limits of some statewide or national survey of nursing hours per patient day. Every director of nursing care needs to have a good understanding of nursing measurement processes so that she can evaluate her own management abilities.

It is the position of this paper that all measurement in nursing care should start with a quality control base. For example, it is unfair to compare the staffing needs of two hospitals on the basis of equal patient census when one hospital is located in a comfortable suburban

Reprinted from Journal of Nursing Administration 2:12-17, Nov.-Dec., 1972.

setting while the other serves a ghetto population. The difference in basic teaching needs alone will radically increase nursing hours in the ghetto hospital, not to mention other factors such as concurrent health problems, lack of family resources, and so forth. Thus, measurement in nursing should start with the quality of care, not only because it is the primary aim in nursing, but because it is essential as a base upon which other meaningful measurements can be made.

Unfortunately, quality control has been the last, not the first, kind of measurement to be made. The reason is relatively simple: It is easier to count patients, nurses, or nursing tasks than it is to identify criteria upon which to determine quality levels. Quality control systems have begun to appear, however, and their formulation will give the director of nursing care a base of support in assessing and justifying her support requirements for her institution's nursing care needs.

COMPONENTS OF A QUALITY CONTROL SYSTEM

What then comprises a nursing care quality control system? Slee identifies three essential components of any quality control program: (1) standards, (2) surveillance, and (3) corrective action.[1] The area of difficulty is the first, that of setting standards. One can choose to appraise any of the following: (1) structure, (2) process, and (3) outcome.[2] If one looks at the format of most accrediting agencies, such as the ANA, the NLN, and the JCAH, it is apparent that these groups have selected structure as the area of concern. The following questions or statements compiled from these three sources will illustrate the point:
1. Is a registered nurse responsible for planning, evaluating, and supervising the nursing care of each patient?
2. Are written care plans used?
3. The nursing department provides training programs and opportunities for staff development.
4. There is a system for recording accurate and objective observations of patients in the clinical record.

These questions and statements identify necessary, but not sufficient, criteria for quality care. Thus it might be necessary for a registered nurse to plan patient care, but because such care is planned by a registered nurse is no assurance that the planning is in fact well done. Written care plans may be necessary for good care, but that such plans are written does not, in and of itself, assure that they are good plans. Criteria based on structure give conditions under which it is likely that good nursing care could take place, but such criteria do not assure that the good care does in fact take place.

Criteria based on outcomes would be ideal, but such criteria are difficult to identify at the present developmental level of nursing research. To use outcomes as criteria, one would have to be able to determine how much of the patient's return to wellness was due to nursing and how much was due to medicine. Documentation is available for intensive coronary nursing care,[3] but little is presently available for the bulk of nursing being done. Some interesting and encouraging data are being developed at health maintenance clinics where selected patient groups are divided between physician and nurse clinics.[4] Generally, however, it appears that nursing outcomes, as standards for quality measurement, will be useful only to nursing divisions operating on a high level of sophistication.

Thus the last criteria to be considered, that of process, offers the most realistic area in which to locate quality control. Many interesting things are presently being done in measuring the nursing process. The director of nursing care should, however, be aware of two distinct forms of analysis, each of which has a different approach and a different aim.

TASK ANALYSIS METHOD

Early in the development of quality control, once nurse leaders had identified process as the area from which to develop quality criteria, there was a great tendency to call in the outside expert to develop the criteria by which to analyze the nursing process. This use of outside personnel, usually systems analysts, led to a task-oriented time analysis route of investigation. The experts, by using time studies, were able to establish time norms for most common nursing tasks. Note, however, that these norms were specific for the institution under investigation. Thus the average bathing time in a research hospital with critically ill patients might logically be longer than that in an average community hospital.

Nevertheless, such studies were of practical value in establishing some criteria for distribution of staff or patients. Nurses have always known that the same unit of thirty patients may be extremely busy one month and not so busy the next month, but never before have they had a scientific base to use as a distribution criterion. Such time studies usually revealed that certain tasks were significant in determining patient nursing care hours and that certain tasks were inconsequential. Drug distribution, for example, seldom affected patient care hours, while presence of a levine tube usually was related directly to increased nursing care hours.

Time studies have contributed greatly to improvements in patient care and staff placement, but certain inherent limitations should be noted. Since most of these original studies were formulated by systems persons rather than by nurses, a great emphasis was placed upon analysis and allocation of specific tasks to specific levels of nursing personnel. Such systems seldom left room, for example, for the patient who needed a registered nurse instead of a nursing assistant because of a high anxiety level (anxiety is not a task). Such studies, also, usually ignored the human need for continuity. If a patient required four levels of activities, then four separate persons should do those tasks.

The primary weakness of these studies, however, is that their data base was always the present practice. Tasks were timed as they in fact took place rather than as they ought to have taken place. Thus these studies must be seen as descriptive rather than as prescriptive of nursing practice.

Studies utilizing the task analysis method are increasing in sophistication. Certain computerized forms can now handle hundreds of specific nursing tasks, and many now include such hard-to-define tasks as patient teaching or relieving patient anxiety. Most nursing divisions have now established their own patient ranking system, usually based on selected tasks to be performed. The PETO system is one such development.[5] This method assigns point values to selected nursing tasks and selected patient states such as: (1) turning every hour rates 12 points, and (2) incontinence with average output rates 8 points. After all criteria have been rated and added, each patient's point value is converted into an estimated number of hours of nursing care. Systems such as this are extremely useful in patient care and staff placement, but they cannot perform a quality control function.

QUALITY CONTROL METHOD

A true nursing quality control system must (1) identify the desired nursing practice criteria, (2) establish a system for comparing the actual nursing practice to that criteria, and (3) use process standards rather than structure standards. The desired nursing practice criteria does not have to be defined in terms of the ideal: it may be defined in terms of the acceptable level of practice. Indeed, criteria can be developed for identifying different levels of excellence in practice.

The primary difference between process and structure standards can be demonstrated by reviewing some of the previous structure standards and converting them to process standards.

Structure sample 2: Are written care plans used?

Related process sample: Is the written care plan appropriate for the patient? Does it demonstrate consideration of his personal needs, disease-related needs, and therapy-related needs?

Structure sample 4: There is a system for recording accurate and objective observations of patients in the clinical record.

Related process sample: The charting shows evidence of relevant observations of patient progress, of patient response to therapy, and of completion of physician's orders. Evidence of the patient's psychic state is also present where relevant.

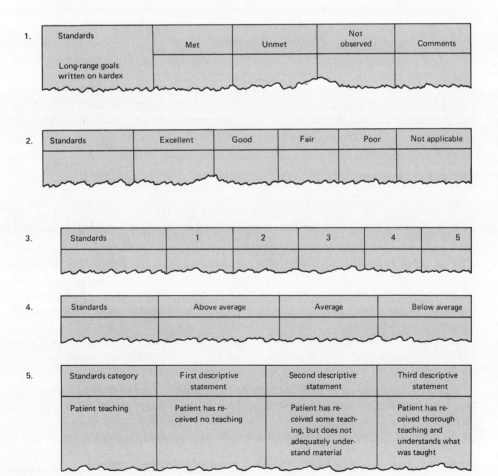

A critical difference between the structure standard and the process standard is that the process standard requires a professional judgment in determining whether each criterion has been met. This element of judgment does afford possibility for some differences in rating, but such differences can be decreased by writing each criterion in clearly defined behavioral terms.

The first step in establishing a quality control system is to identify the areas to be evaluated. These areas may be limited to direct patient care or may be expanded to cover other nursing functions such as recording, assigning, or maintaining equipment. The scope should depend upon the objectives and needs of the institution. Since the evaluating process may be time consuming, quality control is often limited to the evaluation of patient care alone rather than to including nursing administrative functions. Another frequent pattern is to individualize a quality control form to cover all the nursing functions and patient care functions indigenous to a particular unit. A third possibility is that of developing quality control forms specific for particular patients. For example, one could devise a quality control form applicable to all patients with cardiovascular accidents.

Once the scope of the quality control has been determined, a general format for the form itself must be prepared. Since the format will influence the wording of the standards, it must be determined first. The principal rule to follow in selecting a format is to keep it simple, easy to use, and easily interpreted by all users. Some common formats are:

Form 1 is less likely to produce diverse opinions among raters; however, each standard must be defined precisely. Form 2 has the disadvantage of showing greater variation among raters. Form 3 has the same disadvantage, but may be useful if the institution wants to quantify the answers. Quantification has the advantage of promoting competition among nursing units or of permitting the nursing unit to strive to top its previous grade. Form 4 has the advantage of stability, for as the "average" improves in the institution, the form is still applicable. Form 5 is the most difficult to construct, but permits identification of specific levels of nursing care.

SOURCES OF EVIDENCE

Once the scope and format of the quality control system have been determined, the next step is to identify the sources of evidence. Primary and secondary sources are usually combined, but where possible, primary sources are preferable. A primary source gives the rater direct knowledge concerning the standard. For example, if a standard is, "Patient receives adequate oral hygiene," the rater goes to the source, the patient, to observe for this standard. For the standard, "Emergency equipment is complete and ready for use," the observer again goes directly to the source, i.e., evaluates the equipment firsthand.

Not all standards lend themselves to immediate observation techniques. "Promotion of independence" might require a careful evaluation of nursing notes over a period of time. Some standards may combine primary and secondary sources. For example, "Adequate hydration is maintained," might combine direct observation of the skin turgor with secondary observation of the intake and output records.

The patient's chart is a frequent secondary source. Indeed, the evaluation of nursing via the chart is often either included in the quality check or developed separately as a nursing chart audit. Another source often used is the patient's response of satisfaction or dissatisfaction with his nursing care. It is important that a group forming a quality control check determine ahead how relevant patient satisfaction is as evidence of professional care. Wording of questions to patients is quite important. Some questions can be worded so as to give primary responses: "Did the nurse discuss your surgery with you the day before the operation?" Others cannot be given similar weight: "Are you generally pleased with your nursing care?" The following sources are those most frequently used in quality control checks: charts, rounds, records, nursing care plans, patient interviews, nurse interviews, interviews of other health personnel.

After sources of evidence have been selected, the final step in the process is that of constructing the relevant standards. As mentioned previously, the standards should be given in precise behavioral terms so that each rater will give the statement or question the same interpretation. Another factor to consider is proportion. For example, there should not be twice as many questions on psychological aspects as on physical aspects of care unless the group considers psychological aspects twice as important as physical aspects. Thus one should aim for a balanced checklist, with emphasis only on those areas identified as extremely important.

FACTORS THAT INFLUENCE THE QUALITY CONTROL SYSTEM

Many other issues may influence both the quality control form and the implementation policy. The director of nursing care needs to clearly define her purposes in using a quality control system. Formation and implementation of a quality control system can be an educative experience for supervisors and head nurses. If staff development is one of the primary objectives of the quality control system, then the staff should develop its own system. A group can learn much by devising, revising, and testing its own evaluation tool.

If, however, the director is more interested in accurate patient care feedback, then she may wish to have a form evolved with more expertise. Another valid purpose for the quality control system is that of serving as a motivator toward better patient care. Competitive factors have already been discussed. The quality control system also is useful in spotting areas of general weakness and thus may be used as a diagnostic tool by staff education departments.

Still another factor that will influence the form of the quality control system is the department's concept of nursing. The following samples represent divisions of patient care which could be used as a basis for structuring a quality control form.

1. Nursing care[6]
   a. Sustenal
   b. Remedial
   c. Restorative
   d. Preventive
2. Nursing problems[7]
   a. Preserve body defenses
   b. Prevent complications
   c. Reestablish patient with outside world
   d. Detect changes in the body's regulatory system
   e. Implement prescribed therapeutic and diagnostic activity
   f. Provide comfort
3. Nursing care as process[8]
   a. Observation
   b. Inference

c. Validation

d. Assessment

e. Action

f. Evaluation

The particular structure selected is not as important as that a structure *be* selected. Too many control checklists lack organization and simply present a random list of standards.

Finally, after a form is completed, it is important to implement its use in a systematic way. One needs to determine who will evaluate what at what times. Answers to these questions must be based on the institution's needs, but the following guidelines have proved useful in many organizations.

1. Schedule evaluation visits at periodic, but unannounced intervals. The surprise visit is more likely to reflect the normal pattern of nursing care.

2. Not all patients need be evaluated; a sampling technique is quite satisfactory.

3. Patient sampling may be done at random, or patients may be selected on the basis of those requiring challenging nursing care.

4. Persons should serve on the evaluation team long enough to become thoroughly familiar with the evaluation process.

5. If evaluation members split the work, each member should grade the *same* portion of the checklist on all units evaluated.

USE OF QUALITY CONTROL DATA

The third area of quality control identified by Slee was that of corrective action. A quality control system is useless if proper and immediate feedback is not offered to the nursing units involved. It is, however, more productive to have the staff view quality control as a challenge than as a club over their heads. Supervisors and head nurses can be counseled to see the program as a diagnostic tool more easily if they have an integral part in its operation.

For the director, a measure of the quality of nursing care gives a scientific basis upon which to calculate needed nursing personnel. She can measure the point at which increased staffing alone fails to improve care quality. Likewise, she has data to support the point at which care begins to decline due to personnel shortages. The quality control system, as opposed to the time study task analysis approach, has another advantage: it identifies instances when particular nursing teams are more productive of good care than are similar teams in similar circumstances. Thus it may recognize appropriate nursing models for study and imitation. The task analysis method defines all nurses as interchangeable integers. While it will indicate failures of a nursing team to carry the expected number of tasks, it has no means of identifying group excellence in care. The following graph compares some of the critical differences in purpose between the two systems.

	Task Analysis System	*Quality Control System*
Aim of system	Fairly distribute nursing tasks	Evaluate the quality of care
Basic criterion	What *is* being done	What *ought* to be done
Concept of nursing	Nursing is a series of specific tasks	Nursing is process (there is room for various different theories)
What the system points out	Instances when a team produces less completed tasks than the norm	Instances of exceptional nursing, both good and bad
Perspective	What happens in the care delivery system	What happens to the patient

Another factor which makes quality control data even more important is the present financial crisis in health institutions. The director of nursing care is in the difficult position of trying to interpret good nursing care to non-nurse administrators who make decisions vitally affecting nursing resources. Under present economic conditions, administrators may feel justified in decreasing nursing personnel as long as "the job still gets done." Quality control data can help make visible to the non-nurse administrator the price that is paid in such instances. Quality control data provides a guide to staffing needs based upon the quality of nursing care rather than upon less critical issues.

REFERENCES

1. Slee, V. N. How to Know if You Have Quality Control. Hospital Progress **53**(1):38-43, 1972.
2. Donabedian, A. Some Issues in Evaluating the Quality of Nursing Care. American Journal of Public Health **59**(10):1833, 1969.
3. Meltzer, L. E. CCU's Can Save Thousands of Lives: Nurse is Key Factor in Success. Hospital Topics **49**(9):26-27, 1971.
4. Lewis, C., and Resnik, B. Nurse Clinics and Progressive Ambulatory Care. New England Journal of Medicine **277**(23):1236, 1967.
5. Poland, M., English, N., and Thorton, N. et al. PETO—A System for Assessing and Meeting Patient Care Needs. American Journal of Nursing **70**(7):1479, 1970.
6. Pardee, G., Hoshaw, D., Huber, C., and Larson, B. Patient Care Evaluation is Every Nurse's Job. American Journal of Nursing **71**(10):1958, 1971.
7. Brodt, D. F. A Synergistic Theory of Nursing. American Journal of Nursing **69**(8):1674, 1969.
8. Carrieri, V., and Sitzman, J. Components of Nursing Process. Nursing Clinics of North America **6**(1):115-121, 1971.

MEASURING QUALITY OF NURSING CARE
Carol A. Lindeman

Part One

Nursing personnel across the country, it seems to me, are investing significant amounts of time and energy developing procedures and tools to measure the quality of nursing care. It also seems apparent that many of the nurses involved in these efforts have made little progress. They have learned what *not* to do, but not necessarily what to do. Others state their concern that "everyone is inventing the wheel all over again." There is a great duplication of effort at the initial stage of tool development but little activity in reliability and validity testing. Another common reflection is, "If only we'd known what we were getting into!" Meaning, if only we had started with an understanding of measurement and tool development.

In this and the next column, I will present an overview of the major steps and issues in measurement and tool development as they relate to measuring quality of nursing care. This content could serve as a checklist for those already developing tools, or as a frame of reference for those just beginning. The eight steps that will be discussed are:

1. Selection of framework
2. Determination of the goal

Reprinted with permission from The Journal of Nursing Administration 6(5):7-9, 1976; 6(7):16-19, 1976.

3. Identification of the patient group
4. Selection of items or indicators for the tool
5. Quantification of factors comprising the tool
6. Reliability testing
7. Validity testing
8. Scoring

Steps 1 to 4 are discussed in this column. The remaining steps will be discussed in my next column.

SELECTION OF FRAMEWORK

Three major components of the nursing care system have a significant relation to quality of nursing care. These components are (1) the setting in which the care is rendered, (2) the nursing process, and (3) patient outcome. Unfortunately, there is little research information about the relation of these components to each other. Only a few studies link specific nursing actions (such as preoperative teaching) to a specific patient outcome (such as improved ventilatory function in the postoperative period). Furthermore, the studies in the literature have not been replicated in a variety of settings.

This lack of research on the major components of nursing has greatly increased the problems surrounding the measurement of quality nursing care. It means that whichever component is selected as the focus for measurement, it will not be possible to refer to the other two components and their relation to quality. For example, if patient outcome is being measured, assumptions will have to be made about its relation to the nursing process. If process is being measured, assumptions will have to be made about its relation to patient outcome. The same is true if quality is to be measured in terms of the number or preparation of the nursing staff.

Although this view may sound disheartening, it is a true description of our current state of knowledge. It does not mean that nursing cannot proceed to measure quality. We must proceed. Never has there been greater pressure from within and without the profession for systematic assessment procedures and tools. However, it does mean that, as we proceed, we should do so with a clear conceptualization of the nursing care system and an awareness of the limitations of the components selected for measurement.

Some persons have argued that it is "better" or "right" to measure one component of the system (such as patient outcomes) in contrast to another (such as nursing process). In truth, it can be as right to measure quality in terms of outcomes as in terms of process.

The decision to measure any one component of the system will reflect the values, beliefs, and assumptions held by the personnel in that institution. Whatever the decision, it should be made on an *explicit* statement of the values, beliefs, and assumptions, and it should reflect an awareness of the broader framework surrounding the measurement of quality of nursing care. It is also important for later synthesis or contrast of work done at different institutions.

The first step, then, in tool development is conceptualization of the nursing care system and selection of the component to be assessed. The tradeoffs made by selecting one component instead of another should also be stated clearly. One specific outcome of this step is an operational definition of quality of care.

DETERMINATION OF THE GOAL

The second step in tool development is to decide who are the *users* and what are the *uses* of the instrument. As basic as these questions are, and as simple as they seem, they are frequently overlooked. Some of those currently working on procedures for measuring quality of care have assumed that a tool, if it is a "good one," will serve all purposes. That is not true. All tools have limitations. Some of the questions that should be answered about the users are the following: Will they be staff or outsiders? What will be required in terms of background knowledge and experience? Must the user be a nurse? Are interviewing and other skills necessary? Will the user require special training in the application of the tool or will it be possible to collect accurate data without training?

Some of the questions that should be answered about the use of the tool include the following: Is it to be used once only, per patient, or is it to measure change over time? Is it to focus on the individual patient or on groups? Is it to be used with clients covering a broad range of potential scores or a fairly homogeneous section of clients where only a small range of scores is likely? Must the tool be sensitive to variables within a small segment of the potential range of scores or across the whole range? Is it to be used for evaluation of the nursing care as a composite or to determine the quality of specific components as well as the composite? Is it to measure direct as well as indirect components of care? Do you wish to measure input from the nursing team (collectively or separately) or the care from all health professionals? Is it intended for acute conditions, inpatients, outpatients? The result of this second step will be a statement regarding uses of the tool—what it is intended to do or not do and the necessary background and training of the expected user.

IDENTIFICATION OF THE PATIENT GROUP

Most tools are developed to measure the concept within a specific group. For example, an IQ test may be for preschoolers or children age ten, or linked to a certain culture. The items on the test are appropriate for one group but not another. This step in developing tools to measure quality of nursing care has presented great problems.

The two underlying principles of identification of the patient group are (1) the group should be homogeneous in the sense that all items relate equally to all members of the group and (2) variation in scores is due to the concept being measured and not other factors (such as age differences or diagnosis).

In measuring quality of nursing care, approaches to defining a homogeneous group have ranged from being extremely specific to extremely global. One approach calls for the specification of the group in terms of age, medical diagnosis, health care setting, and sex. Although this helps ensure that every item is applicable, it necessitates the development of an endless number of tools. Another example of a popular approach is that of using acuity and medical diagnosis as the deciding factors. A tool would then be developed for the "acutely ill myocardial infarction" group of patients.

Within the coming months, it may be possible to use nursing diagnosis or the results from statistical analysis of nursing care data to create meaningful homogeneous subsets of patients. Unfortunately for the nursing care system, at this time, the best way to create patient groups is not known.

SELECTION OF ITEMS OR INDICATORS

Once you have a clear statement of the what and why of the tool, the next step is to select the specific items or indicators characteristic of the tool. This step involves three stages: identification, definition, and screening. Although some researchers combine these stages into a single process, I would recommend treating them separately. Again, each step will involve value judgments as well as some absolutes.

A common approach to identifying items is to have experts engage in brainstorming.

Using their collective knowledge and experience, the group identifies items that are agreeable to the majority. There are many variations of this basic approach. An expert can be defined differently. To some, it is a nurse with a master's degree in the clinical area under scrutiny; to others, it may be the client. Still others may select nurse researchers as the experts. The group of experts may be all nurses, all health professionals, or a mix of health professionals and clients. The brainstorming may be free association or structured in terms of predefined categories such as physical and psychosocial care or needs. Group process techniques introducing more structure into the discussion could also be used. One such technique is the Delphi in which an anonymous panel is asked to prioritize or rate items. Panel members are given statistical summaries of responses and then asked to respond to each item a second or third time until consensus has developed.

Other approaches for identifying items have included the use of a theory of nursing or of human needs as the basic conceptualization. Still others have used empirical data, case studies, or the body systems to generate the initial set of items.

Regardless of the approach used, important factors at this first stage are that some framework be used to ensure the development of items covering the broad spectrum of the care (or client) to be evaluated and that identification of the items be creative and expansive. Quite often in these first sessions much of the input is criticized as unmeasurable or vague, or "not this" or "not that." Negative comments such as those mentioned usually result in decreased group productivity and a set of items that have been accepted or requested on implicit rather than explicit criteria. Personally, I think it is better to generate as many ideas as possible and then eliminate them at a later point, using an explicit set of criteria.

After this first list is generated, the items must be put into a uniform format and the list evaluated for its comprehensiveness. This can be done by the group that generated the list or a second group of experts.

The second stage involves defining key words and phrases. Before any item can be quantified or measured, it must first have a precise definition. Developing precise definitions is extremely difficult, partially because we speak in clichés and broad generalizations. There is no easy way to develop a definition, but we must be certain to use all the library tools available. Examples of definitions are *length of hospital stay* means "the number of days the patient was hospitalized" (day of admission is counted as a day, day of discharge is not counted as a day). *Effective stir-up regimen* refers to the "conscientious application of the following three precepts at definite intervals during the postoperative period": (1) the patient must inflate his lungs adequately, (2) the patient must cough, and (3) the patient must move and turn.

The next step is to decide the criteria to apply to each item to determine whether it will remain in the tool. Some criteria are mandatory, others are optional. One mandatory criterion is "relevance," or assurance that the item relates to what is to be measured. For example, if quality of nursing care is to be measured, the items must relate to *quality* care and *nursing* care.

Items that reflect the impact of the surgeon or the housekeeper would not be included. Items that reflect unique nursing care would not be included. Because the scope of nursing varies from setting to setting, there is no master list of "relevant" and "inappropriate" items. Knowledgeable people in the setting must determine whether or not nurses routinely perform nursing activities likely to influence the outcomes described in the various items. They must also determine if sufficient time is spent in performing that activity that it is likely to produce a measurable effect.

In addition to selecting items that are clearly related to the operational definition of quality nursing care, the items must meet two other criteria. First, each item must apply to every patient for which the tool is intended. That is, a "not applicable" response should never be possible. If, for example, you are developing items to measure quality of nursing care for adult diabetics, you should have items regarding insulin administration only if they apply to all the patients in the group being measured. If some patients in the group were not insulin-dependent, those items would not apply and therefore should not be included. It is preferable either to have different tools or to word the items so they apply to every patient in the group, rather than to have one set of items, some of which apply to some patients and some of which apply to others.

The second criterion is that every patient being measured should be able to attain a high score. To illustrate this idea, assume you have an item regarding blood sugar level and decide that very high blood sugar levels indicate poor nursing care and normal blood sugar indicates good nursing care. This decision may hold for the majority of your patients. However, it will not hold true for the very brittle diabetic or the individual who does not respond in the predicted way to the prescribed diabetic regimen. Those individuals, even though they follow faithfully and completely the regimen taught to them by the nurse, will not be likely to attain scores on the "good" end of the scale. This situation will result in lower scores for some patients, not because of the quality of nursing care, but because of other factors. To the extent possible, items which favor subsets of patients should be eliminated or the tool not used for those patients where a bias would be evident.

A third mandatory criterion relates to variation on scores on the item. Unless there is variation within a patient, group or overtime, there is no reason to evaluate it. Many first ideas are discarded in terms of this criterion. For example, number of analgesics administered in the recovery room may not be a good item in a tool because most patients receive 0 or 1. There just is not enough variation in the item to discriminate among patients. The lack of variation may not be evident until data are actually collected from patients.

In addition to these three mandatory criteria, others may be specified. For example, one group stated that the items had to be observable and easily obtainable. Another group limited themselves to data from a closed chart. Most groups specify criteria that reflect time, qualifications of data collectors, cost, source of data (patient, chart, relatives).

Once mandatory and optional criteria have been established, they should be applied to each item to determine whether or not the item is to be retained. This step usually necessitates actual data collection from a representative group of patients. Checklists or other data-gathering devices may be developed to facilitate this step. Once the criteria are applied and the information compiled, decisions can be made rather quickly as to whether an item will be retained, discarded, or reconceptualized.

SUMMATION

These first four steps of tool development are probably the most difficult as they require explicit statements of values and assumptions, high-level clinical judgments, and ability to conceptualize. Many researchers or clinicians try to by-pass or hurry through these steps only to discover the seriousness of that error at a later point in time.

Although the steps have been presented as a logical progression, in practice there is movement back and forth throughout the whole process.

In the next column, I will describe the remaining four steps and present an overview of current work in the area of measuring quality of care.

Part Two

In Part I of Measuring Quality of Nursing Care, (*JONA,* June) four major steps for creating a tool were presented. These steps are: (1) selection of a conceptual or theoretical framework, (2) determination of the intended use and users, (3) identification of the patient group, and (4) procedures for generating items and criteria for selecting or rejecting items. In this column, the concepts of quantification, scoring, reliability, and validity will be discussed. The article concludes with a brief overview of several current projects in developing measures of quality of nursing care.

The content in this and the preceding column is intended as a conceptual guideline for the nurse who is attempting to develop a tool to measure quality of nursing care. It is an introduction and not an exhaustive presentation on any of the concepts as they relate to tool development and measurement. Those confronting such issues are advised to consult with experts in tool development or to read extensively before making final decisions.

QUANTIFICATION OF FACTORS

The terms *measurement* and *quantification* are often used interchangeably to designate the process of assigning numbers to objects to represent quantities. A number is used to communicate how much of a given attribute is present at a given point in time. In addition, quantification is essential if the research design requires statistical analysis.

The four most common types of measurement scales are:

Nominal Scale. The nominal scale is a qualitative measurement consisting of a number of discrete, mutually exclusive and exhaustive categories of a variable, each having a distinctive attribute (e.g., sex: female-male; types of illnesses: acute-chronic).

Ordinal Scale. The ordinal scale is a qualitative measurement in which the different persons or items under study are ranked from most to least with respect to a variable (e.g., excellent, very good, average, poor).

Interval Scale. The interval scale is a quantitative measurement in which the distance between the points is equal and can justifiably be broken down into finer subdivisions to provide a refined distinctions among the subjects being measured. An interval scale has no zero point (e.g., scale for body temperature) in contrast to a ratio scale (weight scale) which does.

Ratio Scale. The ratio scale is a quantitative measurement having an absolute zero point. The total absence of the variable makes it possible to determine not only how much greater one measurement is from another, as in an interval scale, but also how many times greater it is (e.g., a scale for the variable "time").

EXAMPLES

Assume there is an interest in measuring contractures as an indication of quality of nursing care. If one is using a nominal scale, the item might read:

Contracture Right Leg
Yes _____ No _____

With an ordinal scale, the item could read:

Contracture Right Leg   Rank _____
Using the numbers from 1 to 7, rank the patient's contracture in terms of other similar patients. "1" refers to greater contracture, "7" to lesser contracture.

An interval scale would require a scaling as follows:

Contracture Right Leg

| 1 | 2 | 3 | 4 | 5 |

Decreased contracture ⟵⟶ Increased contracture

(Place an "X" above the point on the scale that most directly represents the amount of contracture.)

A ratio scale might be used in this instance by asking:

Contracture Right Leg _____
(Express in degrees the nature of the contracture, e.g. $10°$; $30°$)

Although some objects can be measured with all four scales, usually only one or two are suitable. In general, it is better to use an interval or ratio scale because of the type of statistical analysis that can be performed. Time, measurement skills and cost factors may necessitate use of one of the other scales. It is vital that the scale selected be congruent with the stated purpose of the tool, and the nature of the object being measured.

RELIABILITY TESTING

Reliability testing determines consistency and stability of the tool. Reliability of a tool speaks to its dependableness. Reliability itself can be measured in several ways and may refer to 1) scores obtained by different raters for the same object or person, 2) scores for the same object or person at different points in time or 3) scores on different parts of the tool.

Different procedures for determining reliability take account of different problems or concerns. If, for example, a particular tool is to be administered by a number of different persons in one setting or by one person in a variety of situations, it is necessary to determine interrater reliability. An excellent example of the need for this is contained in the report: A Methodology for Monitoring Quality of Nursing Care.[1] The investigators were developing a tool to measure quality of nursing care using process-type items. They reported the following experience.

Following the initial two-day session, the research nurse worked with the observers in each hospital to test for interobserver reliability. We found during these two periods of pretesting that many criteria from other studies were not adequately clarified. A simple example is the statement from the RPSL Nursing Audit: "Are allergies recorded on admission?" Each of three nurse-observers looked at the admissions data under "Allergies," and saw the word "None" written in by the admitting nurse. One observer answered the item as "Yes," one as "No," and one "Not Applicable," the latter two reasoning that none were present, so "Yes" would not be an appropriate response. The item was rephrased later to read: "Is there a written statement about allergies on admission?" The response "Not Applicable" was deleted. Responses of observers then were accurate.

Procedures for determining the consistency and stability of a tool have also been developed. There are two types commonly referred to as split-half reliability and test-retest reliability. Each has several different techniques for determining reliability. To illustrate what is meant by consistency, if items on the tool represent similar observations, the assumption is that scores on those items should be similar. To the extent that they are similar, the tool is reliable. This determination is made through a statistical analysis of those specific items. To illustrate what is meant by stability, if the same individual takes the test at two different points in time, the assumption is that the scores should be similar. To the extent that they are, the tool is reliable. A reliability coefficient is calculated through a statistical analysis of the scores.

Reliability testing is essential in tool development. The results of initial and repeated reliability testing should lead to greater and greater refinement of the items comprising the tool.

VALIDITY TESTING

Validity means the extent or degree to which a tool actually measures what it seeks to measure. Although validity may seem a simple concept, it is extremely difficult and sometimes tedious to determine. Determining validity is as essential in tool development as is reliability; one would not want to use a tool without knowing its validity.

There are three common types of validity, each associated with a major purpose of measurement.

Predictive validity

If a measurement is obtained from which an estimate of some other behavior will be made, then the *predictive* validity of the tool must be established. The question is how well can one predict behavior "Y" from "X," the score on the tool. A common example is predicting success in college from an achievement or intelligence test. Although some nurses may develop tools to measure quality of nursing care in order to predict health at a later point in time, this is currently not a common goal or major intent of most such tools being developed.

Content validity

A second type of validity is called content validity (or logical or sampling validity) and addresses the adequacy with which the items in a tool represent the universe they sample. One common example is a course examination. To what extent, in terms of adequacy and representation, does the examination test course objectives? In measuring quality of nursing care, this may be an important type of validity to determine. The use of a theoretical or conceptual framework to generate items will help in creating a tool with content validity.

Construct validity

A third type of validity is labeled *construct* and has various subtypes. It relates to the trait or concept the tool is to measure and how well the tool measures that particular trait. Construct validity is necessary when the construct cannot be measured directly but must be inferred from other behaviors. For example, anxiety or intelligence cannot be measured directly, but they can be inferred from other behaviors. Construct validity for a tool measuring quality of nursing care would deal with the constructs *quality* and *nursing*. The more abstract the concept, the more difficult it is to establish validity. As pointed out in Part I, precise definitions are basic to sound measurement. Something cannot be measured if it cannot be defined. The need for a precise definition of quality and nursing care is necessary if construct validity is to be determined.

Construct validity can be determined by correlating scores from a new tool with a previously validated measure of the same construct. It can also be determined through discriminatory testing, i.e., testing of patients who received poor nursing care as well as those who received quality nursing care. If the scores discriminate in the expected way, the tool has validity. It is important that several such tests be made. In terms of quality of nursing care, both quality and nursing would have to be tested with relevant groups of patients. Construct validity is never a *proved* issue as it is dependent upon the current state of knowledge about the construct and related constructs.

In selecting the appropriate type of validity to be determined, and the appropriate procedure for doing so, the nature and use of the tool and availability of other tools are factors that should be considered.

Before moving to the next point, a few words should be said about face validity. When experts in the field review a set of items and the items look appropriate the tool is labeled valid. Although this type of validity is helpful during tool construction, it does not assure predictive or construct validity. This type of testing is so ineffective in determining real validity that some investigators refuse to acknowledge that it has any relation to true validity testing.

If face validity is used, it is important to give serious thought to the credentials of the raters. For example, should a nurse clinician or a patient pass judgment on the items of a scale measuring quality of nursing care? In reporting face validity, the credentials and number of raters, the procedures and rater-agreement should be presented.

SCORING

In general, the simpler the scoring procedure, the better. In some instances, however, a more complex procedure is possible or necessary. If the tool has been purposefully developed with several subsections, it may be possible to generate subscores as well as a total score. Again, depending on the theoretical framework, weights may be assigned to the various items or subsections of the tool. The procedure of assigning weights increases the complexity of the scoring procedure and should be done only when there is a sound rationale for it.

The use and scaling of the tool will influence the type of scoring. For example, nominal scales will produce only frequency data in terms of the response categories. Interval or ratio scales will enable the calculation of mean scores. Also, change scores can be computed if that is the intended use of the tool. Scoring, like every other component of tool construction, must be consistent with the assumptions and decisions made at the preceding stages.

OVERVIEW OF SELECTED PROJECTS

Dr. Mabel Wandelt is the primary investigator of the research that led to the development of the Quality Patient Care Scale (QUALPACS).[2] The rating scale consists of 68 items arranged in six subsections: (1) psychosocial: individual; (2) psychosocial: group; (3) physical; (4) general; (5) communication; and (6) professional implications. An experienced observer-rater evaluates the nursing care a patient receives for a two-hour period while the care is in progress. The tool is designed to measure nursing process. Reliability and validity testing have been done and the specific data are available in the literature. The tool has also been used in patient care research.

Rush-Presbyterian-St. Luke's Medical Center, the Medicus Systems Corporation, and The Division of Nursing, DHEW, have developed a methodology to monitor the quality of the patient care system.[3] Although the project is expanding to outcomes, currently the focus is the nursing process.

In this project, the nursing process framework consists of six dimensions. The specific indicators of quality developed for each dimension, or subobjective, were identified from existing methodologies and by expert judgment. Criteria were then examined for interrater reliability. After extensive statistical testing, a final set of 251 criteria was created and categorized by the specific dimensions of the nursing process. The methodology includes random selection of patients for observation and a subset of criteria appropriate to the intensity of the patient's illness. A profile of nursing care along each dimension of the nursing process is produced. The methodology measures quality of care for a group of patients for a circumscribed period of time; it does not measure the quality care for each individual patient.

The final report of this significant contribution to quality monitoring is available through the Government Printing Office. It is to be hoped that progress reports of the extension of this project into outcome measures will also be available in the literature.

Over the past several years, Marie Zimmer and her colleagues at the University of Wisconsin Hospitals have delineated several sets of outcome criteria and a quality review system that has a well-developed rationale and explicit step by step procedures.[4] The methodology emerging from this work is labeled *nursing service evaluation program*. Each set of criteria has a defined patient population in terms of medical diagnosis and other significant factors. This group has made an effort to share their work as it develops so that some sets of criteria have yet to have their reliability and validity established.

Drs. Barbara Horn and Mary Ann Swain[5] from the University of Michigan are currently conducting a project to develop criteria for measuring outcomes. The overall objective of the project is to develop, refine, and validate an approach that will provide measures of the quality of the nursing care process. A model of nursing is being used as a framework. That model describes nursing practice in terms of nine health status domains. Examples of the nine domains are requirements for air, activity, and rest and requirements arising from health deviation.

The major function of the resulting instrument is research, although it will have potential uses such as monitoring of quality. Horn and Swain intend to develop an instrument that can measure the impact of a given change within nursing services on quality of patient care. The focus of the instrument is medical-surgical patients.

Content validity procedures have been implemented, and extensive statistical analysis and reliability testing will be undertaken in the coming months.

Dr. A. C. Bellinger at Wayne State University has recently started a multiphase project to explore relationships between nursing activities and patient outcomes and then to conduct promising experimental studies generated by those data.[6]

Regional Program for Nursing Research Development, Western Interstate Commission for Higher Education, has implemented a program of research in the area of measuring quality of nursing care. One hundred nurses from the 13 Western states have formed 15 workgroups. Each group has selected either tool development or exploration of process-outcome relationships as its focus with a homogeneous group of patients for study. Group members will collect reliability and validity data according to clearly delineated procedures. The stated aims of this research program are:

1. To determine homogeneous groups of recipients of nursing care for purposes of measuring outcomes of care, that is, to create either a conceptual or empirical basis for categorizing recipients of nursing care for purposes of measuring outcomes of care.

2. To establish subsets of valid, reliable outcome measures for each of the homogeneous groups of recipients of nursing care.

3. To determine what outcome measures are the most sensitive indicators of quality of nursing care.

4. To determine when each outcome should be measured in terms of sensitivity to quality of nursing care.

5. To create for selected subgroups of recipients of nursing care tools that consist of valid, reliable outcomes.

6. To establish the relationship between nursing process and outcomes eliminating the effects of health services variables and patient characteristics.

7. To generate hypotheses for future research aimed at establishing cause and effect relationships between nursing care and patient welfare.

The American Nurses' Association has a continuous commitment to quality assurance. Recently, the ANA was awarded a contract by the Bureau of Quality Assurance (BQA), Dept. of Health, Education, and Welfare to develop model sets of criteria for screening the quality, appropriateness, and necessity of nursing care. Experts were used to generate criteria for each of 16 patient groups, or populations. A second group of experts was asked to indicate degree of agreement with the criteria. Apparently there was *not* substantial agreement between the two groups of experts, and high content validity was not demonstrable. Interrater reliability was explored with little training and with a more detailed orientation. Following the validity and reliability testing, a real world testing was conducted. The 16 audit instruments were used in a wide range of hospitals across the country.

It is anticipated that the final report of this project will be released for distribution in the near future.

REFERENCES

1. Jelinek, R. et al. *A Methodology for Monitoring Quality of Nursing Care*. Report of Phase I of PHS Contract NIH 72-4299 July 1972. USDHEW Pub. No. (HRA) 74-25.
2. Wandelt, M. A., and Ager, J. W. *Quality Patient Care Scale*. New York: Appleton-Century-Crofts, 1974.
3. Jelinek, R. et al. 1972.
4. Zimmer, M. *Development of Sets of Patient Health Outcome Criteria by Panels of Nurse Experts*. Final Report of Project #7, Wisconsin Regional Medical Program, University of Wisconsin Hospitals, University of Wisconsin, School of Nursing, Milwaukee.
5. Horn, B. and Swain, M. A. "Health Status Dimensions: A Conceptual Framework for Quality Assessment." Speech presented at the WICHE Research Clinic on Measuring Quality of Nursing Care, August 6, 1975, Denver, Colorado.
6. Bellinger, A. C. "An Overview of Research and Elaboration of Procedure for Generating Subsets of Participants," Speech presented at the WICHE Contact Persons Meeting, September 9, 1975, Denver, Colorado.

THE NURSING AUDIT FOR EVALUATION
OF PATIENT CARE

Maria C. Phaneuf

Nurses in hospitals and public health nursing agencies in New York have only recently begun the formal auditing of nursing service records to appraise the quality of nursing care. The audit method they are using was originated and developed by the Associated Hospital Service of New York (Blue Cross) to evaluate the quality of service to subscribers.

To facilitate use of the audit and to make sure that pertinent information is included, Blue Cross constructed a 3-part schedule, a portion of which was presented in an article describing the development of the method.[1]

Part I, which can be completed by a trained clerk, provides patient identification data and questions pertaining to key administrative policies which safeguard patients and institutions. It has two forms—one for use in hospitals: the other for use in public health nursing agencies. When the audit is to be used in nursing homes, another specific form of Part I may be required. Part II is on the same page as Part I and is identical for hospital, public health nursing agencies, and nursing homes. This is the judgment entry which is made by the nursing audit committee member who has reviewed the record.

Part III deals specifically with the functions of professional nurses as executed in the care of the patient whose record is being reviewed. The functions are those stated by Lesnik and Anderson.[2] The components under each function are the basis for appraising the content and process of care and these components are scored.[3]

Each component stands alone, yet is part of the whole. A "yes" response connotes that there is adequate evidence in the record regarding the component; a "no" means inadequate evidence; "uncertain" indicates *some* evidence toward the affirmative; and a "does not apply" response is self-explanatory. For each component, one of the above responses must be made. The descriptive statements about each component do not focus on the outcome of care, but rather on the process of care. Donabedian has expressed limitations inherent in the use of outcome of care as a measure of quality: "Outcomes might indicate good or bad care in the aggregate; they do not give an insight into the nature and location of the deficiencies or strengths to which outcomes might be attributed."[4]

The statements also show considerable emphasis on disease. The committee who worked with Blue Cross on the development of the audit schedule believed that the greater the nurse's knowledge of the disease process, the greater will be her tendency to individualize patient care. For example, in caring for a patient who has adenocarcinoma treated by surgery and radiation, the nurse needs not only to take care of the operative site as ordered by the physician, but also to look for surgical sequelae, radiation reactions, persistence, spread or recurrence of the cancer, a second primary cancer, or new signs of coexisting, unrelated disease.

It is impossible to make these observations properly without taking careful account of the patient as a unique individual—including his hopes, fears, anxieties, and interpretation of or silence about symptoms. It entails listening responsively and expressing a genuine interest in the patient's well-being or malaise. This helps to deepen the nurse-patient relationship.

Reprinted from Nursing Outlook **14**(6):51-54, 1966. Copyright The American Journal of Nursing Company.

The observations and related impressions as well as nursing judgments must obviously be a matter of record if they are to be useful to all who are professionally responsible for this particular patient. In view of the complexity of modern medical and nursing care and the complexity of the human beings who are the patients, it is difficult to see how quality care can be achieved without an evaluation of the patient care record as an instrument of service and as one important basis for quality appraisal.

The following list of seven functions, with their 50 components and descriptive statements, was developed for our audit committee, but it can be used by any hospital or agency as a guide to the evaluation of nursing care as revealed in the patient's record.

I. APPLICATION AND EXECUTION OF PHYSICIANS' LEGAL ORDERS

1. *Medical diagnosis complete*. The diagnosis is clear enough to permit intelligent nursing care. (Hemiplegia is an incomplete diagnosis: arteriosclerotic cardiovascular disease, cerebral thrombosis, and hemiplegia [left] is an example of a complete diagnosis.) The diagnosis ordinarily conforms to terminology in the *International Classification of Diseases, Adapted for Indexing of Hospital Records and Operation Classification*.[5]

2. *Orders complete*. The physician's orders are clear and inclusive in relation to the patient, his diagnosis, and other clinical data. For example, medication orders are specific—the nature of medications, amount, frequency, and method of administration. It is evident whether the medications are self-administered, or are given by the family or the nurse.

3. *Orders current*. Orders are up to date according to nursing judgment and the institution's policy.

4. *Orders promptly executed*. The record shows reasonable, appropriate timing between the writing of the order and compliance.

5. *Evidence that nurse understood cause and effect*. The records show that the nurse knew what she was doing and why. A nurse performing any function ordered by the physician is legally obligated to understand the cause and effect of that function before she performs it. She is required to understand the basis for the orders, the anticipated therapeutic results, and possible side effects or complications.

6. *Evidence that nurse took medical history into account*. The records show recognition that knowledge of pertinent points in the patient's past pattern of health and illness are vital to intelligent current care. For example, if a nurse knows that a patient on anticoagulants has a past history of gastric ulcer, she will be alert to the specifically increased possibility of gastric hemorrhage. If she knows the patient has diabetes mellitus and is giving him postcholecystectomy care, she will be alert to the diabetic care and cardiovascular symptoms.

II. OBSERVATIONS OF SYMPTOMS AND REACTIONS

7. *Related to course of above disease(s) in general*. There is evidence that the nurse understands the disease in the textbook or classic sense and is observing the patient with the classic picture as a clinical frame of reference.

8. *Related to the course of above disease(s) in this patient*. In addition to knowledge of the disease as in the above component, there is evidence that the nurse observes the patient's individual response to the disease and its treatment.

9. *Related complications due to therapy (each medication and each treatment)*. Recorded observations relate to expected therapeutic results and possible or unexpected untoward side effects.

10. *Vital signs*. When indicated, recording includes temperature; quality of pulse as well as rhythm and rate; blood pressure; quality of respiration as well as rate; tone, temperature, and color of skin; and observations pertaining to feeling tone.

11. *Patient to his condition*. There is evidence that attention was given to the patient's attitude toward his clinical condition and life situation as it influences and is influenced by his condition.

12. *Patient to his course of disease(s)*. There is evidence that attention was given to the demonstrable degree of the patient's understanding and acceptance or rejection of his disease(s) and illness. ("Disease" is interpreted as a pathological process; illness as acute or chronic manifestations of the pathological process.)

III. SUPERVISION OF THE PATIENT

13. *Evidence that initial nursing diagnosis was made*. The record shows that nursing problems were determined and categorized as the basis for nursing care plans directed to solution of the problems. This diagnosis should be made as soon as possible after the first nursing contact with the patient. In some patient care records, nursing care plans strongly suggest that the diagnosis was made. In this event, evidence of the implicit diagnosis should be taken into account.

14. *Safety of patient*. There is recorded evidence of precautions taken to prevent physical injury.

15. *Security of patient*. There is evidence that the nurse is helping to create or maintain a therapeutic environment. This includes supportive interpersonal relations.

16. *Adaptation (support of patient in reactions to condition and care)*. There is evidence of attempts to help the patient adjust to his changing condition, course, and treatment (including termination of treatment).

17. *Continuing assessment of patient's condition and capacity*. The record reflects ongoing evaluation of the current status and situation of the patient and effects of care, with analysis of present nursing problems.

18. *Nursing plans changed in accordance with assessment*. There is evidence that nursing care plans were adapted as indicated by the continuing assessment.

19. *Interaction with family and with others considered*. There is evidence of concern for the people in contact with the patient—family, friends, and others—so that mutual influences can be used to the patient's emotional advantage and those around him.

IV. SUPERVISION OF THOSE PARTICIPATING IN CARE (EXCEPT THE PHYSICIAN)

20. *Care taught to patient, family, or other nursing personnel*. The record reflects what care was taught, what guidance and support were given, to whom, and by whom.

21. *Physical, emotional, mental capacity to learn considered*. The evidence shows that the ability and readiness of those to be taught, guided, and supported were taken into account.

22. *Continuity of supervision to those taught*. The evidence shows that the results of initial and additional teaching were assessed, with appropriate follow-up.

23. *Support of those giving care*. The record reflects the giving of emotional and physical help to those supervised and taught.

V. REPORTING AND RECORDING

24. *Facts on which further care depended were recorded*. Information recorded facilitates continuing physician and nurse management of clinical care.

25. *Essential facts reported to physician.* The record shows that basic necessary information is conveyed to the physician in written or verbal reports. The facts may be major or minor; it is their importance to the physician in his management of the patient's care which makes them essential or nonessential.

26. *Reporting of facts included evaluation thereof.* There is evidence that in reporting facts nursing judgment as to their significance or possible import is included. For example, a report of the fact of wound irrigation should include evaluation of results and the patient's reactions to the procedure.

27. *Patient or family alerted as to what to report to physician.* There is evidence that patient or family members are directed to report to the physician those factors, signs, symptoms, or situations conducive to patient/family-physician rapport. This does not eliminate the nurse reporting the same factors directly to the physician. It includes encouraging the patient or family to ask the physician questions which the nurse cannot properly answer or communicate fears or anxieties which the physician can best allay.

28. *Record permitted continuity of intramural and extramural care.* The record permits an uninterrupted sequence of care—nurse-to-nurse as well as nurse-to-physician and nurse-to-other professionals involved in service to the patient. It is of major importance that the recording indicate succinct reporting to the physician of information which is vital to the patient's therapeutic regimen.

VI. APPLICATION AND EXECUTION OF NURSING PROCEDURES AND TECHNIQUES

29. *Administration and/or supervision of medications.* Whether the nurse gives the medications or supervises the patient or family in process, the record indicates nurse, patient, and family awareness of expected therapeutic results and possible untoward side effects.

30. *Personal care (bathing, oral hygiene, skin, nail care, shampoo).* The record indicates appropriate attention to all aspects of personal hygiene whether the related services are performed by the nurse, patient, family member, or another person.

31. *Nutrition (including special diets).* There is evidence of attention to adequate nutrition, appropriate to the patient's course and condition. If a special diet has been ordered, there is evidence as to whether or not to what extent it is adhered to and appears understood by patient and family.

32. *Fluid balance.* The record indicates consideration of the relationship of intake and output and that this is evaluated in relation to the patient's condition, course of illness, and care.

33. *Elimination.* Evidence that bowel function is considered and appropriate action is taken when the patient's bowels are not functioning normally.

34. *Rest or sleep.* Evidence that the patient's usual or unusual patterns of rest and sleep are taken into account in planning his regimen and supervising his care.

35. *Physical activity.* The record shows the relationship between the amount of activity the patient is permitted and what he is actually doing, as well as what he understands about it.

36. *Irrigations (including enemas).* When ordered, and as indicated, the record shows the procedure done and the results obtained.

37. *Dressings and bandages.* Evidence that these are applied as ordered or indicated, the medication used, if any, and the type of dressing—sterile or clean.

38. *Formal exercise program.* Indication that a treatment plan is carried out as ordered by the physician, or as outlined by a physical therapist at the physician's request.

39. *Rehabilitation (other than formal exercises).* Evidence of teaching or encouragement toward independent living—range of motion (ROM), active and passive exercises, activities of daily living (ADL), uses of aids in ADL. If nursing rehabilitation is not required, there is evidence that the nursing care approach is restorative in nature.

40. *Prevention of complications and infections.* Evidence of good hygiene, early detection of primary or secondary infections, other untoward symptoms, or complications due to therapy. Where possibility of contractures exists, preventive measures should be recorded.

41. *Recreation, diversion.* The record indicates specific attention to the patient's needs for activities which interest and amuse him and take his attention away from disease and illness.

42. *Clinical procedures—urinalysis, B/P.* The record shows the results of urinalyses, blood pressure readings, or other tests done by nurses.

43. *Special treatments (e.g. care of tracheostomy, use of oxygen, colostomy or catheter care, etc.).* Evidence of function performed, indication of results, and evaluation. This includes evidence of observation of patient's reactions and estimated degree of understanding.

44. *Procedures and techniques taught to patient.* Evidence that any treatment the patient needed and could understand or learn was in fact interpreted and taught.

VII. PROMOTION OF PHYSICAL AND EMOTIONAL HEALTH BY DIRECTION AND TEACHING

45. *Plans for medical emergency evident.* Evidence that, by policy or specific teaching, patient, family, and other personnel know what to do in situations which are inherently worrisome or dangerous for the patient, or anxiety or fear aroused in others involved.

46. *Emotional support to patient.* Evidence of helping patient understand and accept his feelings about himself and his condition. This includes helping the dying patient and his family.

47. *Emotional support to family.* The record indicates impressions or evidences of family feeling and reaction to the patient and his condition and, if necessary, work done to help the family toward greater understanding and acceptance of the patient's condition and attitude and their own feelings and attitudes.

48. *Teaching preventive health care.* Evidence of prevention of disease by promotion or protection of health for patient and family. This includes alertness to signs and symptoms of possible new diseases, leading to prompt physician diagnosis and early treatment.

49. *Evaluation of need for additional resources (e.g. spiritual, social service, homemaker service, physical or occupational therapy).* Evidence that, when indicated, the needs for consultation with or request for direct service from other nonphysician professionals are being assessed.

50. *Action taken in regard to needs identified.* Indication that nursing action was taken for needs identified under any one of the above categories, with the knowledge and permission or approval of the patient's physician.

•   •   •

There are two ways of judging quality of nursing care. One is to have an expert nursing practitioner observe directly and regularly the nursing care as it is being provided. Ordinarily this is not possible and will be less so with the expected increase of patients under

Medicare. The other is systematic examination of records to see whether they provide a clear picture of the patient's condition, treatment, and course of illness and whether the content and process of nursing care measure up to the determined standard of practice.

In physician audits of medical care in hospitals, the use of records for assessing quality has been well established in principle and in practice.[6,7] Nursing, as a major part of total patient care, should likewise be assessed—by nurses.

REFERENCES

1. Phaneuf, Maria C. A nursing audit method. Nurs. Outlook **12**:42-45, May 1964.
2. Lesnik, M. J., and Anderson, Bernice E. Nursing Practice and the Law. 2d ed. Philadelphia, Pa., J. B. Lippincott Co., 1955, pp. 247-293.
3. Phaneuf, *op. cit.*
4. Donabedian, Avedis. Evaluating the Quality of Medical Care. Ann Arbor, Mich., School of Public Health. University of Michigan, 1965. (Unpublished paper.)
5. U. S. Public Health Service. International Classification of Diseases, Adapted for Indexing of Hospital Records and Operation Classification. (Publication No. 719) Washington, D.C., U.S. Government Printing Office, 1959.
6. Joint Commission on Accreditation of Hospitals. Five Basic Publications. Chicago, Ill., The Commission, 1964, pp. 11-20.
7. Report on medical review research. Med. Rev. Res. (Albany) Aug. 1965.

AN EVALUATION OF NURSING CARE
BY DIRECT OBSERVATION

Mary Jane Munley

The word "quality" attached to health care services has become a popular adjective to describe the attributes and deficiencies of the present system. Agreement on a definition is difficult to obtain. In the past some nurses have claimed that nursing's unique nature prevented measurement of the activities performed by nurses; hence, the decision that the nursing care given was "quality" care was primarily a subjective observation.

There exists a variety of methods which are currently used to evaluate the quality of nursing care. They include the standards set forth by the Joint Commission on Accreditation of Hospitals, the evaluation of an individual's proficiency, the measurement of deficiencies through the unusual occurrence report, and the audit of discharged patients' clinical records.

In September of 1970, Mercy Hospital began the use of Phaneuf's closed chart audit.[1] This audit measures nursing care records by using the seven standards of nursing care as developed by Lesnik and Anderson.[2] Since its inception, the results of the audit have been used by the Director of Nursing as one basis for planning and developing nursing service. New policies, procedures, and objectives for the department of nursing have been influenced by the audit. This method of auditing evaluates the quality of care in relation to the documentation as found in the patient's closed clinical record. Its results affect the care of patients who are admitted at a later time, but obviously not the care of the patient whose chart was audited.

Reprinted from Supervisor Nurse 2(4):28-39, 1973.

As we used the closed chart audit, it became evident to the author and the Director of Nursing that a tool for direct observation of a patient's nursing care was needed. The purpose of this instrument would be to provide an objective means of evaluating the quality of nursing care with a view toward benefits for the patient whose care was observed. The tool also would provide the consumers of health care, the patients, an opportunity to indicate to us how they perceived the nursing care that they received. The results could influence new procedures and policies and indicate a need for Inservice, but that would not be its primary goal. This idea was given further emphasis in November, 1971, when the Joint Commission on Accreditation of Hospitals visited our organization. It was their recommendation that the closed chart audit be expanded to include the evaluation of the activities and effectiveness of the nursing staff on current individual patients.

A review of the literature failed to provide a measurement instrument which would effectively indicate the level of care given and which would provide the patient an opportunity to participate in the evaluation. Consequently, the accompanying instrument, "The Clinical Evaluation of Nursing Care," was developed here. It is based on the standards of nursing care at Mercy Hospital. It consists of three major components: a patient interview, direct observation of the patient, and an evaluation of his nursing care plan.

The clinical evaluation of the patient's care begins with the patient interview and an explanation to the patient by the nurse evaluator that part of our work includes evaluating the nursing care that he receives. He is also told that he will be requested to answer a few questions. To date, little attention has been given to the patient as a source of valid or useful information, yet it has been indicated that most patients can identify hospital care that is substandard.[3] Perhaps consumers' knowledge of medicine and nursing activities has previously been limited; however, with increased publicity through the communication media, their knowledge has sharply increased and the current inadequacies of health care have been made glaringly apparent. Some of the ten questions asked the patient during the interview include: *Are your needs met? Are your questions answered? Do you receive an explanation of activities and procedures being performed? Do you feel well cared for? Are you lonely?* and *Have you been oriented to your surroundings?*

Although no question directly asks the patient whether his socio-psychological needs are being met, the author feels that the questions "Are your needs being met?" and "Do you feel well cared for?" provide the patient an opportunity to evaluate this aspect of his care. In a short-stay, acute care hospital, we can hope to meet only those socio-psychological needs that directly affect the patient's recovery from his present illness.

Direct observation of the patient and evaluation of the nursing care plan focus on eight categories. The first is the physical needs of the patient. Some examples of items included are: *Is the patient without immediate need of attention?* Upon examination of the patient's skin, *Are there reddened areas on the body from pressure?* If the response is "yes," *Does the nursing care plan indicate approaches taken to decrease pressure?* Several items evaluate what measures are taken to prevent muscular contractures, foot drop, decubiti, and respiratory and circulatory complications of those patients on bed rest. The plan for this individual's care to prevent these complications is measured by observing the nursing care plan. If the patient is ambulatory, these items would be nonapplicable.

Another aspect included is the care given to a patient with an indwelling catheter. *Is the urinary drainage tube above the level of urine? Is the urinary drainage tubing free of kinks and is there straight drainage from the level of the bed to the drainage bag?* On the nursing care plan, if not contraindicated by the medical orders, *Is a plan to force fluids indicated?*

The second component is safety. *Is the patient's signal available to him whether he is in bed or in a chair? Are restraints safely applied?* If this question applies to a patient whose upper trunk is restrained, *Does the nursing care plan include measures taken to maintain adequate pulmonary function?* This would include loosening the restraint every two-three hours and having the patient deep breathe and cough, elevation of the patient's arms over his head, and change in his position. *Are safety measures applied and obvious for the patient who is receiving oxygen? If this is applicable, list the measures taken.* Lastly, *Does the nurse have an unobstructed access to the patient?*

An example of items included in the third component concerning medications is *Does the patient know what medications he is taking?* He should not necessarily be required to know the name of the drug and its dosage, but should be able to describe the drug and its action. For example, a patient may respond that he gets a "hypo" for pain or an antibiotic to prevent infection. A question regarding the nursing care plan is *Are drug allergies indicated?* Also, *Are the untoward side effects of medications the patient is taking listed?* Although it is not feasible to list the side effects of every drug the patient has prescribed for him, possible side effects should be listed for such things as chemotherapeutic agents, insulin, digitalis preparations, and coumadin.

Some examples of questions asked regarding intravenous medications are: *Is the intravenous flowing at the proper rate? If the needle is inserted over a joint, is that part supported by a padded board or splint?*

The fourth category evaluates the social-emotional needs of the patient. *Has the patient been introduced to his roommate? Is the patient encouraged to retain or regain as much independence as possible?* and *Are there diversions at hand for the patient?* The nursing care plan should have a notation regarding the patient's emotional status, including his level of anxiety, and a nursing approach to meet the emotional needs indicated.

The next component evaluates the patient's environment. Observation is made to see if the temperature of the room is comfortable, and if the room is free of unpleasant odors and excessive noise. Direct observations of the bedpan or urinal are made when the patient is on bed rest. For patients in isolation, a sample of the questions asked is, *Does the patient and his family understand the reason for isolation?* and *Does the patient understand his limitations during isolation?*

Measures taken to provide for the spiritual needs of the patient encompass the sixth component. *Are practices of the patient's religion allowed for?* For example, food restrictions, Communion for the Catholic patient, and clergy visits. On the nursing care plan, one question is: *In the event the patient has been seriously or critically ill, has the clergyman's visit been recorded?*

The last two components concern the nursing care plan only. The first is the teaching plan. Questions asked include *Is a teaching plan included? Is notation made of the patient's progress concerning teaching?* and *Does the plan reflect considerations given to family teachings?*

The last section concerns the provisions made for post-hospital care. The question asked is *Are notations made concerning plan for post-hospital care?* If the nursing care plan indicates that the patient will return home, return to a nursing home, or that the Continuing Care Coordinator has been contacted to assist the patient and family in planning his care after discharge, this question can be answered positively.

Each head nurse was introduced to this measurement instrument on an individual basis. The author intended to extend this one-to-one learning experience to all the full-time employed registered nurses, as they function as team leaders in our hospital. However, the amount of time involved made this physically and economically impractical. Consequently, group meetings were held with the team leaders. At this meeting the purpose and need for a clinical evaluation, its comparison to the closed chart audit, and the tool itself were discussed.

A patient's nursing care is currently evaluated on or after the third day of admission. For communication purposes, the nursing care plan is marked "Clinical Evaluation" with the date it was done. Of the head nurses on our three 56-bed units, two have decided that their team leaders will evaluate the nursing care of patients on another team and one has decided that the team leaders will evaluate the nursing care of the patients on their own team.

After measuring a patient's care with this tool, the evaluator then reviews the results with the team leader of that particular patient and the head nurse. They then make the necessary adjustments for the improvement of the patient's care as the evaluation has indicated.

Each head nurse and the team leaders on the day and evening rotation are expected to evaluate the nursing care of one patient per week. The selection of the patient is randomly made by each nurse and each team leader. It is our goal to evaluate approximately twenty per cent of the patients admitted to the hospital which should provide us with a valid indication of the care given.

The average time spent on the "Clinical Evaluation of Nursing Care" is approximately twenty minutes, after the evaluator becomes familiar with the tool. The total possible score is 150. The total of each individual evaluation is equal to the sum of the correct answers plus one-half the sum of the nonapplicable items. Each of the ten questions asked during the patient interview are valued at two points. All other items are equal to one point. This score, representing the quality of care, is assigned a value according to the following scale:

Excellent	(150-116)
Good	(115-85)
Satisfactory	(84-39)
Poor	(38-0)

The results to date do not indicate whether the objectivity of the tool is better maintained when team leaders evaluate the nursing care of patients on their own or another team. Perhaps this will become apparent in another six months to one year.

The response of patients has been favorable. The majority are pleased to participate in this type of evaluation, if that is how it is introduced. However, patients do not respond positively when they are told at the beginning of the evaluation that the nurse is taking a survey or a poll. Patients seem to indicate that they do not want to be categorized into groups of responses. Several of the patients have commented that, by using a tool such as this, it indicated to them a sincerity in wanting to know the truth and that they were confident that if they suggested a needed change it would be made.

How has patient care been improved by use of this tool? A few of the examples are: One patient had no appetite but was to have "fluids encouraged." Once it was determined what the patient's intake was at home and what juices he liked, it became easier to increase his intake. Some patients have received clean utensils as a result, such as water glass, bedpan, and urinal. Another patient indicated that at night he had a difficult time finding the right button on the intercom to call the nurse. A hand control device was obtained for him to use at night. Patients on bedrest who could participate in their care were started on a deep breathing regimen every two hours. A patient who was deformed by arthritis told the evaluator that she could handle cups better if they were half full and could consequently retain some of her independence. This information was communicated to the staff and placed on the nursing care plan.

This method of evaluating the quality of nursing care has undergone two revisions since its inception and continues to be analyzed. Objective measurement of the quality of the nursing care provided the hospitalized patient is one form of self-regulation for the nursing profession. It directly benefits current patients and it emphasizes the responsibility that the nurse practitioner has for providing a high level of quality nursing care to the evermore discriminating patient-consumer.

REFERENCES

1. Phaneuf, Maria C. The Nursing Audit Profile for Excellence. New York, Appleton-Century-Crofts, 1972.
2. *Ibid.*, p. 16.
3. Blumber, Mark S., and Drew, Jacqueline A. "Methods for Assessing Nursing Care Quality," Hospitals, Journal of the American Hospital Association, Vol. 37, November 1, 1963, p. 72.

NURSING CARE PLANS: A SYSTEMS APPROACH TO DEVELOPING CRITERIA FOR PLANNING AND EVALUATION

Betty Jane Ryan

General systems theory offers a strategy particularly relevant to planning nursing care. The planner is provided with new conceptual schemes for analysis, direction, and evaluation of the formal structure which administrates health care efforts. The informal structure is, of course, recognized as also bearing on the problems of health and is necessarily included within the entire system complex. Nursing service administrators, for example, whether conducting the activities of a department or a smaller nursing care unit, daily face problems which they frequently lack the tools to solve adequately.

The major purpose of general systems theory is the design of models embodying the relative complexity necessary to study reality and general enough for use by a variety of knowledge levels. The application of general systems theory to planning nursing care provides a conceptual means for integrating knowledge and action components (nursing assessment, diagnosis, objectives, and prescriptions) of the nursing process so that nursing intervention may not only be forecast but also become a rationally coordinated and measurable product.

Reprinted from Journal of Nursing Administration 3:50-57, May-June, 1973.

CONCEPTUAL MODEL: WHAT IS A SYSTEM?

Universally, a system is defined as a set of elements or units in interaction to achieve a specific goal. System as used here refers to the orderly, logical arrangement of interdependent parts into an interrelated whole to accomplish a given purpose. Implicit in this concept is a degree of wholeness which makes the complete unit something quite different from each part of the unified whole. Systems theory visualizes internal and external environmental factors as an integrated entity.

A system operates to convert or process energy, information, or materials into a planned outcome, product, or information. It is characterized by (1) *input,* the component which receives, stores, or takes in energy in the form of information or material such as time, money, people, equipment, effort, or information; (2) *throughput,* the processor, convertor, or assimilating means of changing the energy received into (3) *output,* the outcome, result, or product, and (4) *feedback,* a regulating mechanism which functions as a monitor, evaluator, or control to insure that the planned goals are obtained. Feedback has the additional task of reintroducing a part of the output to the input at the proper phase.

As a system moves from a relatively fixed, mechanistic structure, it becomes a less-closed system. A closed system is one which operates with fixed, automatic, ritualistic relationships requiring little or no outside intervention or interaction. It tends to lose its essential organizational characteristics when information from outside itself enters the system. On the other hand, an open system interacts with its environment. This type of system continuously gathers and receives information about the environment and behavioral reactions to events occurring within and between component relationships, using this information as the means for signaling directions or adaptations toward the goals of the system.

In an open system, the whole is considered in terms of flow. The flow process involves input as the energizer (or starting force), throughput as the process activity, and output as the result of the action. Feedback is that part of the flow which serves as a control by continually monitoring and evaluating all component actions and interactions. The flow process is cyclic in operation; it strives for balance and seeks to sustain the life of the system.

Essential elements of a viable system. At least three essential elements constitute a viable system having both the capacity and potential to induce change and to survive. The first is *goal direction.* In nursing, these goals must be operational so as to enable continuous evaluation and determination of the degree or extent of goal achievement. It is begging the problem to state general goals such as "to restore to self-independence" or "to optimize well-being." Such statements are more directional than operational and are not conducive to credible evaluation. Goals must of necessity be as quantitative as possible. Quantitative standards can then be factored to produce criteria as tests and indices of the more general, qualitative goals. Goals should be as operational as possible and should not be confused with the methods determined to achieve the goals.

A second factor necessary to the viability of a system is *feedback,* which represents the analysis of information about the system as a guide for future behavior. The existence of feedback presupposes (1) information-gathering capability and (2) ability to evaluate information. Planning for feedback by establishing standards and determining criteria for evaluation in a nursing care system should be built on both capabilities and be carefully related to the goals set by the system.

A third important factor is the *ability to change* or adapt. Goals and feedback are meaningless if the system has no potential for change. Adaptability is necessary for a system to maintain its goal direction. The primary reason for change is found in the challenge that system goals be continuously sought and advanced. Change may be focused on any combination of (1) methods for achieving outcomes or goals, (2) the goals themselves, and (3) the feedback capabilities. A powerful attribute of systems theory is its ability to solve problems according to a planned methodology. The problem is analyzed as a total process, and the conclusions drawn are then utilized as information in making decisions. Another attribute of systems theory is its potential to focus on a multiplicity of relations because it operates independently, though not in mutual exclusion of any discipline or content area; indeed, it is more often multidisciplinary in application than otherwise.

Definitions of terms. Before proceeding with the presentation of a strategy, it is necessary to clarify and define pertinent terminology. The specific words to be discussed are *project, planning, control,* and *systems analysis.* All of these terms are related to and are employed in an activity which is consuming more and more of the energies of professional nurses in the preparation and implementation of evaluation techniques.

Borrowing from Paul Gaddes: "A project is an organization unit dedicated to the attainment of a goal, generally the successful completion of a development product on time, within budget, and in conformance with predetermined specifications."[1] While this definition relates specifically to industry, it provides an essential description of a nursing care plan as a development *project.* A nursing care plan can be said to have a definite goal; it is complex in that a mix of human, material, and informational resources is used in interdependent and interrelated jobs; it is homogeneous in the sense that one nursing care plan can be differentiated from another; and it is nonrepetitive since one nursing care plan is designed for a given patient in a given time period and cannot be applied to another patient or to the same patient at another time.

Planning, in its most general connotation, outlines the future and announces decisions in advance of what must be done. The output of a nursing care planning process may take the form of procedures, schedules, orders, or prescriptions. The purpose of any plan is to bring about behavior that will lead to desired outcomes. To accomplish its purpose the nursing care plan must (1) describe actions—some synonyms are objectives, goals, and behavioral specifications, and (2) serve as a formal tool or guide for directing nursing care.

Broadly viewed, *control* functions as a monitor to insure the achievement of specified objectives. As a feedback mechanism the control formula of noting deviations from the plan, taking necessary corrective actions, and recycling the program is included within the concept for purposes of this discussion.

System analysis presents no difficulty in being defined since the term was previously ascertained to signify an array of component parts interacting interdependently to accomplish a particular purpose according to plan. So defined, it is assumed that any system can be factored into a series of subsystems and that each subsystem can be further factored. Once factored (analyzed), the system can be reconstructed and unified (synthesized). A definition of analysis is described by Martin Starr in terms of the principle of disassembly.[2] Following this principle, analytic behavior consists of operations that involve division, dissection, classification, partitioning, and similar actions. In contrast, the principle of assembly applies to synthesis with related operations of integration, unification, and summation. Simply stated, analysis breaks the system down into operative parts whereas synthesis puts it back together as a whole unit.

OPERATIONAL MODEL

The nursing care plan viewed as a system is characterized as being made up of several interrelated parts, units of activities that belong exclusively to the whole project; hence, one can describe the nursing care plan as an entity having structural and functional boundaries that distinguish it from the rest of the environment. Although it can be demarcated, the nursing care plan still operates within an environment which affects it and which the plan itself affects. With this characterization the concepts of open system and system analysis assume validity and become useful tools for planning nursing care, fixing the responsibility for that care, and evaluating the same care. To demonstrate the application of the concepts, the first step is to establish the goal, or objectives, of the nursing care plan. The subsequent steps are to define the nursing care plan, to identify its components and elements, and finally to establish criteria for measuring results of the plan for care.

Stated or written objectives declare expected outcomes or intended results of an action. Nursing care plan objectives are to collect and communicate information about a specific patient which will guide and direct nursing intervention toward correction of a health problem or maintenance of a designated level of health. Within this statement can also be found the definition, purpose, and standards for evaluating the effectiveness of a nursing care plan.

To define a nursing care plan without prior reference to the nature of nursing and a philosophy of nursing care is tantamount to committing a sin of omission. Basically, nursing is herein considered a process involving the functions of nurturing, sustaining, teaching, and advocacy. It is generally recognized that the nurse's principal role is to make decisions regarding each of these functions. A nursing care plan is one device evolved to expedite and facilitate the delivery of health care within the purview of the professional nurse practitioner. Operationally, the nursing care plan is defined as follows: A *nursing care plan* is an information receiving, processing, sending, and evaluating center initiated by the professional nurse through the use of specialized assessment, diagnostic, communication, and judgmental skills and compiled as a guide for directing nursing activities toward the fulfillment of health needs of the patient and the achievement of related nursing goals.

Again, the purpose of a plan is extracted from the definition of the plan. It also answers the question "What are we trying to do?" In this circumstance, the nursing care plan is expected to (1) bring a broad area of information to bear on the health problems of an individual patient and (2) control the operations or performance of the nursing care team in the coordinated manner of a single mind.

The next step requires use of the principle of disassembly, because several tasks to be done to reach the stated objectives must be identified, described, and classified. The results of this analysis usually take the form of a hierarchical scheme or chart ranking several cognition levels of prime and supporting activities. Both analysis and synthesis focus upon definitions of who, what, when, where, and how. It should be noted that the same definitions integral to the system as a process are also integral to the system as a complete unit.

Figures 1 and 2 schematically diagram the concepts, components, elements, and activities of a nursing care plan system and how these defining characteristics are synchronized in time and synthesized in the relative space of a goal-oriented entity.

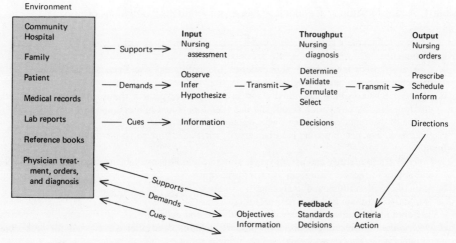

Figure 1. Conceptual design for planning and evaluating nursing care.

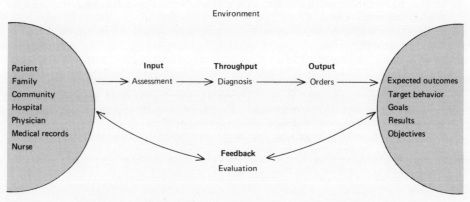

Figure 2. Flow diagram of nursing care plan system.

EVALUATION OF NURSING CARE

The ubiquitous problem of determining and selecting criteria for evaluating nursing care is extensive and critical. To date the efforts to develop a nursing care evaluation system have followed a general educational model involving instructional, contextual, and criterion variables. A major emphasis has been on identifying rules, principles, concepts, and knowledge which attempt to explain outcomes as cause-effect relationships between variables. Planning a nursing care evaluation system should concentrate on measuring outcomes in comparison with input as informational data, since desirable or expected outcomes generate from input. It is important to note also that behavioristic variables and other background data enter the system as givens, becoming a part of the system not to be manipulated or acted upon by the organization but to serve as energy to initiate action and provide information for possible corrective action to improve future outcomes.

Table 1. A classification of feedback strategies for evaluating outcomes of nursing care plans

1. Environment
   a. *Objectives:* To define operational boundaries, to identify and assess needs in that context, and to delineate problems underlying needs
   b. *Method:* By describing individually and in relevant perspective the major subsystems of the environment, by comparing actual and intended inputs and outputs, and by analyzing possible causes of discrepancies between what should be and what is
   c. *Decisions:* For deciding who is to be served, what needs are to be met, when and where
2. Input
   a. *Objectives:* To identify and assess target system capability, available change system resources, and ability to receive, store, and sort information
   b. *Method:* By describing and analyzing:
      1. Available human and material resources
      2. Solution alternatives for relevance, feasibility, and economy
   c. *Decisions:* For selecting sources of support, solution, and alternatives, and for prescribing actions for deciding how change will be brought about
3. Throughput
   a. *Objectives:* To process information that will predict defects in the change procedure. To maintain a record of what was done, to and by whom, when, and where
   b. *Method:* By monitoring anticipated barriers to goal achievement and remaining alert to unanticipated or unplanned ones
   c. *Decisions:* For putting the plan in operation and refining the design; i.e., for insuring the attainment of objectives
4. Output
   a. *Objectives:* To relate outcome information to objectives, environment, input, and throughput information
   b. *Method:* By operationally defining criterion measures associated with the objectives, by comparing these measures with predetermined standards or comparisons, and by interpreting the recorded behavior outcomes with input and process information
   c. *Decisions:* For continuing, modifying, terminating, or refocusing a change activity and for lending that to other major phases of the change process. That is, for recycling the change activities

Table 2. The total nursing plan

Objective: To communicate information and direct nursing action toward continuous progression of the individual patient's nursing care
Criteria:
   1. Initiated on admission of patient to the health service
   2. Initiated, compiled, and written by a professional nurse
   3. Contains the following components:
      a. Nursing assessment
      b. Nursing diagnosis
      c. Nursing orders
      d. Nursing objectives
   4. Updated periodically at specified times in response to changes in patient care needs and nursing objectives
   5. Readily available to nursing staff
   6. Used in nursing care rounds, team conferences, and change-of-shift reports

Table 3. Nursing assessment

Objective: To identify factors that will influence nursing care
Criteria:
1. Permits the immediate development of a beginning, individualized plan of care
2. Contains personal identifying information
3. Describes the patient's perceptions of his needs and problems
4. Includes patient's expectations about his illness and therapy
5. States patient preferences regarding:
   a. Hygienic needs
   b. Dietary practices
   c. Fluid needs
   d. Elimination
   e. Sleep and rest pattern
   f. Self-care
6. Does not duplicate information gathered by other members of the health team

Table 4. Nursing diagnosis

Objective: To determine patient problems related to health and decide solutions
Criteria:
1. Contains statements of patient's current and potential problems arranged in order of immediacy
2. Identifies strengths and deficiencies of coping responses
3. Shows discrepancies between current behavioral responses and expected outcomes of plan of care
4. Considers lack of health information as a problematic area
5. Translates needs and problems into nursing objectives

Table 5. Nursing objectives

Objective: To identify and describe target behaviors and/or desirable outcomes or nursing intervention
Criteria:
1. Identifies specific target behavior
2. Desirable outcomes are derived from identified needs and problems
3. Statements are phrased clearly, concisely in action terms

Table 6. Nursing orders

Objective: To direct and coordinate nursing activities so that each patient's health deficits can be corrected or ameliorated in a continuous progression toward optimum health
Criteria:
1. Describes specific actions necessary to achieve objectives and/or solve problems
2. Considers patient preferences
3. Plans for teaching health care
4. Prescribes timing—date, hour, and/or minutes
5. Orders are revised, based upon changes in patient's behavior as determined by the professional nurse and/or members of the health team
6. Includes patient, family, and/or community participation in plans for discharge and aftercare
7. Includes initials of author

Evaluation, within the context of systems theory, is characterized as the feedback capability of the system. It identifies deviations or deficiencies within the system and moves the system toward fixing responsibility and controls. As a feedback and control process it involves measurement and the comparison of resulting measures against standards. Standards may be desired outcomes, expected outcomes, predicted outcomes, norms, and other forms of criteria. The selection of measures is based upon explicit objectives. Measurable objectives are mirrored in outcomes, and all relevant outcomes should properly be included in the set of measurable criteria to be used. Evaluation thus becomes not an end in itself but an additional means to achieve the purpose. Generally, this purpose is to promote and facilitate decisions affecting the cycling and recycling of the system (Table 1).

Having considered nursing care plan objectives and the definition and purpose of the nursing care plan, thus disclosing the reciprocity inherent among standards, expected outcomes, objectives, and criteria, the final step is to delineate criteria by which both the quantity and quality of a plan for nursing care can be assessed accurately. The following tables list the structural and functional criteria required to operationalize a nursing care plan system (Tables 2 to 6).

CONCLUSION

Planning nursing care need not be bound by traditional means of gathering, assessing, and processing information. Creative, innovative approaches offer problem-solving methodologies that permit the light of new reason to untie knotty problems of the past. General systems theory offers a comprehensive and lucid formulation for nursing administrators to plan, direct, and control effective nursing service.

One goal for planning nursing care should be a search for valid and reliable tools for measuring information, decisions, and directions as well as outcomes in terms of stated objectives and their operational criteria. An assessment device for measuring the efficacy of a plan of nursing care has been developed, illustrating the application of general systems theory to nursing care planning (Table 7). Designed primarily as an educational guide,

Table 7. Strategy for planning and evaluating nursing care plans

Units in sequence	Elements	Activities	Standards (expected outcomes)	Criteria	Frequency Yes	Vague	No
Total nursing care plan	Nursing assessment Nursing diagnosis Nursing objectives Nursing orders	Analyze Synthesize Decide Direct Coordinate Instruct	Communicates information about individual patient and his environment which guides nursing team in care of that patient	Initiated on admission of patient Initiated, compiled and written pencil by professional nurse Contains these components: Nursing assessment, diagnoses, objectives, orders Readily available to nursing staff Used in nursing rounds and team conferences Updated periodically			

Table 7. Strategy for planning and evaluating nursing care plans—cont'd

Units in sequence	Elements	Activities	Standards (expected outcomes)	Criteria	Frequency		
					Yes	Vague	No
Nursing assessment	Personal identifying factors about patient Orientation to environment Perceptions Expectations Preferences Habits of daily living	Interview Observe Describe Sort Classify Report Record	Records identifying information permitting immediate development of a plan for nursing care including patient's perceptions, preferences and expectations.	Permits immediate development of beginning individualized care plan Contains personalized identifying information Describes patient's perceptions of his own needs and problems Includes patient's preferences Includes patient's expectations about his illness and therapy Is not duplicated in medical records			
Nursing diagnosis	Statements describing patient's current and potential problems, strengths, and deficits	Analyze data Predict outcomes Make inferences Hypothesize Determine needs Identify problems Establish priorities Record	In terse statements describes patient's current and potential problems	Contains short statement of patient's current and potential problems Statements are arranged in order of immediacy Identifies strengths and deficits of coping responses Considers lack of health information a problematic area Shows discrepancies between current behavior and expected outcomes			
Nursing objective	Statements identifying desirable behavioral changes, treatment goals, or intended results of intervention	Translate needs/problems into target behaviors Formulate goals Determine conditions which must exist to precipitate change	Concise statements describing target behavior, treatment goals, or intended results of nursing intervention	Identifies target behaviors Desirable outcomes are derived from identified needs/problems Statements are phrased succinctly in action terms			
Nursing orders	Directions Schedules Procedures Principles	Specify nursing actions Determine when, who and where Translate principles into concrete directions	Prescribes nursing intervention in action terms formulated to carefully direct the nursing team toward progressive, continuous and personalized nursing care	Describes nursing intervention techniques behaviorally Considers patient preferences Plans for teaching health care Schedules treatment events Revised as behavioral change indicates Includes patient, family, community participation in current and aftercare plans Initialed by author			

general systems theory has been used to teach nurses how to construct a plan of nursing care and how to test the efficacy of that plan. Its guidelines are simple to follow, although detailed. As a comprehensive measuring tool it can be utilized by auditing committees to correlate nursing prescriptions for intervention with patient responses as found in written records or charts. The tool also lends itself easily to planning a problem-oriented system of charting.

SUGGESTED READINGS for Chapter 5

BOOKS

Beyers, M., and Philips, C.: Nursing management for patient care, Boston, 1971, Little, Brown & Co. Describes the framework of management—hospital organization, role of manager, nurse as manager, manager's relationship to organization, expectations of nurse-managers in hospital, and challenge of management—motivation, development of staff, introducing change, devising and using plan of care, appraising staff performance, discipline, and communication. Presents three case studies.

Blood, D. F., and Budd, W. C.: Educational measurement and evaluation, New York, 1972, Harper & Row, Publishers. Presents a discussion of validity, relevance, reliability, objectives, observation tests—anecdotal records, checklist, rating scale, development and use of checklists and rating scales, participation charts; paper-and-pencil tests, assembling and scoring objective examinations; item analysis, standardized tests, statistical treatment of test scores, grading, and reporting.

Brook, R. H.: Quality of care assessment: a comparison of five methods of peer review, Washington, D.C., 1973, U.S. Department of Health, Education, and Welfare. A study of five methods of care assessment.

Byrne, M. L., and Thompson, L. F.: Key concepts for the study and practice of nursing, ed. 2, St. Louis, 1978, The C. V. Mosby Co. Discusses the following concepts: organismic behavior, basic human needs, level of wellness, adaptation, behavioral patterning, steady state, stress, behavioral stability continuum, structural variable, consequences of an act; presents working model for assessing patient's needs and predicting effects of nursing care.

Carter, J. H., et al.: Standards of nursing care: a guide for evaluation, New York, 1972, Springer Publishing Co., Inc. Discusses the development of standards and indices and the utilization of staff for implementing them. Presents indices.

Davidson, S. V. S., editor: PSRO: utilization and audit in patient care, St. Louis, 1976, The C. V. Mosby Co. A collection of articles about quality assurance.

Doughty, D. B., and Mash, N. J.: Nursing audit, Philadelphia, 1977, F. A. Davis Co. Discusses how to construct and conduct a nursing audit and presents sample sets of criteria for numerous conditions.

Douglass, L. M., and Bevis, E. O.: Nursing leadership in action: principles and application to staff situations, St. Louis, 1974, The C. V. Mosby Co. Discusses the principles of leadership, teaching, learning, group dynamics, delegation of authority, effective conference, and evaluation of personnel.

Froebe, D. J., and Bain, R. J.: Quality assurance programs and controls in nursing, St. Louis, 1976, The C. V. Mosby Co. Discusses quality control and assurance programs.

Kron, T.: The management of patient care, Philadelphia, 1971, W. B. Saunders Co. Discusses leadership, management, planning for patient care, conducting team conference, team nursing, use of care plan, staff relationships.

Mager, R. F., and Pipe, P.: Analyzing performance problems, Belmont, Calif., 1970, Fearon Publishers, Inc. A programmed text on analyzing performance problems; contains quick reference checklist.

Mayers, M. G., Norby, R. B., and Watson, A. B.: Quality assurance for patient care: nursing perspectives, New York, 1977, Appleton-Century-Crofts. Discusses the evaluation process, quality assurance mechanisms, documentation of patient care, and implementation of quality assurance programs. Presents record forms and criteria for several conditions.

Nicholls, M. E., and Wessells, V. G., editors: Nursing standards and nursing process, Wakefield, Mass., 1977, Contemporary Publishing Co. A collection of articles about nursing standards and quality control.

Phaneuf, M. C.: The nursing audit profile for excellence, New York, 1972, Appleton-Century-Crofts. Discusses some problems of evaluating quality of nursing care, what an audit is and is not, the audit instrument, planning for auditing, orientation of the audit committee, auditing process, influences of auditing; appendices contain table of random numbers, suggested readings, explanations of audit schedule components, and audit forms.

Tucker, S. M., et al.: Patient care standards, St. Louis, 1975, The C. V. Mosby Co. Lists observations, acute care, ongoing care, teaching, and discharge activities for numerous conditions through the use of a systems framework.

Wandelt, M. A., and Stewart, D. S.: Slater nursing competencies rating scale, New York, 1975, Appleton-Century-Crofts. Presents and discusses the Slater Nursing Competencies Rating Scale.

Yura, H., and Walsh, M. B., editors: The nursing process, Washington, D.C., 1967, The Catholic University of America Press. Discusses assessing patient needs, planning to meet those needs, implementing, and evaluating the plan of care.

Yura, H., and Walsh, M. B.: The nursing process: assessing, planning, implementing, evaluating, New York, 1973, Appleton-Century-Crofts. Discusses components of the nursing process.

PERIODICALS
Evaluation

Anderson, M.I.: Development of outcome criteria for the patient with congestive heart failure, Nurs. Clin. North Am. 9(2):349-358, 1974. Uses congestive heart failure as a model for developing outcome criteria.

Anderson, N.: Audit of care processes and patient outcome: one facet of QA, Nurs. Adm. Q. 1(3):117-128, 1977. Presents samples of outcome criteria.

Bailit, H., et al.: Assessing the quality of care, Nurs. Outlook 23(3):153-159, 1975. Discusses structure, process, and outcome in relation to assessing the quality of care with special mention of the nurse practitioner.

Beard, J. M.: Quality care: administration's concern, AORN J. 23(7):1326-1336, 1976. Discusses quality control in the operating room.

Benedikter, H.: Assessing the status of a nursing audit process, Nurs. Adm. Q. 1(3):129-137, 1977. Describes how to evaluate a nursing audit.

Berg, H. V.: Nursing audit and outcome criteria, Nurs. Clin. North Am. 9(2):331-335, 1974. Discusses the use of outcome criteria for the nursing audit.

Bille, D. A., and Jurkovic, J.: Nursing process audit: the style is individual, Nurs. Adm. Q. 1(3):85-115, 1977. Presents a comprehensive audit tool, a nurse interview audit tool, a bedridden patient audit tool, and a patient teaching audit tool.

Bloch, D.: Evaluation of nursing care in terms of process and outcome: issues in research and quality assurance, Nurs. Res. 24(4):256-263, 1975. Organizes previous work into a framework and recommends the process-outcome type of evaluation.

Bloch, D.: Criteria, standards, norms—crucial terms in quality assurance, J. Nurs. Adm. 7(7):20-29, 1977. Presents a hypothetical model that helps clarify the relationship of criteria, standards, and norms.

Clinton, J. F., et al.: Developing criterion measures of nursing care: case study of process, J.

Nurs. Adm. 7(7):41-45, 1977. Describes the development of patient-outcome criteria.

Corn, F., and Magill, K.: The nursing care audit—a tool for peer review, Superv. Nurse 5(2):20-28, 1974. Presents a nursing care audit used in obstetrics at the Bronx Municipal Hospital Center.

Correlates of the quality of nursing care, J. Nurs. Adm. 6(9):22-27, 1976. A research report indicates that numerous interrelated variables influence the quality of nursing care.

Costanzo, G. A., and Vertinsky, I.: Measuring the quality of health care: a decision oriented typology, Med. Care 13(5):417-431, 1975. A comprehensive discussion of classification of methodologies for measuring the quality of health care.

Curtis, J., Rothert, M., and Christian, B.: A practical evaluation of nursing care as part of the nursing process, J. Nurs. Educ. 13(3):11-15, 1974. Indicates that the effects can be evaluated for significance and in relation to patient needs.

Daubert, E. A.: A system to evaluate home health care services, Nurs. Outlook 25(3):168-171, 1977. Describes an evaluation of records with the use of defined criteria.

Davis, A. I.: Measuring quality: development of a blueprint for a quality assurance program, Superv. Nurse 8(2):17-26, 1977. Describes the development of a quality assurance program.

Diddie, P. J.: Quality assurance—a general hospital meets the challenge, J. Nurs. Adm. 6(6):6-16, 1976. Discusses the implementation of a quality assurance program at the Veterans' Administration Research Hospital in Chicago, Illinois.

Donabedian, A.: Quality of care: problems of measurement. II. Some issues in evaluating the quality of nursing care, Am. J. Public Health 59:1833-1836, Oct., 1969. Discusses technical and operational issues of the nursing audit.

Dunham, G. W.: A quality of patient care project, Superv. Nurse 7(4):34-38, 1976. Discusses the development of a patient care audit.

Durham, R. C.: How to evaluate nursing performance, Hosp. Management 109:24-25, 28, 32, May, 1970. Discusses development of the rating form.

Eddy, L., and Westbrook, L.: Multidisciplinary retrospective patient care audit, Am. J. Nurs. 75(6):961-963, 1975. Recommends that retrospective audits be multidisciplinary.

Estes, M. D.: Introducing the nursing audit, Am. J. Nurs. 64(9):91-92, 1964. Discusses the rationale for a nursing audit.

Ethridge, P. E., and Packard, R. W.: An innovative

approach to measurement of quality through utilization of nursing care plans, J. Nurs. Adm. 6(1):25-31, 1976. Nursing care plans serve as a basis of documentation for evaluation of the nursing process at St. Mary's Hospital and Health Center in Tucson, Arizona.

Falls, M. E.: Collaboration for quality: as seen by the nurse, Superv. Nurse 7(11):49-51, 1976. Indicates that participation on a manufacturer's panel is an aspect of quality assurance.

Felton, G., et al.: Pathway to accountability: implementation of a quality assurance program, J. Nurs. Adm. 6(1):20-24, 1976. Discusses implementation of a quality assurance program at Children's Hospital National Medical Center in Washington, D.C.

Finkelman, A. W.: The standards of nursing practice and the supervisor, Superv. Nurse 7(5): 31-34, 1976. Identifies and discusses the standards of practice as a guide for professional practice.

Fuller, M. E.: A nursing director looks at quality control, Superv. Nurse 4(4):56-59, 1973. Author maintains that the quality of patient care can be improved through a combination of the nursing audit, an instrument for evaluating current care of hospitalized patients, in-service education, and new policies.

Gassett, H.: "Q for Q"—quest for quality assurance, Superv. Nurse 8(2):29-35, 1977. Describes efforts to implement quality assurance at Presbyterian Hospital in Albuquerque, New Mexico.

Glasson, P. L.: The struggle for total quality, Superv. Nurse 8(2):36-40, 1977. Discusses measurement of quality.

Gordon, P.: Evaluation: a tool in nursing service, Am. J. Nurs. 60(3):364-366, 1960. Discusses staff evaluation.

Greenough, K.: Determining standards for nursing care, Am. J. Nurs. 68(10):2153-2157, 1968. Discusses how and by whom standards for practice can be developed. Standards should be defined in terms of action and behavior that are visible and measurable.

Greenspan, J.: Medical audit: an effective aim of quality assurance, Hosp. Community Psychiatry 28(12):901-903, 1977. Describes the audit system developed by the Joint Commission on Accreditation of Hospitals for retrospective reviews.

Griffith, E. I.: A rational approach to patient service review, Nurs. Outlook 17(4):49-51, 1969. Discusses the evaluation of public health nursing services.

Gruendemann, B.: Evaluating nursing care: an

interim AORN report, AORN J. 20(8):232-236, 1974. Describes components of the nursing process and elaborates on evaluation.

Hagen, E.: Appraising the quality of nursing care. In Jacobi, E., and Notter, L. E., editors: American Nurses' Association Eighth Nursing Research Conference, Washington, D.C., 1972, U.S. Department of Health, Education, and Welfare. Suggests using patient outcomes, processes and activities, and working conditions to direct evaluation of nursing care.

Hanna, K. K.: Nursing audit at a community hospital, Nurs. Outlook 24(1):33-37, 1976. Outlines the audit process and discusses the steps.

Harman, R. J.: Nursing services information system, J. Nurs. Adm. 7(3):14-20, 1977. Discusses how a data base and Nursing Services Information System instruments are used to improve the quality of patient care.

Haussmann, R. K. D., and Hegyvary, S. T.: Field testing the nursing quality monitoring methodology: phase II, Nurs. Res. 25(5):324-331, 1976. Presents the design, analysis, and findings of a field test of a method for monitoring quality of nursing care. Lists criterion objectives and subobjectives.

Hegyvary, S. T., and Haussmann, R. K. D.: Monitoring nursing care quality, J. Nurs. Adm. 5:17-26, June, 1975. Presents a pilot program and discusses the problems of quality monitoring.

Hilger, E. E.: Developing nursing outcome criteria, Nurs. Clin. North Am. 9(2):323-330, 1974. Presents outcome criteria for colostomy care.

Holle, M. L.: Retrospective nursing audit—is it enough? Superv. Nurse 7(7):23-29, 1976. Discusses the standards of the American Nurses' Association and the Joint Commission on Accreditation of Hospitals.

Huckabay, L. M. D.: The significance of administrative control in quality assurance, Nurs. Adm. Q. 1(3):51-55, 1977. Discusses the role of the nurse administrator in quality assurance.

Hunter, A. R.: Nursing audit pinpoints needs, AORN J. 20(8):241-244, 1974. Discusses use of the nursing audit in the operating room.

Hurwitz, L. S., and Tasch, V.: Developing a quality assurance program in nursing, Superv. Nurse 8(6):50-51, 54-55, 58-59, 1977. Discusses the evolution from a nursing audit to interdisciplinary audit and presents outcome criteria for asthma patients.

Jenkinson, V. M.: Select the right yardstick to measure nursing quality, Dimens. Health Serv. 52(2):40-41, 1975. Recommends which tool to use for various situations.

Johnson, M.: Outcome criteria to evaluate post-operative respiratory status, Am. J. Nurs. **75**(9): 1474-1475, 1975. Temperature, cough, respirations, and lung condition were the outcome criteria used to evaluate postoperative respiratory status.

Jones, M. C.: An analysis of a family folder, Nurs. Outlook **16**(12):48-51, 1968. Study of two public health nurses' services to same family revealed differences in nursing care given.

Kabot, L. B.: Objective evaluation for clinical performance, Superv. Nurse **8**(11):16-18, 1977. Recommends the use of a performance checklist for the evaluation of orientees.

Keeler, J. D.: The process of program evaluation, Nurs. Outlook **20**(5):316-319, 1972. Identifies purposes, objectives, activities, and resources as the main components for the planning and evaluation of public health nursing programs.

Kelley, L., and Jones, M. K.: Quality control in medical records—an internal system, Med. Record News **48**(5):45-52, 1977. Describes the use of medical records for documentation of quality of care.

Kirchhoff, K. T.: Let's ask the patient: consumer input can improve patient care, J. Nurs. Adm. **6**:36-40, Dec., 1976. Presents a questionnaire administered to patients and discusses the results.

Klonoff, A., and Cox, B.: A problem-oriented system approach to analysis of treatment outcome, Am. J. Psychiatry **132**(8):836-847, 1975. Evaluated the outcome by the number of problems identified by clients and the amount of distress associated with them.

Langford, T.: Nursing evaluation—necessary and possible, Superv. Nurse **2**:65+, Nov., 1971. Discusses the planning of a systematic evaluation of nursing care. Presents an evaluation instrument.

Laros, J.: Deriving outcome criteria from a conceptual model, Nurs. Outlook **25**(5):333-336, 1977. Uses Roy's model of four primary modes—physiological needs, self-concept, role function, interdependent relations—and man's adaptation to a changing environment as the conceptual model for developing outcome criteria.

Lewis, W. R.: Health behavior and quality assurance, Nurs. Clin. North Am. **9**(2):359-366, 1974. Presents a case study and discusses categories of health behavior and the historical and social background of health beliefs.

Lohmann, G.: A statewide system of record audit, Nurs. Outlook **25**(5):330-332, 1977. Discusses different systems used in different regions and the problems and results of record audits.

Marram, G. D.: Patients' evaluation of their care: importance to the nurse, Nurs. Outlook **21**(5): 322-324, 1973. Study indicates that nurses say patient's opinion of his care is important but should not influence nurse's performance rating or hospital's system of rewards and penalties.

McCaffrey, C.: Performance check lists: an effective method of teaching, learning, and evaluating, Nurse Educ. **3**(1):11-13, 1978. Discusses the use of checklists and presents a performance checklist for routine neurological vital signs.

McClure, M. L.: ANA standards for nursing services: consideration in evaluation, Superv. Nurse **7**(8):27-31, 1976. Discusses the ANA standards for nursing service as a tool for self-examination.

McGuire, R. L.: Bedside nursing audit, Am. J. Nurs. **68**(10):2146-2148, 1968. Describes the nursing audit done at bedside.

McNally, F.: Nursing audit: evolution without pain, Superv. Nurse **8**(6):40, 45-46, 1977. Discusses the evolution of the nursing audit at one hospital.

Nadler, G., and Sahney, V.: A descriptive model of nursing care, Am. J. Nurs. **69**(2):336-341, 1969. Group of industrial engineers plan to identify factors that affect the quality of patient care, develop measurement scales, and develop a mathematical model that interrelates all factors into measure of quality. Describes an approach to identifying factors.

Nehring, V., and Geach, B.: Patient's evaluation of their care: why they don't complain, Nurs. Outlook **21**(5):317-321, 1973. Study found patients are reluctant to make any negative or critical comments about their care.

Newmark, G. L.: Can quality be equated with cost? Hospitals **50**(7):81-86, 1976. Discusses the utilization review system mandated by HEW as a condition of participation under Medicare and Medicaid because of the limited funds for implementing the professional standards review organization program nationwide.

Nicholls, M. E.: Quality control in patient care, Am. J. Nurs. **74**(3):456-459, 1974; In Nicholls, M. E., and Wessells, V. G., editors: Nursing standards and nursing process, Wakefield, Mass., 1977, Contemporary Publishing Co., pp. 87-93. Discusses the quality control process and criteria for standards.

Nursing profession review, J. Nurs. Adm. **6**:6-12, Nov., 1976. Presents a framework for review of professional nursing and discusses issues and problems related to the evaluation process.

On the scene: the Duke University Hospital experience in QA, Nurs. Adm. Q. **1**(3):7-50, 1977.

A collection of papers describing the Duke University Hospital experience with quality assurance.

Pardee, G., et al.: Patient care evaluation is every nurse's job, Am. J. Nurs. **71**(10):1958-1960, 1971. Presents and discusses an evaluative checklist to assess care of patient at different times.

Perkins, D. J.: Setting standards for care, Nurs. Homes **19**:22-24, 31, March, 1970. Stresses the importance of balancing desire for higher standards with the politics and economics of the situation.

Phaneuf, M. C.: A nursing audit method, Nurs. Outlook **12**(5):42-45, 1964. Discusses the purposes and method of auditing patient care records.

Phaneuf, M. C.: Analysis of a nursing audit, Nurs. Outlook **16**(1):57-60, 1968. Discusses the nursing audit.

Phaneuf, M. C.: Quality of care: problems of measurement. I. How one public health nursing agency is using the nursing audit, Am. J. Public Health **59**:1827-1832, Oct., 1969. Describes how nursing audit was used to evaluate nursing care and findings.

Phaneuf, M. C.: Model for quality: a matrix, AORN J. **23**(5):759-765, 1976. Discusses an ethical-moral framework.

Phaneuf, M. C., and Wandelt, M. A.: Quality assurance in nursing, Nurs. Forum **13**(4):328-345, 1974. Identifies the characteristics of a quality assurance program and control methods.

Pridham, K. F.: Assessing the quality of well child care: components of care and selection of outcomes, Nurs. Clin. North Am. **9**(2):367-379, 1974. Presents the criteria for assessing the parent's plan for feeding infants.

Ramey, I. G.: Setting nursing standards and evaluating care, J. Nurs. Admin. **3**:27-35, May-June, 1973. Defines philosophy, standards, and objectives; gives examples of professional nursing standards; presents an evaluation tool.

Ramirez, M. S.: Auditing of nursing care plans, Superv. Nurse **6**(6):29-38, 1975. A nursing care plan audit committee functions at St. Luke's Hospital in New York City. Presents forms used by that committee.

The relationship of nursing process and patient outcomes, J. Nurs. Adm. **6**(9):18-21, 1976. Study reports that the relationship between the nursing process and patient outcomes is inconsistent and may differ with diagnosis. Recommends the use of both process and outcome measures.

Rinaldi, L.: Managing a hospital audit committee,

Superv. Nurse **8**(6):60-62, 1977. Discusses management of a hospital audit committee.

Rotkovitch, R.: The heartbeat of nursing services—Standard IV, J. Nurs. Adm. **6**(4):32-35, 1976. Discusses the need for nurses to participate on committees.

Routhier, R. W.: Tool for the evaluation of patient care, Superv. Nurse **3**(1):15-27, 1972. Describes the development of a tool for the evaluation of patient care.

Rubin, C. R., Wallace, C., and Hill, R.: Auditing the POMR system, Superv. Nurse **6**(10):23-31, 1975. Describes the process for evaluating problem-oriented records. Presents audit forms.

Rubin, C. R., Rinaldi, L. A., and Dietz, R. R.: Nursing audit—nurses evaluating nursing, Am. J. Nurs. **72**(5):916-921, 1972. Illustrates how auditing a patient's chart can indicate what care ought to be included and how to assure that care given was documented.

Schick, D.: Steps for evaluating patient care, AORN J. **20**(8):237-239, 1974. Outlines ten steps of the process review.

Schwartz, D. R.: Toward more precise evaluation of patients' needs, Nurs. Outlook **13**(5):42-44, 1965. Discusses the importance of patient progress record and nursing care plan to the evaluation of patient care.

Selvaggi, L. M., et al.: Implementing a quality assurance program in nursing, J. Nurs. Adm. **6**(7): 37-43, 1976. Discusses implementation of a quality assurance program at Jackson Memorial Hospital in Miami, Florida.

Spicer, J. G., and Lewis, E. M.: Intensive care staff nurses develop peer review criteria, Nurs. Adm. Q. **1**(3):57-61, 1977. Describes the development of peer review criteria for an intensive care staff.

Stevens, B. J.: Analysis of trends in nursing care measurement, J. Nurs. Adm. **2**(2):1-6, 1972; In Nicholls, M. E., and Wessells, V. G., editors: Nursing standards and nursing process, Wakefield, Mass., 1977, Contemporary Publishing Co., pp. 77-84. Identifies the components of a quality control system, task analysis, and quality control methods and discusses factors that influence the quality control system.

Stevens, B. J.: ANA's standards of nursing practice: what they tell us about the state of the art, J. Nurs. Adm. **4**(5):16-18, 1974. Discusses each of the eight standards of nursing practice.

Stevens, B. J.: ANA's standards for nursing services: how do they measure up? J. Nurs. Adm. **6**(4):29-31, 1976. Compares the 1973 Standards for Nursing Services with the 1965 version.

Taylor, J. W.: Measuring the outcomes of nursing

care, Nurs. Clin. North Am. **9**(2):337-348, 1974. Report of the pilot project to test the feasibility of developing criteria for patient outcomes in a neurological unit.

Thomas, M.: Implementing the criteria for evaluating a hospital department of nursing, Nurs. Outlook **16**(2):49-51, 1968. Hospital used National League for Nursing's "Criteria for Evaluating a Hospital Department of Nursing Service" to improve nursing service.

Tyler, J. D.: Change through new graduates, Superv. Nurse **4**(4):41-49, 1973. Describes the use of portable desks from which eight patients are served; evaluates the results.

Wallace, R. F., and Donnelly, M.: Computing quality assurance costs, Hosp. Prog. **56**(5): 53-57, 1975. Costs are calculated for the medical audit, utilization review, and nursing audit programs at Little Company of Mary Hospital in Evergreen Park, Illinois. Benefits are believed to outweigh the costs.

Watson, A., and Mayers, M.: Evaluating the quality of patient care through retrospective chart review, J. Nurs. Adm. **6**(3):17-21, 1976. Discusses clerical criteria development, analysis of data, corrective action, and reevaluation of retrospective chart review.

Weinstein, E. L.: Developing a measure of the quality of nursing care, J. Nurs. Adm. **6**(6):1-3, 1976. Discusses tool development for the instrument used at the Hospital for Sick Children in Toronto.

Wiggins, A., and Carter, J. H.: Evaluation of nursing assessment and intervention in the surgical ICU, Nurs. Clin. North Am. **10**(1):121-144, 1975. Discusses methods of evaluating nursing care and establishment of criteria. Presents a nursing care index.

Wiseman, J.: A nursing audit of basic care, or nursing A.B.C. Part 1, Nurs. Times **72**(48):169-172, 1976. Discusses the Blackpool Nursing Service audit consisting of checklists for the various levels of nursing staff and presents tools.

Wiseman, J.: A nursing audit of basic care, or nursing A.B.C. Part 2, Nurs. Times **72**(49):173-174, 1976. Identifies the advantages and disadvantages of audits.

Wolfe, H.: Can nonnurses make qualitative observations of nursing care? Nurs. Outlook **13**(2): 52-53, 1965. Study finds nonnurses are not able to recognize and record the details of nursing care as accurately and completely as nurses.

Woolley, A. S.: The long and tortured history of clinical evaluation, Nurs. Outlook **25**(5):308-315, 1977. Presents a historical development of evaluation.

Zimmer, M. J.: Quality assurance for outcomes of patient care, Nurs. Clin. North Am. **9**(2):305-315, 1974. Discusses the need for quality assurance, what it is, the role of registered nurses, the clinical nurse specialist, the director of nursing, and steps in the development of a quality assurance program.

Zimmer, M. J.: Guidelines for development of outcome criteria, Nurs. Clin. North Am. **9**(2): 317-321, 1974. Lists characteristics of outcome criteria, formation of sets of criteria, application of criteria, and participation in establishing outcome criteria.

Systems analysis

Archer, S. E.: PERT: a tool for nurse administrators, J. Nurs. Adm. **4**:26-32, Sept.-Oct., 1974. Explains the program evaluation review technique.

Benson, C., Schmeling, P., and Bruins, G.: A systems approach to evaluation of nursing performance, Nurs. Adm. Q. **1**(3):67-75, 1977. Describes a systems approach to evaluation.

Finch, J.: Systems analysis: a logical approach to professional nursing care, Nurs. Forum **8**(2): 176-189, 1969. Discusses the systems analysis theory and its potential for development of science of nursing.

Freibrun, R. B.: Operations analysis applied to a drug distribution system, Am. J. Hosp. Pharm. **33**(4):452-458, 1976. Discusses the philosophy and process of systems analysis in relation to a drug distribution system.

Howland, D.: Approaches to the systems problem, Nurs. Res. **12**:172-174, Summer, 1963. Discusses scientific management, industrial and human engineering, operations, and systems research.

Howland, D.: A hospital system model, Nurs. Res. **12**:232-236, Fall, 1963. Conceptualization of hospital systems model.

Howland, D., and McDowell, W. E.: The measurement of patient care: a conceptual framework, Nurs. Res. **13**:4-7, Winter, 1964. Discusses development and use of hospital systems model for measurement of patient care.

Kraegel, J. M.: A system of patient care based on patient needs, Nurs. Outlook **20**(4):257-264, 1972. Systems approach was used to design demonstration model of patient-centered care in patient's room.

Messick, J. M., Singh, A. J., and May, P. R. A.: A systems analysis approach to planned change in a clinical psychiatric program, J. Psychiatr. Nurs. **13**(4):7-11, 1975. Describes how systems analysis was used to plan change for an outpatient treatment program. Presents a case study.

O'Malley, C. D.: Application of systems engineering in nursing, Am. J. Nurs. **69**(10): 2155-2160, 1969. Discusses how consultant service in systems engineering helped improve nursing services.

Pierce, L. M.: A patient-care model, Am. J. Nurs. **69**(8):1700-1704, 1969. Discusses methodological problems and goals of systems analysis of the patient-care model.

Poland, M., et al.: PETO: a system for assessing and meeting patient care needs, Am. J. Nurs. **70**(7):1479-1482, 1970. PETO system is an acronym of the authors' surnames; the system emphasizes coordinating time needed to give care with nursing time available.

Robinette, T.: What is health planning? Nurs. Outlook **18**(1):33-35, 1970. Discusses steps for health planning.

Rushworth, V.: Manpower planning at district level, Nurs. Times **71**:2032-2033, 1975. Outlines the steps in manpower planning.

Salvekar, A.: Management engineering reduces cost/improves care, Hosp. Prog. **56**(1):28-30, 1975. Suggests that management engineering can be used to control costs and improve care through improved effectiveness.

Vogt, M. T., Mickle, M. H., and Vogt, W. G.: The role of current modeling techniques in planning for future needs in allied health, J. Allied Health **4**(2):7-16, 1975. Presents a model that can be used to evaluate health manpower.

INDEX